Evidence-Based Practice in Complementary and Alternative Medicine

Sanjeev Rastogi
Editor

Francesco Chiappelli • Manisha Harish
Ramchandani • Ram Harsh Singh
Co-Editors

Evidence-Based Practice in Complementary and Alternative Medicine

Perspectives, Protocols, Problems, and Potential in Ayurveda

Springer

Editor
Assoc. Prof. Sanjeev Rastogi
PG Department of Kaya Chikitsa
State Ayurvedic College
Lucknow University
Lucknow, Uttar Pradesh
India
rastogisanjeev@rediffmail.com

Co-Editors
Prof. Francesco Chiappelli
Division of Oral Biology and Medicine
UCLA School of Dentistry
Los Angeles, CA
USA
fchiappelli@dentistry.ucla.edu

Dr. Manisha Harish Ramchandani
Division of Oral Biology and Medicine
UCLA School of Dentistry
Los Angeles, CA
USA
rmanisha@ucla.edu

Prof. Ram Harsh Singh
Department of Kaya Chikitsa
Institute of Medical Sciences
Banaras Hindu University
Varanasi
India
rh_singh2001@yahoo.com

ISBN 978-3-642-44561-3 ISBN 978-3-642-24565-7 (eBook)
DOI 10.1007/978-3-642-24565-7
Springer Heidelberg Dordrecht London New York

Softcover reprint of the hardcover 1st edition 2012

Printed on acid-free paper

Springer is part of Springer Science+Business Media (www.springer.com)

Foreword I

After visiting the Central Institute of Research in Indigenous Systems of Medicine at Jamnagar on November 2, 1955, Pandit Jawaharlal Nehru had observed—"a fascinating inquiry is going on in this research institute and it may well lead to very fruitful results. The only right approach has to be one of science, that is, of experiment, trial and error. In whatever type of medicine we may deal with, we cannot profit by its study unless we apply the method of science. Nothing should be taken for granted. Everything should be tested and proved and then it becomes a part of scientific medicine—old and new."

In other words, Pandit Nehru was championing the cause of (scientific) evidence based medicine.

In the Mahatma Gandhi Memorial Oration that I delivered at the Indian Institute of Management, Kolkata on October 16, 2001, I had said

> It is only by fusing the ancient wisdom and modern science that India can create world class products, because new products cannot compete with products, which have only tradition and empirical observation as the knowledge base. The knowledge to be integrated into the traditional products has to emerge from modern science, especially modern biology and chemistry.

In other words, again I was championing the cause of (scientific) evidence based medicine.

I am delighted to see that this book represents the spirit of these foregoing sentiments. More specifically, it champions the creation of evidence based Ayurveda (EBA).

Ayurveda is one of the earliest frameworks which systematized knowledge of health and healthcare. Its framework is not only self-consistent, but also uses cause and effect arguments to correlate manifestations of sickness, its causes and its treatments. When this framework was developed in ancient India—the notion of a molecule did not exist, nor was the cell and the role it plays in the life process known. The discoveries of DNA and functional genomics lay more the 3,000 years in the future, yet in spite of all this Ayurveda offered effective treatments for many disorders, particularly those with multiple causes. For some degenerative diseases, most Indians consider it to be the treatment of last resort. Despite this, why has there not been a universal acceptance of Ayurveda? The book argues that such evidence based approach is a first step towards global acceptability of Ayurveda.

Dr. Sanjeev Rastogi and his colleagues have addressed the importance of evidence in this book in a very comprehensive manner. The book addresses an often raised question as to why do we need an evidence base for a health care practice, which is prevalent for ages. This book brings together the collective knowledge and insights of leading experts from the *vaidya* community. It logically emphasizes the extended benefits of establishing EBA by addressing the need of better and dependable health care and prospective recognition and growth of Ayurveda as a contemporary science.

The authors emphasize that EBA is quite achievable within its own purview, without compromising its fundamentals. Indeed, it can be done by essentially utilizing its own tools of generation of evidence. This emphasis is supported by very appropriate elaborative and convincing examples.

The book outlines the protocols for research synthesis in the context of Ayurveda. It covers important topics like evidence based clinical practice, diet and nutrition concepts, clinical evidence in the tradition, concept of *prakriti* (constitution), *panchakarma*, Ayurvedic approach to cardiovascular diseases, *rasayana* and rejuvenation and oral diseases. I was particularly happy to see the comprehensive contribution on the most discussed safety issues of Ayurvedic drugs in the purview of EBA with a recommendation that we should strengthen the pharmacovigilance system for Ayurvedic products to find out the rare side effects.

The book not only outlines the challenges towards EBA but also suggests possible solutions. The need of reporting single case studies and case series is very well highlighted. The example of *Amavata* defines the need for reappraisal of basic principles of Ayurveda. By giving an example of reappraisal of salivary diagnostics from the point of view of Ayurveda, it is shown as to how truly innovative ideas can be generated. Elaborative flowcharts provided in the book makes it especially easy to understanding the concepts.

I appreciate the commitment, energy and enthusiasm of Dr. Sanjeev Rastogi and his team in making this most valuable contribution, since evidence based Ayurveda could indeed be a powerful frontline solution, which will help mankind's continuing quest in the twenty-first century to fulfil the dream of "health for all."

National Research Professor & President Global Research Alliance,
National Chemical Laboratory,
Pune 411 008, India

R.A. Mashelkar

Foreword II

Over the last few decades, Ayurveda was mainly known in the West as a wellness intervention. However, Ayurveda is clearly making its way into medical health care: Ayurveda clinics are getting established, and research projects are starting up. As a perceived newcomer to the field of medical care in Western countries, it is important to develop and improve the scientific knowledge base and to continue to foster further research. Firstly, we need to understand why Ayurveda has become so popular in the West, and secondly, we need better evidence about its safety, effectiveness, efficacy, and cost-effectiveness in order to make rational decisions about its public and private provision. On the basis of positive evidence, Ayurveda may become integrated as an additional element within patient-centered medicine in the West.

The bringing together of traditional knowledge and concepts of evidence-based medicine is clearly a step in the right direction, which has to be taken with great care. This is something the authors of this book, when writing their contribution, have taken into account in a thoughtful manner. Ayurveda is a traditional, whole medical system that has a unique and complex diagnostic and interventional approach. Complex treatments follow the theory that the combination of the different treatment elements exerts synergistic effects relevant for the outcome. Evaluation of whole medical systems within the methodological framework of conventional clinical research results in fragmentation of the interventions. For example, comparing an Ayurvedic medicine such as Yogaraja Guggulu with a placebo for osteoarthritis of the knee would provide information on the safety and the specific effect of Yogaraja Guggulu but not on Ayurveda as a whole treatment system. Ayurveda, as typically applied for the treatment of osteoarthritis of the knee, would entail a complex intervention that is individualized according to the constitution of the patient (dosha). Aside from Ayurvedic medicines, the intervention could include dietary and lifestyle advice, yoga, abhyanga, local bastis, and performance of basti-karmas. To understand if Ayurveda is noninferior or superior to a complex conventional treatment, it would be necessary to compare both treatment approaches against one another.

One has to bring together traditional and clinical research, ideally by involving the relevant stakeholders—the patient, the practitioner, researchers, producers, and health policy decision makers—in order to carry out useful comparative effectiveness research. Both the evidence on safety and efficacy of single medicines as well as the evidence on the effectiveness of a complex and individualized Ayurveda intervention are needed to convince decision makers in the West that Ayurveda can play a role in medical health care.

This book provides an excellent overview about the theoretical framework of Ayurveda and gives insight into its evidence base. It helps to better understand what it is about Ayurveda that people perceive as helpful and provides explanations on the healing properties by drawing on traditional Ayurveda theory. I hope this book will be widely read and valued by practitioners and researchers interested in this particular area of medicine.

Claudia M. Witt, M.D., M.B.A.
Professor of Medicine, Vice Director
Carstens Foundation Distinguished
Professor for Complementary Medicine Research,
Institute for Social Medicine, Epidemiology
and Health Economics,
Charite University, Berlin,
Germany

Preface

It is almost 5 years back, when I came in touch with Prof Francesco Chiappelli. A foundation to this book was laid at that time, although it took almost 5 years for the preliminary thoughts to get refined and mature in the shape of a book.

A clinical practice based upon evidences of comparative effectiveness, safety, efficacy, and cost-effectiveness of chosen interventions and also upon reliability and validity of diagnostic tools which were used to make a diagnosis is mandatory to give prevailing health care a realistic face. Accountable decision making in terms of disease diagnosis and in choosing the most appropriate medical care in light of best available evidences is an utmost requirement to give rise to transparency and accountability in medical care ultimately aiming to provide the best possible care to everyone. This had been a well-cherished dream sought long back at the Alma-Ata declaration of "Health for All."

It is beyond the scope of discussion any more that CAM should also be brought into the purview of evidence-based practice of medicine (EBPM). Any medical intervention where a patient is given hope of betterments in terms of improvements of quality of life or through changing end point measures should essentially be brought under the purview of regular monitoring to prevent substandard practices and eventually to maximize the prospective benefits from a chosen therapy. The same would also be important to give rise to a uniform status to health care for its impacts spreading beyond the geographical boundaries or the type of care involved.

It is important to understand here that an evidence-based practice in CAM is not as straightforward as it is seen in conventional medicine. Paucity of secondary documentary evidences (in the form of published research documents) and treatment protocol variations reflecting the caregiver's or patient's preferences, inclinations, needs, or beliefs together make decision making in CAM a unique exercise which is difficult to be replicated at any other similar situation. It should therefore be clearly understood that applying evidence to CAM would have to be a novel exercise at its own, requiring a cautious introspection into all of its resources and practice styles including the subjective methods of decision making in intervened clinical conditions.

Evidences in Ayurveda (to CAM in general) would require to be crafted carefully and diligently while keeping each such subset population of clinical entity in mind, where a differential decision making would warrant, based upon the specifications observed on account of *Roga* (disease) or *Rogi* (patient). A whole system research (WSR) brings a beautiful model to evaluate such interventions in the true spirit of their practice in real-life situations. It is however important to understand that a WSR should again be fractioned in various subsets of practices to make it a real representative to the CAM practices. Ayurvedic diagnostics are found lagging behind in the evidence synthesis when the same is compared to its interventions. It is again important to reiterate that an evidence-based diagnostic decision making is rather more important in CAM compared to their efficacy evidences based upon contemporary end point measures. As therapeutic decision making in Ayurveda relies solely upon the *dosha, dushya,* and *prakriti* status of the patient, it is imperative to develop tools for such diagnoses, which may eventually help decision making referring to the choice of suitable intervention.

Finally, the rapid emergence of CAM globally is partly in repercussion to complexities associated with conventional therapy for their over-reliance upon technical breakthrough, making them more mechanical and less human. CAM, through its holistic principles and patient-centered approach, offers more solace in conditions where conventional medicine is unable to offer any. A resurgence of CAM therefore lies in its simplicity, accessibility, affordability, and humanistic and cultural bindings. Any approach to make it more standardized (eventually making it more complex) should always be weighed against the benefits and losses it may cause. It is mandatory to care for the basic attributes of CAM while approaching for any exercise to amend its practice style.

It is clear that practicing evidence-based Ayurveda (EBA) in view of such intricacies and limitations is an uphill task which would require Herculean efforts. The present work is a modest compilation of works from different streams of thoughts in Ayurveda and evidence-based medicine aiming to bring more accountability in Ayurvedic practice through synthesizing the evidences initially and disseminating these evidences eventually to help Ayurvedic practice for optimizing its impacts. Being first of its kind, the book represents innumerable ideas and thoughts as foundation, upon which a strong EBA can be built in future if the same vigor and zeal to "bring the best of Ayurveda before the world" is continuously sustained.

Sanjeev Rastogi
PG Department of Kaya Chikitsa,
State Ayurvedic College,
Lucknow University, Lucknow,
Uttar Pradesh,
India

Acknowledgments

This work has been the result of dedication and untiring efforts of innumerable scientists and vaidya-scientists (Ayurvedic physicians with scientific zeal) working since long to bring an equitable, affordable, sustainable, and dependable form of health care with due respect to the traditional wisdom of health care.

We are able to cite only a few of them in the entire work, but we acknowledge them all for their contributions which ultimately have paved the way to the thought of evidence-based Ayurveda, of which this book emerged.

Prof Francesco Chiappelli, an icon in the field of evidence-based medicine, dentistry, and complementary medicine, has been the principal motivator for me to take up this project. He not only has encouraged me to come forward with the idea of evidence-based Ayurveda but also has assured me of his help at any time of need. I am proud to have worked with him at many occasions earlier and to have him as a coeditor to the team which finally has shaped this book.

Prof RH Singh, the other coeditor to the book, has been a legendary vaidya-scientist in contemporary sense. My thoughts of Ayurveda got nurtured and refined in Banaras Hindu University where I worked as an associate to Prof Singh. He has been the vital force behind all my works related to bringing Ayurveda on scientific footings. His constant encouragement and visionary touch is reflected throughout in this work. I am honored to have him as another coeditor to this work.

Dr Manisha Harish Ramchandani, the final coeditor to this book, represents the new age science. Through her cutting-edge approach, as a coeditor, she did admirably to improve the quality and content of the book to every extent.

It is the hard work of all our contributors which shaped this book. They represent the most refined and open-minded strata of people with an equal flair for science as well as for Ayurveda. Undoubtedly, the work represents the thoughts on Ayurveda in tune to the need of science.

Ms Irmela Bohn from Springer (Berlin Heidelberg) deserves utmost praise for her unconditional and continuous support to this project from the time of conception till delivery. It was her rigorous support only which metamorphosed a mental exercise into a concrete book.

I specially thank my wife, Dr Ranjana, and my son, Shashwat, who permitted me for months together to remain absconded from family matters to complete this task. Without their constant support, love, and admiration, this work would not have been possible.

I dedicate this work to *Charaka*, the nomadic saint physician of Ayurveda, who enabled us to share from his treasure house of wisdom the eternal *Charaka Samhita*. It is still mesmerizing to read through *Charaka Samhita* for the more we see, the more we find it relevant to the contemporary sense.

Contents

Part I: Evidence-Based and Comparative Effectiveness Analysis

1 **Fundamentals: Evidence-Based Practice in Complementary and Alternative Medicine—Perspectives, Protocols, Problems, and Potentials** 3
Francesco Chiappelli

Part II: Evidence-Based Medicine and Ayurveda

2 **Transforming Ayurveda: Stepping into the Realm of Evidence-Based Practice** 33
Sanjeev Rastogi and Ram Harsh Singh

3 **Diet and Nutrition Concepts in Ayurveda: Gleaming into Opportunities for Evidence-Based Applications in Health Care** 51
Devesh Rastogi, Shalini Gupta, Ranjana Rastogi, and Rajiv Rastogi

4 **Clinical Evidence in the Tradition of Ayurveda** 67
P. Ram Manohar

5 **Evidence-Based Traditional Persian Medicine** 79
Mahsa Dousti, Manisha Harish Ramchandani, Andre Barkhordarian, Sohrab Danaei, and Francesco Chiappelli

Part III: Substantiating Ayurvedic Theory and Practice Toward Evidence-Base

6 ***Prakriti* Analysis in Ayurveda: Envisaging the Need of Better Diagnostic Tools** 99
Sanjeev Rastogi

7 ***Panchakarma*: Ayurvedic Detoxification and Allied Therapies—Is There Any Evidence?** 113
Sivarama Prasad Vinjamury, Manjusha Vinjamury, Sobhana Sucharitakul, and Ingebritt Ziegler

8 Gut and Joint Interconnections: A Reappraisal to Ayurvedic Understanding of Joint Diseases 139
Sanjeev Rastogi and Ranjana Rastogi

9 Ayurvedic Approach to Cardiovascular Diseases: Delineating the Literary and Clinical Evidences 159
Sanjeev Rastogi, Rajiv Rastogi, and P.S. Srivastav

10 *Rasayana* Therapy and Rejuvenation 177
Ram Harsh Singh and Sanjeev Rastogi

11 Translational Effectiveness in Ayurvedic Medicine: Implications for Oral Biology and Medicine 191
Manisha Harish Ramchandani, Mahsa Dousti, Andre Barkhordarian, and Francesco Chiappelli

Part IV: Towards Future Perspectives of Evidence-Based Ayurveda

12 Safety Aspects of Ayurvedic Drugs 211
K.K. Pant, C.K. Katiyar, and Arun Gupta

13 Toward Evidence-Based Practice of Ayurveda: Extrapolating the Challenges in the Current Decade 233
Sanjeev Rastogi

Index 247

Part I
Evidence-Based and Comparative Effectiveness Analysis

Chapter 1
Fundamentals: Evidence-Based Practice in Complementary and Alternative Medicine—Perspectives, Protocols, Problems, and Potentials

Francesco Chiappelli

1.1 Introduction: Evidence-Based Decision-Making in Health Care

1.1.1 The Primary Cause of Things

In an early publication over a decade ago [1], we proposed that it was necessary to approach the then novel and emerging field of evidence-based dentistry from a teleological perspective. To state it in brief, the Aristotelian concept of teleology proposes that we must look for the primary causes of things, acts, or events, and that when such things, acts, or events are initiated and sustained toward a clear and definable end, then they are "teleological." In simpler terms, a process or action is teleological when it is driven and conducted for the sake of an end that can be outlined; that is to say, a teleological process is one that displays a articulated finality, that has a cogent final cause, a "telos" (Greek for final cause, τελοσ).

Aristotle (384 BC–322 BC) identified and discussed two types of final causes. He proposed that:

- A process endowed of an "external" final cause was one driven for the sake of, and dependent upon, a primary reason external to itself, such as for example a parent acting for ensuring the well-being of the child.
- By contrast, a process is said to have intrinsic telos (intrinsic cause of finality) when it operates for itself, and not for the sake of something external to itself. One could cite the example of the crook taking advantage of the rich widow for

F. Chiappelli
Division of Oral Biology and Medicine,
UCLA School of Dentistry,
Los Angeles, CA, USA
e-mail: fchiappelli@dentistry.ucla.edu

S. Rastogi (ed.), *Evidence-Based Practice in Complementary and Alternative Medicine*,
DOI 10.1007/978-3-642-24565-7_1, © Springer-Verlag Berlin Heidelberg 2012

the simple outcome of enriching himself by tricking her into bestowing upon him expensive gifts.

Contemporary philosophy of science errs in dismissing the fundamental tenets of teleology, since it is evident that its principles could significantly contribute to the interpretation of existing observations in a range of fields, from behavioral neuroscience to clinical psychology. Furthermore, teleological propositions could help advance the field of health care by providing sound emphasis to novel models toward increasing the health literacy of the patients, and their compliance to treatment, and well as toward yielding more powerful,[1] valid, and reliable modes of treatment intervention.

Whether one consults the tradition of what has now been called "Western medicine," or the traditional medical models found in innumerable cultures and societies around the world, which are subsumed in the term "alternative medicine," and whether one considers either of these medicines alone or in combination to each other, in a "complementary" mode as we now call it, it is clear that there is a fundamental finality to the action of he who provides health care to another: to assist and to cure, causing no harm, while grounded in a moral of conduct that strives to respect, to celebrate and to benefit the life of the person being cared for [2].

Clearly, the actions of those who provide health care, be they physicians, dentists, nurses, or clinical psychologists, have a certain, clear, and distinct extrinsic teleological finality: the health-care provider actions, decisions, and interventions are driven for the sole purpose[2] of ensuring that the patients regain, sustain, or maintain his or her physical, mental, and psychoemotional well-being. The health-care provider's action may therefore be either predominantly interventional in nature – that is to say, there is a disease process or an illness that needs to be countered so that the patient can *regain* physical and mental well-being; or it can encompass largely preventative measures that are meant to assist the patient *to sustain and to maintain* health and well-being.

The finality of Western medicine is principally intervention, although clearly not totally so— many Western medical interventions (increasingly, one should note in fact) are directed toward preventive medicine, but it is the case that the Western health-care tradition is called on, predominantly, to cure disease rather than to prevent it. By contrast, non-Western health-care traditions—"alternative medicines," such as the traditional Indian Ayurvedic corpus of medical interventions—generally aim to prevent illness primarily, and secondarily, when necessary, to intervene to regain the state of non-illness.

In part because of this fundamental divergence in the extrinsic teleological primary cause of Western and "alternative" health care, and because of the distinct philosophical traditions, Western medicine has come to rely more on continual

[1] The term "power" is intended here from the perspective of statistical significance and clinical relevance.

[2] Of course, assuming that the fundamental tenets of ethical behavior are verified and enforced.

novel developments in experimental evidence than on rigid and outdated tenets. By contrast, "alternative" medicines are grounded primarily on centuries-old knowledge and tradition, which now are tested, characterized, and confirmed by sound experimental designs.

Thus has evolved the misgiving that whereas Western medicine is based on research evidence, "alternative" medicines are not. Indeed, it has also been charged that "alternative" medicines cannot, perhaps can never be based on research evidence for the simple reason that "alternative" medical procedures and protocols have not, and in some instances cannot be subjected to "mainstream" experimental methods [3]. That is, of course, a fallacy of the like of proving that something cannot be proven not to be round because it is not round to begin with.

What we know today in the Western world as Western medicine has grown and evolved from our Western scientific tradition, and it is what it is because of its foundations in Western culture and the Western view on science, health, and disease. It gathers experimental evidence to prove or to disprove hypotheses in support of further growth and evolution that particular—one could say biased—view of health and illness.

By contrast, "alternative" medicines have arisen from distinct philosophical tradition and are ground in views and tenets of health and illness that are different, sometimes diametrically opposed to the Western view. To subject "alternative" medicines to the criteria of the Western tradition is as ill-conceived as the reverse: to subject the Western medical tradition to the test of "alternative" medical schemata. Whereas we, in the West, will seek to characterize molecular pathways, proteomic signatures and profiles, and cell lineages; "alternative" scientific traditions will seek to capture the essence of the totality of the balance among the multiple aspects—mind and body—that constitute the individual and determine his/her state of health or ill-health, ease or disease.

To be overly simplistic, one could state that the Western view on the health sciences might be that the primary cause of a disease process might be certain cellular, biochemical, or molecular events gone wrong. Therefore, the primary cause of health care might be to identify, by means of stringent experimental work, what the responsible biological events might be so that then, based on that research evidence, they can be targeted in focused and directed therapeutic interventions.

By contrast and by opposite, the "alternative" medicines view would suggest that the primary cause of a disease might be the imbalance among certain energies (cf. Qi in Traditional Chinese Medicine) among certain organs or bodily regions or systems. Therefore, the teleological drive behind health-care intervention might be a complex and well-articulated, individualized program, which might include certain manipulations (e.g., acupuncture), medicaments (e.g., infusions), or self-directed interventions (e.g., Tai Chi).

Recent decades have witnessed an attempt by many to bring together these two fundamentally distinct tradition for the ultimate benefit of the patient. The Western tradition has become increasingly well-versed in "integrative medicine" and "systems biology," in an effort to elucidate, based on the traditionally Western hypothesis-driven "scientific process" the fundamental tenets of mind–body interaction.[3]

Be that as it may, what is clear is that health care is an evolving science. Whether we consider it from the current Western perspective, or the "alternative" views held in non-Western cultures, the challenge of procuring interventions to our fellow humans, for the purpose of preventing disease, maintaining and sustaining health, or countering an illness and regaining health, is always dependent upon our training, skill, and expertise. Whereas we receive our training during our formative years, we are called to sharpen our skills and expertise continuously through a process of continuing education. We continued improvement of our clinical judgment rests upon our sustained effort to update our knowledge base with the best newly available information, and our continuously improved clinical decisions depend upon the extent to which we utilize the informational evidence at our disposal to ensure effective and efficacious preventive or treatment interventions.

In other words, and to return to the primary cause of the point brought forth here, the extrinsic teleologic determinant of our service to our fellow human beings, the external final cause of our providing health care, whether in the Western medicine context or in the context of "alternative" medicine, is to proffer benefit to them in the form of maintaining, sustaining, or regaining health. That is achieved, regardless of the medical tradition we espouse, depending to a large extent on our training, and on how well we keep sharpening our skills and expertise by ensuring updates of the best and most reliable new information and evidence.

We could say therefore that, whether we are trained in Western health care or in "alternative" health care, we must update our skills and expertise continuously only with the best available evidence in order to ensure that we provide effective and efficacious care to our patients. The external final cause, the *prima causa*,[4] from a teleological viewpoint, of our updating our skills and expertise with the best available evidence is to perfect our clinical decision-making.

---

[3] It is interesting to note that Ancient Rome, which signifies the foundations of the cultural traditions in the West, already recognized the need to consider the health of the mind and the health of the body (cf. *mens sana in corpore sano*, a healthy mind in a healthy body). Of course, the medicine of Rome (e.g., Galen, 129 AD–ca. 210 AD) rested upon the medicine of ancient Greece (e.g., Hippocrates 460 BCE–ca. 370 BCE) and was sustained throughout the Middle Ages and the Renaissance in Europe. It was perhaps not before the Swiss scientist Paracelsus (1493–1541) that a movement against this tradition began to be clearly articulated in the West, despite the fact that his hermetical views were that sickness and health in the body relied on the harmony of man (microcosm) and Nature (macrocosm). While, Paracelsus is considered by many as one of the "fathers" of Western medicine, his views that because everything in the universe is interrelated, beneficial medical substances are to be found in herbs, minerals, and various alchemical combinations thereof that will be benefit in preventive disease, and in regaining health. We are part of, Paracelsus argued, the universe, one coherent organism that permeates with one uniting life-giving spirit, and our health derives from and depends upon our interrelationship with its entirety. Within the span of a hundred years, Western thought underwent a remarkable transformation, leading to the work of Malpighi, Tissot, Jenner, Koch, Pacini, and many others that paved the way to today. The point to note, however, is that the drive to reductionism, which appears to be predilected in the West at present, is not the only valid perspective upon the health sciences, and in fact was not the Western approach to health care a few hundred years ago, when indeed it was considerably more affine to the modes of health care we today label as "alternative."

[4] The primary cause.

1.1.2 Based on the Evidence Versus Evidence-Based

It is argued that the Western view of delivering health care is superior because it rests on research evidence. This, one might argue is a fallacy as well, simply because there is good research evidence and there is bad research evidence. If research evidence is tainted by a suboptimal research methodology, if bias and error abound, if data are misanalyzed and misinterpreted, then it is possible and even probable that the utilization and integration of that evidence in the clinical decision-making process will result in, at best, a useless and, at worst, a harmful intervention for the patient. It is critical that the research evidence we utilize to sharpen our skills and expertise be the best available.

That, in and of itself, seems self-evident and routine: do we not have a reliable, albeit complex, responsible, albeit overburdened, efficient, albeit imperfect system of peer review to assess and to determine the quality of the research evidence, which we might eventually integrate in our clinical decision? Indeed, we do—but, it is precisely because of its inherent complexity that our system overburdens the reviewers and more often than not leads to imperfect reviews, incomplete assessments, and biased evaluations of research, that we face the real risk of encountering all too often peer-reviewed published evidence that is laced with errors, bias, and weaknesses.

Should we be so fortunate to have the time materially to scrutinize each report so as to eliminate what is not acceptable due to excessive error and bias, and keep only what is the best available evidence to update and to sharpen our skills and expertise, then we would indeed do great service to our patients. Short of that, short of ensuring that we only integrate into our clinical decisions the best available evidence, we put our patients at risk, and we contradict the very oath we hold dear of "do not harm."

The medical literature is gargantuan. Even if we had the expertise to do so, we could not exhaustively peruse the published reports in the manner just outlined, and still have the material time to take care of our patients. Therefore, we would become selective on which report we are going to peruse. By doing so, inevitably, we insert into the very process the gravest fault of all research: the bias of selection. By selecting what report we shall consider in our perusal, we de facto select the kind of evidence we will be willing to utilize in the process of sharpening our skills and expertise: we de facto taint the very process of our clinical decision-making with a bias that is inappropriate because it is not related to the condition of the patient, to the intervention we are considering, or to the outcome sought.

That is to say, health care based on the evidence suffers from an unalienable bias. It is thus inappropriate and can even be dangerous to the well-being of our patients. By contrast, when a systematic process of synthesis is applied to the entire body of the available evidence, such that the acceptable evidence can be obtained, from which a consensus of the best available evidence can be derived, evidence-based health care is procured, which the optimal and safest manner to update skills and expertise to provide effective and efficacious health care. In brief, the best available evidence emerges from a concerted process of systematically synthesizing and analyzing all of the available evidence that pertains specifically to the patient under consideration, the interventions under consideration, and the clinical outcome under consideration.

Evidence-based Western medicine, therefore, entails making fully informed clinical decisions that integrate not only the patient's medical history and clinical test results but also the training of the clinician, and his/her skills and expertise updated by the consensus of the best available research evidence, itself derived from a systematic process of research synthesis. To exactly the same extent, evidence-based complementary and alternative medicine (CAM) [4] utilizes and integrates the patient's information, with the clinician's training, skills and expertise, as well as the consensus of a research synthesis process that yields the best available evidence for judicious clinical decision-making that relies upon comparative effectiveness and efficacy research and analysis for practice (CEERAP) [5].

1.2 Research Synthesis

1.2.1 Introduction

The essence of the science and role of research synthesis in the context of CAM can be rendered by the following two quotes:

- The French moralist and essayist, Luc de Clapiers, Marquis de Vauvenargues (August 6, 1715 to May 28, 1747), stated in his *Réflexions et Maximes* that …*il est plus aisé de dire des choses nouvelles que de concilier celles qui ont étés dites*: that is to say—it is easier to say new concepts than to reconcile those things that have been said. That is precisely the purpose and ultimate goal of research synthesis for evidence-based medical practice: to reconcile research evidence toward obtaining the best available evidence for effective and efficacious treatment intervention.
- The British physicist John William Strutt, the 3rd Baron and Lord of Rayleigh (November 12, 1842 to June 30, 1919) also said that "… the work which deserves, but I am afraid does not always receive, the most credit is that in which discovery and explanation go hand in hand, in which not only are new facts presented, but their relation to old ones is pointed out…". In the vast and complex domain of alternative and complementary medicine, that is particularly the case: that is, the clinical importance and relevance of juxtaposing new facts and evidence to century-old non-Western medical tradition.

1.2.2 Protocol

Research synthesis follows the scientific method [6–10], which can be outlined in brief as follows:

- Statement of the hypothesis and research question
- Crafting of the research approach to test the hypothesis and answer to the research question (i.e., research design, sampling issues, tools of measurement)

- Presentation of the findings and summary of the results by means of descriptive statistics
- Statistical analysis of the data
- Inferences, discussion of limitations and intervening variables, identification of future research toward further testing the hypothesis and answering the research question in greater details

1.2.2.1 The Question

Firstly, it is critical to set the question of the research at hand and to realize that a research question, when stated in the affirmative, is nothing but the study hypothesis. Thus, for instance, one could set out to test the research query of whether or not Ayurvedic intervention can prevent the onset of ulcerative colitis by stating the following research question:

- *Is Ayurvedic intervention effective and efficacious in preventing the onset of ulcerative colitis?*

In the same vein, the research hypothesis will become:

- *Ayurvedic medicine is effective and efficacious in preventing the onset of ulcerative colitis.*

When a piece of research is built and crafted to answer specifically one such research question, it is qualified as a hypothesis-driven study. The search for the best available evidence, which is obtained through the research synthesis design, is hypothesis-driven because it addresses a specific type of research question that is rendered by the acronym P.I.C.O. (patient, interventions under consideration, outcomes). The more specific nature of the comparative effectiveness question as it entertains as well timeline and settings considerations engenders a more specific acronym from those studies: P.I.C.O.T.S. [5, 10, 11].

The P.I.C.O. and P.I.C.O.T.S. research questions direct the search for evidence about the which intervention under consideration may, or may not be more effective or efficacious[5] for the particular patient population targeted in the study, and in light of the specific clinical outcome of interest. In that regard, the P.I.C.O. and P.I.C.O.T.S.

[5] The distinction between the "effectiveness" and the "efficacy" of a clinical intervention is critical at this juncture. The US Federal Coordinating Council for Comparative Effectiveness Research Report to the President and the Congress, dated June 30, 2009, stated that "…because it (comparative *effectiveness* research) …[applies]… to real-world needs and decisions faced by patients, clinicians, and other decision makers [generally including assessment of risks, costs vs. benefits]…". By contrast, in "…*efficacy* research, …the question is typically whether the treatment is efficacious [i.e., works clinically] under ideal, rather than real-world, settings …[and]….[t]he results … are … not necessarily generalizable to any given patient…." Simply stated, whereas the former pertains to risk, benefits and cost assessment, the efficacy pertains to whether or not a given clinical intervention works clinically, and brings about the clinical outcome sought.

questions drive the process of search and analysis of the *best available* evidence by means of the research synthesis design.

In brief, the P.I.C.O. and P.I.C.O.T.S. questions define and determine the sample of publication to be scrutinized to obtain the *available* evidence, the tools of evaluations that serve to assess the *best* evidence, the statistical analysis required to establish reliability and validity of the results, and the inference of the findings for immediate implication to clinical practice. The P.I.C.O. and P.I.C.O.T.S. questions also set the criteria for deductive reasoning leading incremental progress of research in the future.

The question is crafted based on descriptors of:

- The clinical problem and patient population (P)
- The clinical interventions (I) under
- Consideration/comparison/contrast (C), and
- Clinical outcome (O) of interest: PICO. The PICO question may undergo minor changes and alterations, as per the specific research question: it may examine a
- Predictive (P), rather than a comparative model (hence, PIPO); or it may incorporate
- Elements of time (T) and
- Settings (S) (hence, PICOTS, PIPOTS)

In brief, the method of science instructs that the creation of new knowledge that is obtained through research is driven by the scientific method. The scientific method consists of a series of sequential steps that arises from a theory, a hunch, or a simple observation.

1.2.2.2 The Methodology

Secondly, it is important to note the two principal domains of methodology, as they pertain to the research synthesis process. On the one hand, the sample of a research synthesis design consists in the peer-reviewed and non-peer-reviewed published research literature, as well as unrecorded observations. Thus, the term "available" underscores the fact that we limit the subjects of study in a piece of research synthesis investigation, in the same manner as any other piece of research, to the accessible sample: that is to say, the accessible research literature that specifically targets[6] the question under study.

Unpublished evidence and evidence that is published in non-peer-reviewed journals are often excluded from a research synthesis design, in part, because it is exceedingly difficult to obtain these types of evidence in a valid and reliable manner. The literature available through the proceedings of scientific meetings, dissertations, and non-peer-reviewed journals is termed "gray literature" and is likewise most often excluded from research synthesis endeavors. In brief, it is argued that the

[6] This approach to sampling is in no way different than what is done in a clinical trial, where the investigator determines and establishes before hand what is the accessible and what is the target sample of the study.

evidence that has not been sifted through the widely accepted peer-review process is likely to be fraught with issues of validity, quality, and bias, which will interfere with the research synthesis process.

The research synthesis process is most often focused, otherwise indicated, on peer-reviewed literature. The search for that sample is obtained by utilizing the medical subject headings (MeSH terms) and keywords that can be derived from the P.I.C.O./P.I.C.O.T.S. question. That is, the attention given to crafting a superior P.I.C.O./P.I.C.O.T.S. will determine the quality of the sample.

The search is actualized by accessing the National Library of Medicine (Pubmed-Medline, www.ncbi.nlm.nih.gov/pubmed), and usually at least two other search engines (e.g., Cochrane, www.cochrane.org; Bandolier, www.jr2.ox.ac.uk/bandolier; EMBASE, www.embase.com; Center for Review Dissemination; www.york.ac.uk/inst/crd; Google scholar; etc.).[7] The purpose of the multiple search is to ensure comprehensive inclusion of all of the available literature within the confines of the inclusion/exclusion criteria dictated by the research synthesis process, while at the same time minimizing as much as possible dangers of selection bias and systematic sampling errors.

It must be underscored that some degree of publication bias cannot be avoided simply because, as a general rule, papers that are statistically significant, whether they demonstrate clinical relevance or not, tend to be preferentially published in the scientific literature, compared to reports that demonstrate clinical relevance but fail to reach statistical significance. The problem of publication bias is inherent to our present system of scientific literature and is an unavoidable issue of the research synthesis process, which is generally discussed as a limitation of the utilization of the best available evidence in considerations of the clinical relevance of the findings, and clinical decision-making [5–10].

As noted, a well-stated P.I.C.O./P.I.C.O.T.S. question will reveal imbedded keywords for the literature of interest. When the sample of literature thus obtained is very small, a reconsideration of the P.I.C.O./P.I.C.O.T.S. question will be required to make them broader, and therefore encompassing of a larger segment of the available research bibliome.[8] That is so, principally, because a research synthesis protocol on a sample of literature that is less than 5 may lead to meaningless analyses and interpretations. By contrast, when the resulting sample of literature is very large, then inclusion and exclusion criteria must be set to restrict the search outcome in order to make it more specific to the P.I.C.O./P.I.C.O.T.S. question.

It actually may occur that the sample of literature that is produced by the initial search remains gargantuan, following and despite stringent inclusion and exclusion criteria. Then, a process of random sampling of the resulting literature subpopulation may be confidently entertained, and the research synthesis design may be conducted on a random sample, in a process akin and identical to that used to obtain a random sample of subjects in an experimental design or a clinical trial.

---

[7] The following section "resources" list a few search engines specific to complementary and alternative medicine.

[8] The bibliome is the body of pertinent research literature available for any given systematic review (SR): the term systematic review indicates the report produced from a research synthesis.

Furthermore, the sampling process in research synthesis suffers from the same threats and limitations as the process of sampling in other research designs (i.e., observational designs, experimental designs, randomized clinical trials). For example, the threat of selection bias adulterates the sampling process in experimental studies when sampling is driven by convenience rather than by chance. Sampling of the literature suffers likewise from selection bias, when, for instance, our evaluation capabilities (i.e., critical reading, assessment tools) fail to be all-inclusive, including such barriers as include language, search engine, library availability, among others. That is another facet of the publication bias noted above.

On the other hand, the second major domain of methodology in the research synthesis designs pertains to the assessment of the level and quality of the evidence. As the sample process described above yields the *available evidence*, the assessment of the quality of the evidence uncovers the *best evidence*.

The goal of research synthesis is to obtain the best research evidence pertaining to any given scientific question, and making available and accessible. At issue, therefore, lie the specific definition and the practical quantification of the term "best." Two contemporary schools of thought can be succinctly described as such:

- On the one hand, there are those who defend the original proposition that a ranking system can be arbitrarily devised to evaluate the strength of the results of a study purely on the basis of the nature of the design.
- On the other hand, some argue that the best research is that which most strictly adheres to the fundamental tenets and standards of research methodology, design, and analysis.

The first system inevitably establishes one research design as superior, and another as inferior, and has evolved in a pictorial representation, that is, as we have stated elsewhere [7–10], as ludicrous as it is useless to the pursuit of the *best available* evidence.

To represent a ranking system graphically, such as a pyramid, which places clinical trials about the top, and animal studies about the bottom, is to ignore two important facts about health-care research:

1. Animal studies are a sine qua non to clinical trials—every and any intervention clinical trial on a group of patient cannot be initiated unless the proper safety and toxicity studies have been run on animal models.
2. Clinical trials encompass in fact a family of research protocols that begin with fundamental mechanistic studies on human materials, that is why, even at that very early stage, the National Institutes of Health[9] refers to this research as

[9] NIH in fact categorizes several types of clinical trials, including *Prevention trials*: prevent a disease, prevent a disease from returning; *Screening trials*: better detect certain diseases or conditions; *Diagnostic trials*: find better tests or procedures for diagnosing a particular disease or condition; *Treatment trials*: test experimental treatments, new drugs, surgery, or radiation therapy; *Quality of life trials*: improve comfort and quality of life for individuals with a chronic illness (i.e., Supportive Care trials); *Compassionate trials*: (Expanded Access trials): provide partially tested, unapproved therapeutics to patients with no other options.

"clinical research" continue on testing with animal subjects and, only when deemed safe, are tested for efficacy and for effectiveness with human normal subjects first, only then is a sample of patients tested (clinical trial, Phase III), and ultimately with a larger group of patients across study centers (Phase IV).[10]

The level of evidence pyramid simply ignores these facts, and in a wantonly oversimplified approach—some would say—assigns a rank close to the best to any study that tests an intervention on patients. This is achieved by means of a checklist, the consolidated standards of reporting trials (CONSORT) [5–11, 13]. Originally developed over a decade ago [13], it continues to suffer from its fundamental flaws even in its most recent upgrade and revision [14], and varied applications and modifications, including the 22-item checklist for evaluating the conduct of randomized controlled trials in livestock with production, health and food-safety outcomes (REFLECT) [15], the statement developed to ensure the developed the strengthening the reporting of observational studies in epidemiology (STROBE) [16, 17], or for strengthening the reporting of genetic association studies (STREGA; strega-statement.org) [18–20].

In the exact same mode, the STandards for Reporting Interventions in Clinical Trials of Acupuncture (STRICTA) were developed, published in the original format about a decade ago [21], and revised recently [22]. To this end, a collaboration between the STRICTA Group, the CONSORT Group, and the Chinese Cochrane Centre was established, and a panel of experts consulted. A consensus was obtained for the revised the STRICTA checklist to include 6 items and 17 subitems, which probe the acupuncture rationale, the details of needling, the treatment regimen, other components of treatment, the practitioner background, and the control or comparator interventions. The revised STRICTA benefits from a set of clear explanations of the criteria for each item, as well as examples of good reporting for each item. The revised STRICTA checklist is intended for use in conjunction with both the CONSORT statement and its extension for non-pharmacological treatment [22].

In the case of Ayurvedic medicine, concerted efforts have been deployed to utilize and to integrate CONSORT criteria [23, 24], but they have met with fundamental difficulties because of the characteristic complexities of the multimodal facets of

[10] According to Pocock [12], at least five different degrees or levels of clinical trials can be identified, the first two of which, certainly, fit in the descriptive narrative of experimental mechanistic-type research, and thus consistently fall short a ranking above observational studies in the pyramidal representation of the "level of evidence": Phase 0—human microdosing studies, designed to test whether or not the drug or agent behaves in human subjects as was expected from preclinical studies; Phase I—first stage of testing in a small sample of human healthy volunteer subjects ($n<100$) to verify the treatment's safety (pharmacovigilance), tolerability, pharmacokinetics, and pharmacodynamics; Phase II—larger, but still limited, study ($n<300$) with volunteer normal subjects and patients to test how the efficacy of the treatment (IIA studies test dose requirements; IIB verifies efficacy at the prescribed dose[s]); Phase III—large multicenter studies ($n>3{,}000$) aimed at being the definitive assessment of *efficacy and effectiveness*, usually in comparison with current "gold standard" treatment; Phase IV—"post marketing surveillance" trial, aimed at detecting rare or long-term adverse effects over a much larger patient population and longer time period than possible in a Phase III trial.

this mode of integrative medicine. As of late, it was recognized[11] that individual standards of a nature similar to CONSORT, STROBE, and STRICTA are needed for all systems of traditional complementary and alternative medicine, including Ayurveda [25, 26].

In the assessment of the level of evidence, the very top level of the pyramid is given to the systematic reviews, perhaps because early on in the establishment of research synthesis in evidence-based and comparative effectiveness research, it was presumed that systematic reviews in the health sciences ought to incorporate clinical trials exclusively.

The level of evidence is established on the basis of the type of study design that was used to generate the evidence under evaluation. Typically, a hierarchy is generated as follows (cf. US Preventive Services Task Force):

- *Level I*: Evidence obtained from at least one properly designed randomized controlled trial.
- *Level II-1*: Evidence obtained from well-designed controlled trials without randomization.
- *Level II-2*: Evidence obtained from well-designed cohort or case–control analytic studies, preferably from more than one center or research group.
- *Level II-3*: Evidence obtained from multiple time series with or without the intervention. Dramatic results in uncontrolled trials might also be regarded as this type of evidence.
- *Level III*: Opinions of respected authorities, based on clinical experience, descriptive studies, or reports of expert committees.

The UK National Health Service uses a similar system with categories labeled A, B, C, and D:

- *Level A*: Consistent Randomized Controlled Clinical Trial, cohort study, with clinical decision rule validated in different populations
- *Level B*: Consistent Retrospective Cohort, Exploratory Cohort, Ecological Study, Outcomes Research, case–control study; or extrapolations from level A studies
- *Level C*: Case-series study or extrapolations from level B studies
- *Level D*: Expert opinion without explicit critical appraisal, or based on physiology, bench research or first principles

In more recent years, since the fast emergence of systematic reviews, it is generally accepted that systematic reviews have a level of evidence that is even higher than I or A—a level "super-I/A." The complication of course arises at present, when one considers that the science of research synthesis continues to evolve, such that

[11] The Institute of Ayurveda and Integrative Medicine (I-AIM) collaborated with the South Asian Cochrane Network to organize a workshop to develop standards for reporting Ayurveda clinical trials (cf. South Asian CONSORT meeting, Christian Medical College, Vellore, India, January 12, 2010; Professor Darshan Shankar, Hon. Adviser for Indian Systems of Medicine to the Member (Health), Planning Commission of India, Chair). STRACT was proposed as the possible name for the CONSORT-like checklist of standards for reporting Ayurveda clinical trials.

multiple systematic reviews on a given clinical questions can now be pooled into what has been referred to as complex systematic reviews, and as clinically relevant complex systematic reviews (CRCSR) [27].

The initial attempt to quantify the CONSORT checklist was the Jadad scale [28], which overwhelmingly suffers from low reliability (i.e., unsatisfactory inter-rater and intra-rater reliability, unsatisfactory Cohen k coefficient of agreement) and construct or content validity, as discussed elsewhere [7–10]. Nevertheless, proponents of the assessment of the level of evidence purport to establish the *best available* evidence based on those criteria alone.

We and others have proposed that the *best available* evidence is not what stands atop a pyramid, but rather the research evidence that emerges from top-quality research: that is, research that satisfies the fundamental and widely accepted standards of superior research methodology, design, and data analysis. High-quality research answers the research question and tests the hypothesis in a scientific approach that is the most sound possible, considering all the limitations, intervening variables, and other possible confounders. Therefore, high-quality research, whether it is a clinical trial, an observational study, or an experimental design, whether it addresses Western medicine, Chinese medicine, or Ayurvedic medicine, will be of high-quality if it satisfies the criteria and standards of sound research methodology, design, and analysis; and in that regard, it promises to generate the *best* evidence.

What really is important is not so much *what* type of research was done, but *how* it was conducted. That only determines the excellence of the evidence produced [7–11, 13].

That is the view espoused by the second school of thought about how to obtain the best available evidence. The best evidence is not to be inferred by a checklist, but rather quantified on the basis of stringent and commonly shared criteria of excellence.

Increasingly, systematic reviews address the concern of the quality of the evidence. Usually, it is obtained by means of an in-house tool developed ad hoc, and only briefly described. Increasingly, however, well-constructed instruments to assess the quality of the evidence are used that are psychometrically tested for reliability and for validity and that generate continuous, or semicontinuous, score measurements [29–31].

Specifically with respect to evaluating the quality of systematic reviews, Shea and colleagues developed and characterized the assessment of multiple systematic reviews instrument (AMSTAR), through a process of factor and cluster analyses of previously existing instruments for this purpose (e.g., Overview Quality Assessment Questionnaire, OQAQ; Sacks' checklist; quality assessment of studies of diagnostic accuracy included in systematic reviews, QUADAS) [32, 33]. This process resulted in the identification of 11 domains that are essential for high-quality systematic reviews:

- "A priori" design provided
- Duplicate study selection and data extraction
- Comprehensive literature search
- Status of publication (i.e., gray literature) used as an inclusion criterion

- List of studies (included and excluded) provided
- Characteristics of the included studies provided
- Scientific quality of the included studies assessed and documented
- Scientific quality of the included studies used appropriately in formulating conclusions
- Methods used to combine the findings of studies
- Publication bias
- Conflict of interest

The AMSTAR was recently updated, revised, and made stringently quantifiable [31].

1.2.2.3 The Design

The third main point of the protocol of a scientifically driven research process is the design. The design of studies aimed at obtaining the best available evidence for the effectiveness and efficacy of clinical interventions are, by definition, research synthesis designs. The elements of these designs are the very components we have outlined to this point. When research designs in general and research synthesis designs in particular are planned and conducted correctly, they must produce quantifiable measures, which can be analyzed statistically.

1.2.2.4 The Analysis

Thus, the fourth and critical step in the pursuance of comparative effectiveness and efficacy is the analysis of the data. Over a decade ago, it became apparent that standards must be established for the appropriate reporting of meta-analytical analyses, especially when these pertained to the identification of the best available evidence for health care. The Quality of Reporting of Meta-analyses (QUOROM) statement [34] presented in 1999 as a checklist, and a flow diagram to outline the optimal flow of presentation of the abstract, introduction, methods, results, and discussion sections of a report of a meta-analysis. They were structured and organized into 21 headings and subheadings, which had the advantage of providing a set of guidelines for investigators, but were often arduous to understand and follow for the neophytes. In a recent development, QUOROM was revised and improved, and presented as the Preferred Reporting Items for Systematic Reviews and Meta-analyses (PRISMA) statement in 2009 [35, 36]. Whereas longer and more complex than CONSORT, PRISMA[12] consists of a 27-item checklist and a four-phase flow diagram, which is actually more user-friendly than QUOROM.

It is customary to think of research synthesis and meta-analysis as one and the same. But, whereas research synthesis is the structure by which the investigator

[12] prisma.org

obtains the systematic review, the meta-analysis is one of the protocols that the investigator will utilize judiciously to obtain one specific aspect of analysis of the data of the systematic review. There may be instances where a meta-analysis is not needed, or impossible to conduct in a given systematic review. That, in and of itself, does not diminish the value of the systematic review product, and the strength of the evidence it presents [6, 7].

In and of itself, meta-analysis is simply a statistical protocol, a combinatorial process of analysis that is extraordinary sensitive to several properties of the data. Two principal properties deserve mention in the context of this discussion are heterogeneity/homogeneity of outcome, and data quality

1. Clinical outcomes, whereas they may seem to clear and crisp measurable entities, more often than not can be quantified in more than one way. The heterogeneity in outcome measure is one clear danger for the validity of any meta-analytical reasoning, because it speaks directly to what, really, are we combining together, what really are we making overall inferences about. There are statistical tests that we must run on the outcome measurements that establish whether or not homogeneity is verified (cf. Cochran Q and its transformation as the I^2 test)—that is to say, whether or not the extent of outcome measure heterogeneity is within the level of confidence and is, in fact, not statistically significant [37].
2. The data pooled together into a meta-analysis be from reports that are deemed of good quality. If the data in the input are all of high quality, then the variability due to residual inexplicable error will be small, and the effect, if there is one, will be apparent and clearly statistically significant. If, on the other hand, the data that are used in the meta-analysis originate from studies that are fraught with serious quality issues, then each of these sets of data will carry into the meta-analysis its contribution of residual inexplicable error, and the total overall variability will be large and negate the ability of a statistically significant overall effect to become apparent over this residual error "noise." Similarly, albeit not as dramatically, if a meta-analysis should incorporate some solid and good studies and a few studies with serious quality issues, the contribution of the former to the variability due to residual inexplicable error will be small, but the contribution of the latter to the overall error will be disproportionately large. That will, more often than not, mask a statistically significant overall effect.

For that reason, many—most, but not all—investigators argue in favor of a two process of data analysis for systematic reviews:

- One school of thought that argues in favor of including all—bad and good—studies in a meta-analysis, akin perhaps to including all—good and bad—materials in the construction of a skyscraper. Should we be surprised if a high proportion of meta-analyses conducted in this manner evince no statistical significance overall?
- The other school of thought proposes to establish first the quality of the research evidence by acceptable sampling analysis [6, 7, 31]. Then, based on these assessments, eliminate the studies that demonstrate excessive flaws, as determined by the score of the quality of evidence assessment tools (i.e., acceptable sampling analysis). For the studies that remain, test for homogeneity, and if no significant

heterogeneity is noted with the accepted studies, then run the meta-analysis. The forest plot thus generated has the best likelihood of evincing overall significance, if there is one to be shown. Stated in statistical terms, it is necessary to perform both acceptable sampling and homogeneity analyses in order to ensure power of a meta-analysis.

The question remains as to what might be the recommended statistical approach to follow when performing a CRCSR, a synthesis of several systematic reviews. Following assessment of quality (e.g., R-AMSTAR, 30), and acceptable sampling, the CRCSR must be tested for homogeneity, as noted. If homogeneity is established, then meta-analysis will be permissible. But, from a purely statistical standpoint, our current conceptualization of the meta-analytical protocol pertains to coalescing data obtained from primary studies (e.g., clinical trials), not secondary studies (i.e., systematic reviews) that themselves present their own individual meta-analyses. The current attempts to generate "cumulative meta-analyses" as the simplistic additive product of a new meta-analysis generated every time a new piece of evidence emerges[13] [38, 39] appear to be incongruent with statistical theory on several grounds [40]. For example, the suggested approach implies repeated analytical testing of data set (n), as the data set grows to include the new piece of evidence ($n+1$). As stated, the principles do not proffer any limit to these repeated testing events, which seem at prima facie to incorporate the same bias[14] one finds upon performing repeated t tests. Further exploration of the theoretical tenets that impinge upon cumulative meta-synthesis is urgently needed, and lest cumulative meta-analyses accumulate in the literature needlessly.

1.2.2.5 The Consensus Inference

The question that researchers ask pertains to whether statistically significant differences obtain. Then, somehow, forest plot summary data and confidence intervals, which are coalesced and analyzed group data, are transformed by means of the magical—it may seem—process of interpretation and inference into clinical relevance, a consensus inference.

[13] In cumulative meta-analysis studies are added one at a time in a specified order (e.g., according to date of publication or quality) and the results are summarized as each new study is added. In a graph of a cumulative meta-analysis each horizontal line represents the summary of the results as each study is added, rather than the results of a single study. That is to say, a cumulative meta-analysis is actually a series of meta-analyses, where each analysis in the sequence incorporates one additional study. While cumulative meta-analysis is most often used to track evidence over time, it is also be used to show how the evidence shifts and changes in time.

[14] In the case of repeated t test, this bias lends the analysis increasingly less powerful, by "chipping away" from the level of significance, α as follows: $p(\text{Type I error}) = 1-(1-\alpha)^c$, thus when $c=1$ (one comparison) then $p=1-(1-0.05)^1=1-(0.95)1=0.05$; but if we were to perform 3 "cumulative" t tests, then $c=3$ and $p=1-(0.95)^3=0.14$. It is probable that the level of significance of a cumulative meta-analysis would be biased in a similar manner, based on probability distributions.

The consensus statement must be clear statement of the clinical implication and relevance of the research synthesis and meta-synthesis. It must present clearly the strength of the clinical recommendation thusly conceptualized. The GRADE (Grades of Recommendation, Assessment, Development, and Evaluation) approach is an instrument for grading the quality of underlying evidence and the strength of clinical recommendations [31, 32]. In a similar vein, the AGREE (Appraisal of Guidelines and Research and Evaluation, Europe) is an instrument developed to provide a basis for defining steps in a shared development approach to produce high-quality clinical practice guidelines revised based upon the best available evidence [33, 34].

Case in point is a recent systematic review of clinical trials and quasi-experimental studies aimed at testing certain among the plethora of the Ayurvedic medicine pharmacopoeic herbs that might contribute to a decrease in cholesterol and therefore reduce the risk of ischemic heart disease (P.I.C.O.). For this particular investigation, the pertinent literature was searched in the National Library of Medicine, the National Center for Complementary and Alternative Medicine, Ovid, and EBSCO Information Services at three time points (T). Three standardized reviewers were used to ascertain the inter-rater reliability of the quality of evidence assessments. Both issues of effectiveness and efficacy were examined and led to the overall consensus inference that Ayurvedic herbs can significantly benefit patients with hyperlipidemia [41]. In a similar vein, a retrospective meta-analysis of observation studies conducted on 85 Ayurvedic herbal interventions with reported anticancer efficacy pointed the fact that herbs with *Katu*, *Tikta*, *Kasāya Rasa* (i.e., bitter, pungent, and astringent taste), *Usna Virya* (i.e., hot biopotency), and *Katu Vipāka* (i.e., catabolic active metabolites), and herbs with dry, coarse, light, and sharp biophysical properties are endowed with both effective and efficacious anticancer properties [42].

In brief, perhaps the single most important use of the science of research synthesis and research meta-synthesis in the health sciences, including complementary and alternative medicine, pertains to empowering the clinician to make fully informed decisions for treatment that rest not only on the patient's wants and needs, clinical tests and history, or the clinician's experience and personal awareness of the available research, but, as well, on the best available evidence. It is important to stress the summative quality of this sine qua non: in addition to all the previous, which equate the best current clinical practice, reliance on the science of research synthesis and meta-synthesis signifies adding to the decision-making process the best available evidence. Hence, the need to have reliable instruments to assess and to establish the strength of the clinical relevance and recommendations for the uncovered *best available* evidence.

Whereas both the GRADE and the AGREE instruments are laudable efforts in the direction of fostering the growth and expansion of research synthesis and meta-synthesis, they also suffer from inherent psychometric weaknesses. Therefore, we have endeavored in the process of expanding the GRADE tool (Ex-GRADE[15]) in an

---

[15] Chiappelli et al. [5]; Phi et al. [45].

effort to emphasize not only in dual applicability to systematic reviews and to CRCSR but also in the solid conceptualization it offers of the strength of the clinical recommendation the instrument proffers. The information produced by the research synthesis process, and by the Ex-GRADE evaluation of the thusly obtained *best available* evidence, can then be safely utilized in clinical decision-making for effectiveness and efficacy [9, 10].

As stated above and in absolute terms, efficacy refers to whether or not a clinical intervention tested in the context of a clinical trial yielded valid and replicable outcomes. In lay language, we might say that efficacy tells us whether or not the treatment "worked," and it does so because of its inherent dependence upon the effort the investigator in constructing the research project correctly, and fractionating as much as the random error as possible. In that regard, efficacy establishes the replicability of the clinical outcome. By contrast, effectiveness relates to the experiential reality of the clinical practice and pertains to whether or not the intervention minimizes risk, maximizes benefit, and yields these outcomes at the lowest (or at least the most reasonable) cost. It is fair to say that effectiveness does not pertain to a clinical trial study per se, but rather to the pragmatic implementations of its findings to the intricate complexities of clinical treatment. Considerations of effectiveness seeks to evaluate costs, benefits, and harms of clinical interventions, such as complementary and alternative medicine in general and Ayurvedic medicine in particular to prevent, diagnose, treat, and monitor a clinical condition or to improve the delivery of care. Its purpose of is to assist consumers, clinicians, purchasers, and policymakers to make informed decisions that will improve health care at both the individual and population levels [43, 44].

1.2.3 Resources (Appendix) for Complementary and Alternative Medicine

It should be evident from the discussion above that, as the body of scientific information in health care and in complementary and alternative medicine grows, and because of differing criteria of establishing the quality of research reports, the scientific literature is becoming replete with multiple systematic reviews that pertain to the same original clinical question, but that may differ in their conclusions. This observation leads to the realization that the science of research synthesis is itself growing. Therefore, it is important that resources be identified that guide the search for, and the interpretation of the *best available* evidence.

One such resource is CAMline is an evidence-based website on complementary and alternative medicine (CAM) for health-care professionals and the public. It represents a successful collaboration of conventional and CAM organizations, interests, and expertise (www.camline.ca/index.html). Other similar resources are provided in the Appendix.

1.3 Conclusion

In the preceding paragraphs, we have touched upon the salient fundamental elements of the evidence-based process in complementary and alternative medicine. We have proposed that in the domain of the science of research synthesis, we must engage in the gargantuan task of establishing methodologies, designs, modes of statistical analysis, and appropriate inferential criteria for the process of synthesis of systematic reviews into "meta-systematic" reviews. We need to go beyond the current protocols of research synthesis that pertain to primary research reports, and develop and validate new and effective procedures for "research meta-synthesis" for the evaluation of the best available evidence now existing in the form of systematic reviews. We have identified established protocols, and uncovered new and novel avenue of emergence of this rich and active field.

Specifically, we have proposed the thesis of this chapter is that CAM is enriched by the systematic approach of comparative effectiveness and efficacy research and analysis for practice (CEERAP). We discussed the implications and applications of EBDM in CAM, the systematic nature of the CEERAP process toward EBDM, and the pitfalls and limitations of this approach as it pertains specifically to Ayurvedic medicine.

Appendix

Evidence-Based Complementary and Alternative Medicine Online Resources Prepared by Linda Murphy and Jennifer Hoock for W8 at STFM 2007 (available from www.fmdrl.org/index.cfm?event=c.getAttachment&riid=1487)

Free Online Full-Text and/or Bibliographic Databases on CAM

- AGRICOLA (Agricultural Online Access) AGRICOLA is created by the US National Agricultural Library. It includes citations about herbs and medicinal plants and includes references from the Herb Research Foundations' HerbalGram. Production of electronic records began in 1970, but the database covers materials in all formats, including print works from the fifteenth century. Some records are linked to online full-text documents. URL: http://agricola.nal.usda.gov/
- CAM on PubMedCAM on PubMed was developed jointly by NLM & NCCAM. CAM on PubMed provides journal citations related to complementary and alternative medicine (CAM). It is a subset of all citations found on the NLM's PubMed. The subset contains over 220,000 citations from mid-1950 to the present. The subset restricts retrieval to specific CAM topics. Individual citation displays holding

information, and some of which provide direct access to free full-text of articles. URL: http://www.ncbi.nlm.nih.gov/entrez/query.fcgi?db=PubMed&itool=toolbar

- Cochrane Collaboration Complementary Medicine Field Funding was awarded in 1996 to the University of Maryland Program of Complementary Medicine to establish the Cochrane Collaboration Complementary Medicine Field. Their main function is to construct a database of all the known RCTs (published or unpublished, in all language) that pertain to CAM. Approximately 5,800 CAM RCTs and over 230 systematic reviews have been identified. URL: http://www.campain.umm.edu/ris/risweb.isa
- HerbMed The public site of HerbMed is a free, searchable database produced by the Alternative Medicine Foundation, Inc. It is updated only two times a year. The new herbs and updates of existing herbs are only available on the professional version, HerbMedPro, and it is available for licensing or subscription (http://www.herbmed.org/licensing.asp). HerbMed aims to provide access to the scientific data underlying the use of herbs for health. Information is provided for each herb on evidence for activity, warnings (including contraindications, adverse effects, and interactions), preparations, mixtures, mechanisms of action, and other information. URL: http://www.herbmed.org/
- ICL (Index to Chiropractic Literature) This is a free web-based database funded by the Association of Chiropractic Colleges. Librarians from 13 different chiropractic colleges contributed to its indexing. This database indexes 41 chiropractic journals using terms from MeSH and CHIROSH from 1985 to the present. URL: http://www.chiroindex.org/#results
- Memorial Sloan-Kettering Cancer Center This information resource, presented by our Integrative Medicine Service, provides evidence-based information on herbs, botanicals, and other products. URL: http://www.mskcc.org/mskcc/html/11570.cfm
- NIH The Office of Dietary Supplements (ODS) The ODS provides a web-searchable database of funded research and scientific papers on dietary supplements. It contains two databases called CARDS and IBIDS. The International Bibliographic Information on Dietary Supplements (IBIDS) database provides access to bibliographic citations and abstracts from published, international, scientific literature on dietary supplements. Computer Access to Research on Dietary Supplements (CARDS) is a database of federally funded research projects pertaining to dietary supplements. URL: http://dietary-supplements.info.nih.gov/index.aspx
- OSTMED: The Osteopathic Literature Database A bibliographic index to the osteopathic medicine literature. Sponsored by the American Osteopathic Association and the American Association of Colleges of Osteopathic Medicine, OSTMED is produced by the Gibson D. Lewis Health Science Library of the University of North Texas Health Science Center at Fort Worth and the A.T. Still Memorial Library of the Kirksville College of Osteopathic Medicine. OSTMED® contains selected journal and book citations from the 1800s through 2003. Unfortunately, since financial support ceased January 31, 2004, citations are no longer being added to the database. URL: http://ostmed.hsc.unt.edu/ostmed/index.html

- The Trip Database: "It is produced by TRIP Database Ltd." The TRIP database searches sources of medical information, including publications on evidence-based medicine, query-answering services, guidelines, E-textbooks, medical images, patient information leaflets, and peer-reviewed journals in PubMed. URL: http://www.tripdatabase.com/index.html

Systematic Reviews

- Bandolier Complementary and Alternative Therapies Bandolier Complementary and Alternative Therapies provides EBM health-care-related issues to medical professionals and consumers. Health topics include the nature of evidence, herbal medicine and supplements, acupuncture, homeopathy, massage, and safety concerns. The site provides abstracts of systematic reviews, meta-analyses, or other studies about CAM. The content is "tertiary" publishing, distilling the information from secondary reviews of primary. Currently it contains over 100 summaries on the effectiveness of CAM. URL: http://www.jr2.ox.ac.uk/bandolier/booth/booths/altmed.html
- The Cochrane Library Developed by the Cochrane Collaboration, the Cochrane Library supplies high-quality evidence to inform people providing and receiving care, and those responsible for research, teaching, funding, and administration at all levels. The database is updated quarterly on the Internet. The Library consists of Systematic Reviews, Abstracts of Reviews of Effectiveness, Register of Controlled Trials, the Methodology Reviews, and the Cochrane Methodology Register. The Library contains over 5,700 reports of RCTs and over 80 systematic reviews in CAM. URL: http://www3.interscience.wiley.com/cgibin/mrwhome/106568753/HOME
- PEDro: an initiative of the Centre for Evidence-Based Physiotherapy (CEBP) PEDro is the Physiotherapy Evidence Database. It has been developed to give rapid access to bibliographic details and abstracts of randomized controlled trials and systematic reviews in physiotherapy. Most trials on the database have been rated for quality to help users quickly discriminate between trials that are likely to be valid and interpretable and those which are not. Reliability of the PEDro scale for rating quality of randomized controlled trials has been published in Physical Therapy 83(8):713–721, 2003 August. Abstract can be viewed at http://www.ptjournal.org/info/pt_abs.cfm. PEDro also contains evidence-based clinical practice guidelines. URL: http://www.pedro.fhs.usyd.edu.au/index.html

Fee-Based EBCAM Online Resources

- The Natural Medicines Comprehensive Database A comprehensive database that provides evidence-based, clinical information on natural products. It is designed for medical professions and updated daily. Product Search is available at the top of every page. It can be browsed or find general data on a selected product. It can also be searched by scientific name, common name, brand name, or by ingredient. URL: http://www.naturaldatabase.com

- Natural Standard (electronic resource): the authority on integrative medicine The database provides evidence-based information about complementary and alternative therapies. It contains three subdatabases: herbs and supplements, condition center, and alternative modalities. For each therapy covered by Natural Standard, a research team gathers scientific data and expert opinions. Validated rating scales are used to evaluate the quality of available evidence. Information is incorporated into comprehensive monographs designed to facilitate clinical decision-making. All monographs undergo blinded editorial and peer review prior to inclusion. URL: http://www.naturalstandard.com/

CAM Curriculum Resources

- EDCAM: Educational Development for Complementary and Alternative Medicine Provided CAM curriculum resources that were developed and reviewed by the EDCAM grant team and advisory panel along with expert consultants in the field of CAM and medical education. URL: http://www.amsa.org/humed/CAM/index.cfm
- Stress reduction, relaxation, and wellness: "This module describes a workshop that would provide medical students with healthy coping skills and introduce lifelong self-care techniques for stress reduction, relaxation, and wellness. Both didactic and experiential learning are emphasized, particularly in the area of mind-body medicine." URL: http://www.amsa.org/humed/CAM/A.doc
- Introduction to Evidence-Based Complementary and Alternative Medicine: "This module provides guidelines and resources for basic introduction to the various medicines practiced around the world, collectively referred to as complementary and alternative medicines (CAM). Epidemiology, usage, and terminology are emphasized." URL: http://www.amsa.org/humed/CAM/B.doc
- The Core Curriculum CAM Integration in ten categories: "The curriculum resource materials were developed and reviewed by the AMSA Foundation's EDCAM Grant Team and Advisory Panel along with expert consultants in the field of CAM and medical education." URL: http://www.amsa.org/humed/CAM/resources.cfm
- Nutrition and Lifestyle: "This module provides guidelines and resources for education to medical students about the medical aspects of nutrition and lifestyle and their effects on health." URL: http://www.amsa.org/humed/CAM/C1.doc
- Mind–Body Medicines: "This module provides guidelines and resources for education to medical students about mind-body medicines and the scientific and clinical basis for their usage." URL: http://www.amsa.org/humed/CAM/C2.doc
- Alternative Systems of Medical Thought: Traditional Chinese Medicine, Kampo, Tibetan Medicine, and Acupuncture: "This module provides guidelines and

resources for education to medical students about alternative medical paradigms evolving in Asia and the clinical practice of traditional Chinese medicine (TCM), kampo, Tibetan medicine, and acupuncture." URL: http://www.amsa.org/humed/CAM/C3.doc

- Alternative Systems of Medical Thought: Yoga, Ayurveda, Native American, and Yoruba-Based Medicines: "This module provides guidelines and resources for education and background on alternative systems of medicine including Yoga and Ayurveda, and also introduces other systems that emphasize attunement with the environment such as Native American medicines and Yoruba medicine." URL: http://www.amsa.org/humed/CAM/C4.doc
- Alternative Systems of Medical Thought: Homeopathy and Flower Essences (updated 5/03): "This module provides guidelines and resources for education to medical students about homeopathy and provides a brief introduction to flower essence therapy." URL: http://www.amsa.org/humed/CAM/C5.doc
- Bioenergetic Medicines: "This module provides guidelines and resources for education to medical students about medical therapies using low-level energetic fields known commonly as energy medicine." URL: http://www.amsa.org/humed/CAM/C6.doc
- Pharmacologic/Biologically Based: Herbal Medicines: "This module provides guidelines and resources for education to medical students about plants used as medical therapies in herbal medicine, and introduces basic principles of naturopathy and aromatherapy." URL: http://www.amsa.org/humed/CAM/C7.doc
- Pharmacologic/Biologically Based: Nutrition, Dietary Supplements and Vitamins: "This module provides guidelines and resources for education to medical students about nutrition from a biochemical aspect. It includes background on dietary supplements, vitamins, and minerals." URL: http://www.amsa.org/humed/CAM/C8.doc
- Manipulative Therapies: Chiropractic and Osteopathy: "This module provides guidelines and resources for education to medical students about osteopathy and chiropractic, practices employing manipulative therapy." URL: http://www.amsa.org/humed/CAM/C9.doc
- Manipulative Therapies: Therapeutic Massage: "This module provides guidelines and resources for education to medical students about manual therapies including touch therapy, massage, and other medicinal approaches using hands, touch, and/or body awareness. It includes background on other movement and/or educational approaches such as Feldenkrais, Trager, Alexander Technique, deep fascial realignment like Rolfing, and massage therapies used in other systems such as Ayurveda and traditional Chinese medicine." URL: http://www.amsa.org/humed/CAM/C10.doc
- CAM Clinical Interviewing: "This outline describes suggested activities for students to learn how to incorporate holistic principles into their clinical skills of interacting with patients. Divided into four main categories, the CAM clinical interviewing components of the curriculum should emphasize CAM history taking, holistic interviewing, patient-centered care, and cultural competency.

An additional introduction to alternative medical methods of clinical diagnosis is also provided." URL: http://www.amsa.org/humed/CAM/D.doc

- Integrative Medicine Field Study: "This module provides suggested activities and resources for students interested in moving beyond didactic and experiential work in CAM. As part of the integrative medicine field study course, AMSA suggests four independent and self-directed exercises to complement the existing curricula: CAM research, literature searches, community service, and mentorship." URL: http://www.amsa.org/humed/CAM/E.doc
- The Consortium of Academic Health Centers for Integrative Medicine (CAHCIM): The Center is supported by a grant from the Philanthropic Collaborative for Integrative Medicine. Their membership currently includes 36 highly esteemed academic medical centers http://www.imconsortium.org/cahcim/members/home.html. Their mission is "to help transform medicine and health care through rigorous scientific studies, new models of clinical care, and innovative educational programs that integrate biomedicine, the complexity of human beings, the intrinsic nature of healing, and the rich diversity of therapeutic systems." URL: http://www.imconsortium.org/
- Core competencies in integrative medicine for medical school curricula: a proposal. Acad Med. 2004 Jun;79(6):521–531. Review.PMID: 15165971 [PubMed—indexed for MEDLINE]
- Curriculum in Integrative Medicine: A Guide for Medical Educators. May 2004 "The Consortium of Academic Health Centers for Integrative Medicine Education Working Group developed a set of competencies for undergraduate medical education (medical school level) that was published in the June 2004 issue of Academic Medicine: Core Competencies in Integrative Medicine for Medical School Curricula: A Proposal URL: http://www.imconsortium.org/img/assets/20862/AcademicMedicine1.pdf As a follow-up, the EWG project leaders developed and disseminated a curriculum guide that provided specific examples and illustrations from Consortium institutions regarding how medical schools can approach the implementation of the recommended competencies. The Guide for Medical Educators is no longer available in print, but all materials may be downloaded. The EWG is presently writing a follow-up article to this guide that will highlight these innovative curricula and provide additional examples from newer Consortium member schools." URL: http://www.imconsortium.org/img/assets/20825/CURRICULUM_final.pdf
- Northwest AHEC Online Professional Curriculum on Herbs and Dietary Supplements These online courses specifically designed for Physicians, physician assistants, nurses, advanced practice nurses, pharmacists, dietitians, nutritionists, other interested health-care professionals and health professions students-in-training (including residents, fellows, and postdoctoral students). The goal is to improve knowledge, confidence, and communication with the use of herbs and dietary supplements. The curriculum has been approved for a maximum of 14 h of continuing education credit. URL: https://northwestahec.wfubmc.edu/learn/herbs_ce/index.cfm

Free Online Journals and Newsletters

- Alternative Health News Online, URL: http://altmedicine.com/FrameSet.asp
- BMC Complementary and Alternative Medicine from Vol. 1, 2001 to the present. URL: http://www.pubmedcentral.nih.gov/tocrender.fcgi?journal=10&action=archive
- British Medical Journal: As of March, 2007, it published and collected over 140 articles on Complementary Therapies. URL: http://bmj.com/cgi/collection/complementary_medicine
- Dietary Supplements/Food Labeling Electronic Newsletter, URL: http://www.cfsan.fda.gov/~dms/infonet.html
- Evidence-based Complementary and Alternative Medicine from Vol. 1, 2004 to the present. URL: http://www.pubmedcentral.nih.gov/tocrender.fcgi?journal=241&action=archive
- Natural Standard Monthly Newsletter URL: http://www.naturalstandard.com/
- NCCAM Newsletter, URL: http://nccam.nih.gov/news/newsletter/

References

1. Chiappelli F, Prolo P (2001) The meta-construct of evidence based dentistry: Part I. J Evid Based Dent Pract 1:159–165
2. Chiappelli F, Prolo P, Cajulis OS (2005) Evidence-based research in complementary and alternative medicine I. Evid Based Complement Altern Med 2:453–458
3. Kopelman LM (2004) The role of science in assessing conventional, complementary, and alternative medicines. In: Callahan D (ed) The role of complementary and alternative medicine: accommodating pluralism. Georgetown University Press, Washington, DC, pp 36–53
4. Chiappelli F, Prolo P, Rosenblum M, Edgeron M, Cajulis OS (2006) Evidence-based research in complementary and alternative medicine II: the process of evidence-based research. Evid Based Complement Altern Med 3:3–12
5. Chiappelli F, Cajulis C, Brant XMC (2011) Applications for comparative effectiveness and efficacy research and analysis for practice (CEERAP) in developing patient-centered optimal treatment interventions in health care for the next decade. In: Chiappelli F, Brant X, Cajulis C (eds) Comparative effectiveness and efficacy research and analysis for practice (CEERAP): applications for treatment options in health care. Springer, Heidelberg
6. Littell JH, Corcoran J, Pillai V (2008) Systematic reviews and meta-analysis. Oxford University Press, New York
7. Chiappelli F (2008) The science of research synthesis: a manual of evidence-based research for the health sciences—implications and applications in dentistry. NovaScience, Hauppauge
8. Chiappelli F, Cajulis OC, Oluwadara O, Ramchandani MH (2009) Evidence-based based decision making—implications for clinical dentistry. In: Columbus F (ed) Clinical dentistry: diagnostic, preventive, and restorative services. NovaScience, Hauppauge
9. Chiappelli F (2010) Sustainable evidence-based decision-making. Monograph. NovaScience, Hauppauge
10. Chiappelli F, Brant XMC, Oluwadara OO, Neagos N, Ramchandani MH (eds) (2010) Understanding evidence-based practice: toward optimizing clinical outcomes. Springer, Heidelberg
11. Whitlock EP, Lopez SA, Chang S, Helfand M, Eder M, Floyd N (2009) Identifying, selecting, and refining topics. In: Methods guide for comparative effectiveness reviews. Agency for

Healthcare Research and Quality, Rockville, MD. http://effectivehealthcare.ahrq.gov/healthInfo.cfm?infotype=rr&ProcessID=60. Accessed 1 September 2011
12. Pocock SJ (2004) Clinical trials: a practical approach. Wiley, New York
13. Moher D, Schulz KF, Altman DG (2001) The CONSORT statement: revised recommendations for improving the quality of reports of parallel-group randomized trials. Ann Intern Med 134(8):657–662
14. Moher D, Hopewell S, Schulz KF, Montori V, Gøtzsche PC, Devereaux PJ, Elbourne D, Egger M, Altman DG, Consolidated Standards of Reporting Trials Group (2010) CONSORT 2010 explanation and elaboration: updated guidelines for reporting parallel group randomised trials. J Clin Epidemiol 63:e1–e37
15. Sargeant JM, O'Connor AM, Gardner IA, Dickson JS, Torrence ME, Dohoo IR, Lefebvre SL, Morley PS, Ramirez A, Snedeker K (2010) The REFLECT statement: reporting guidelines for randomized controlled trials in livestock and food safety: explanation and elaboration. J Food Prot 73:579–603
16. Vandenbroucke JP, von Elm E, Altman DG, Gøtzsche PC, Mulrow CD, Pocock SJ, Poole C, Schlesselman JJ, Egger M, STROBE Initiative (2007) Strengthening the Reporting of Observational Studies in Epidemiology (STROBE): explanation and elaboration. Epidemiology 18:805–835
17. von Elm E, Altman DG, Egger M, Pocock SJ, Gøtzsche PC, Vandenbroucke JP, STROBE Initiative (2007) The Strengthening the Reporting of Observational Studies in Epidemiology (STROBE) statement: guidelines for reporting observational studies. Lancet 370:1453–1457
18. von Elm E, Moher D, Little J, STREGA Collaboration (2009) Reporting genetic association studies: the STREGA statement. Lancet 374:98–100
19. Little J, Higgins JP, Ioannidis JP, Moher D, Gagnon F, von Elm E, Khoury MJ, Cohen B, Davey-Smith G, Grimshaw J, Scheet P, Gwinn M, Williamson RE, Zou GY, Hutchings K, Johnson CY, Tait V, Wiens M, Golding J, van Duijn C, McLaughlin J, Paterson A, Wells G, Fortier I, Freedman M, Zecevic M, King R, Infante-Rivard C, Stewart A, Birkett N (2009) STrengthening the REporting of Genetic Association studies (STREGA): an extension of the STROBE Statement. Ann Intern Med 150:206–215
20. Thelle DS (2009) STROBE and STREGA: instruments for improving transparency and quality of reporting scientific results. Eur J Epidemiol 24:7–8
21. MacPherson H, White A, Cummings M, Jobst KA, Rose K, Niemtzow RC, STRICTA Group (2002) Standards for Reporting Interventions in Controlled Trials of Acupuncture: the STRICTA recommendations. J Altern Complement Med 8:85–89
22. MacPherson H, Altman DG, Hammerschlag R, Li Y, Wu T, White A, Moher D, STRICTA Revision Group (2010) Revised STandards for Reporting Interventions in Clinical Trials of Acupuncture (STRICTA): extending the CONSORT statement. Acupunct Med 28:83–93
23. Narahari SR, Ryan TJ, Aggithaya MG, Bose KS, Prasanna KS (2008) Evidence-based approaches for the Ayurvedic traditional herbal formulations: toward an Ayurvedic CONSORT model. J Altern Complement Med 14:769–776
24. Rastogi S, Chiappelli F (2010) Bringing evidence basis to decision making in complementary and alternative medicine (CAM): prakriti (constitution) analysis in Ayurveda. In: Chiappelli F, Brant XMC, Oluwadara OO, Neagos N, Ramchandani MH (eds) Understanding evidence-based practice: toward optimizing clinical outcomes. Springer, Heidelberg, Chap 7
25. Mathur A, Shanker V (2010) Standards of reporting Ayurvedic clinical trials—Is there a need? J Ayur Integr Med 1:52–55
26. Tillu G (2010) Workshop on a CONSORT statement for Ayuveda. J Ayur Integr Med 1:158–159
27. Chiappelli F, Avila J, Chai DY, Dimaano C, Kudaverdian A, Park SH, Peng S, Sahhal S (2010) Evidence-dentistry in the XXI century: toward clinically relevant complex systematic reviews (CRCSRs). Open Dent J 4:1–3
28. Jadad AR, Moore RA, Carroll D, Jenkinson C, Reynolds DJM, Gavaghan DJ, McQuay HJ (1996) Assessing the quality of reports of randomized clinical trials: is blinding necessary? Control Clin Trials 17(1):1–12

29. Chiappelli F, Navarro AM, Moradi DR, Manfrini E, Prolo P (2006) Evidence-based research in complementary and alternative medicine III: treatment of patients with Alzheimer's disease. Evid Based Complement Altern Med 3:411–424
30. Systematic Reviews: CRD's guidance for undertaking reviews in health care (2009) Center for Reviews and Dissemination, York University (www.york.ac.uk/inst/crd/index.htm)
31. Kung J, Chiappelli F, Cajulis OS, Avezova R, Kossan G, Chew L, Maida CA (2010) From systematic reviews to clinical recommendations for evidence-based health care: validation of revised assessment of multiple systematic reviews (R-AMSTAR) for grading of clinical relevance. Open Dent J 4:84–91
32. Shea BJ, Hamel C, Wells GA, Bouter LM, Kristjansson E, Grimshaw J, Henry DA, Boers M (2009) AMSTAR is a reliable and valid measurement tool to assess the methodological quality of systematic reviews. J Clin Epidemiol 62:1013–1020
33. Shea BJ, Grimshaw JM, Wells GA, Boers M, Andersson N, Hamel C, Porter AC, Tugwell P, Moher D, Bouter LM (2007) Development of AMSTAR: a measurement tool to assess the methodological quality of systematic reviews. BMC Med Res Methodol 7:10
34. Moher D, Cook DJ, Eastwood S, Olkin I, Rennie D, Stroup DF (1999) Improving the quality of reports of meta-analyses of randomised controlled trials: the QUOROM statement. Quality of reporting of meta-analyses. Lancet 354:1896–1900
35. Moher D, Liberati A, Tetzlaff J, Altman DG, PRISMA Group (2009) Preferred reporting items for systematic reviews and meta-analyses: the PRISMA statement. PLoS Med 6:e1000097
36. Liberati A, Altman DG, Tetzlaff J, Mulrow C, Gøtzsche PC, Ioannidis JP, Clarke M, Devereaux PJ, Kleijnen J, Moher D (2009) The PRISMA statement for reporting systematic reviews and meta-analyses of studies that evaluate health care interventions: explanation and elaboration. PLoS Med 6:e1000100
37. Bartolucci AA, Hillegas WB (2010) Overview, strengths, and limitations of systematic reviews and meta-analyses. In: Chiappelli F, Brant XMC, Oluwadara OO, Neagos N, Ramchandani MH (eds) Understanding evidence-based practice: toward optimizing clinical outcomes. Springer, Heidelberg, Chap 2
38. Lau J, Schmid CH, Chalmers TC (1995) Cumulative meta-analysis of clinical trials builds evidence for exemplary medical care. J Clin Epidemiol 48:45–57
39. Moles DR, Needleman IG, Niederman R, Lau J (2005) Introduction to cumulative meta-analysis in dentistry: lessons learned from undertaking a cumulative meta-analysis in periodontology. J Dent Res 84:345–349
40. Janket SJ, Moles DR, Lau J, Needleman I, Niederman R (2005) Caveat for a cumulative meta-analysis. J Dent Res 84:487
41. Singh BB, Vinjamury SP, Der-Martirosian C, Kubik E, Mishra LC, Shepard NP, Singh VJ, Meier M, Madhu SG (2007) Ayurvedic and collateral herbal treatments for hyperlipidemia: a systematic review of randomized controlled trials and quasiexperimental designs. Altern Ther Health Med 13:22–28
42. Singh RH (2002) An assessment of the Ayurvedic concept of cancer and a new paradigm of anticancer treatment in Ayurveda. J Altern Complement Med 8:609–614
43. Agency for Healthcare Research and Quality (AHRQ) report: creating a framework for "best evidence" approaches in systematic reviews, review protocol (2010) Agency for Healthcare Research and Quality, Rockville, MD. http://www.ahrq.gov/clinic/tp/bestevtp.htm. Accessed 1 September 2011
44. Higgins JPT, Green S (eds) (2008) Cochrane handbook for systematic reviews of interventions. The Cochrane Collaboration 2008. Wiley, Chichester. www.cochrane.org
45. Phi L, Ajaj RA, Ramchandani MH, Brant XMC, Oluwadara O, Polinovsky O, Moradi D, Barkhordarian A, Sriphanlop P, Ong M, Giroux A, Lee J, Siddiqui M, Ghodousi N, Chiappelli F (2011) Expanding the Grading of Recommendations Assessment, Development, and Evaluation (Ex-GRADE) for Evidence-Based Clinical Recommendations: Validation Study. Open Dent J (in press)

Part II
Evidence-Based Medicine and Ayurveda

Chapter 2
Transforming Ayurveda: Stepping into the Realm of Evidence-Based Practice

Sanjeev Rastogi and Ram Harsh Singh

2.1 Introduction

Before we start a discussion about the need of transforming Ayurveda through adoption of evidence-based approaches, a theme of this book, it needs to be clarified that by no means, it challenges the classical principles or practice of Ayurveda but rather supplements it in light of best available evidences to the tune of conventional understanding. Where these evidences are not available due to the paucity of tools or due to the inadequacy of work done, this provokes us to search, create, and amend the existing pieces of clues from clinical practice of Ayurveda and transform them into the nitty-gritty of evidence-based research upon which evidence-based Ayurveda (EBA) as a discipline can successfully be erected.

For selecting a treatment, previously, it was considered sufficient to know about the pathophysiological process of a disease and to understand what a drug might be doing to interrupt such a process [1]. Such pieces of information were often collected independently in pathology and pharmacology labs and were clubbed together to determine a clinical application. More often, these experiments were done through isolated pharmacologically active compounds on in vitro or animal models where a disease was produced artificially.

Only later, it was realized that experiments done on synthesized model cannot simulate the real-life situation of a pathogenesis in a human being and also the behavior of a drug compound studied in such models cannot be replicated in a

S. Rastogi (✉)
PG Department of Kaya Chikitsa, State Ayurvedic College, Lucknow University, Lucknow, Uttar Pradesh, India
e-mail: rastogisanjeev@rediffmail.com

R.H. Singh
Department of Kaya Chikitsa, Institute of Medical Sciences, Banaras Hindu University, Varanasi, India
e-mail: rh_singh2001@yahoo.com

S. Rastogi (ed.), *Evidence-Based Practice in Complementary and Alternative Medicine*, DOI 10.1007/978-3-642-24565-7_2, © Springer-Verlag Berlin Heidelberg 2012

human object where a number of confounding factors operate simultaneously to affect the net outcome of the drug effect.

It is because of this reason; such experimental medicines often fail to produce the holistic effects against a pathogenesis or are often accompanied with a variety of undesired effects which might not be welcomed by all.

Randomized clinical trials intervened at this moment, by offering to study the effects of certain drugs upon human subjects with defined pathogenesis. Randomization offered a reduction of bias related to sample selection which might have influenced the results in case of a stratified sample [2]. Further addition of controlling mechanism to randomized study has given an additional edge to these studies by identifying its superiority, noninferiority, or equivalence to the comparator [3]. Placebo (a compound mimicking the therapeutic compound in appearance, taste, and smell but not having any therapeutic value) which was identified as a strong influencing factor to determine the net outcome of any therapeutic intervention was also added later to these studies to find if the intervention is substantially different than no treatment or placebo.

This gradual awakening about the necessity of unbiased and therefore dependable information as a compulsive paraphernalia to make a decision making regarding the diagnosis, treatment selection, or prognosis projected randomized controlled trials (RCT) as gold standard in the field of clinical research methods. An addition of blinding to the whole trial to avoid any personal influence offered by patient, physician, or the data analyzer has given it the final punch.

For the purpose of clinical application of medicine, RCT has erupted as a tool to validate the information obtained through an explicit clinical examination and its interpretation in order to procure best possible outcome through application of interventions having a sound evidence basis. It is easy to understand that an availability of such evidences has drastically reduced the time and experience required by a physician to make a clinical judgment.

The continued use of RCTs, however, in a range of studies during last 50 years has exhibited certain significant inbuilt weaknesses in this approach warranting rethinking that RCT is no more the gold standard giving way to the emergence of many other alternative ways of testing the truth through observational studies and pragmatic trials.

2.2 Evidence-Based Medicine: What Is This All About?

In efforts to define the EBM, we find people variously explaining and elaborating it. For a common purpose, we can propose EBM as a process of systematically appraising the available evidences in order to help a decision making regarding diagnosis, treatment, or prognosis of a disease aiming to aid to the delivery of optimal care to patients [4].

A movement of evidence-based practice in medicine does not have a long history. It begun in its preliminary form as an small activity at Mc Master University in

Canada with an objective to improve the learning and decision-making skills of their graduates [5]. A better and stable decision-making skill was observed among those medical graduates who received EBM learning in comparison to those who were receiving the convention learning [6]. Beginning as a small activity localized to a specific institute and its people, it gradually was accepted by many as a new discipline since it aimed at optimizing the net outcomes through a continuous and rigorous process of introspection of all the evidences helping in making decision in a particular field. A simple outcome of this process was extending the benefits of research from laboratory to patients and a translation of theory into practice, an objective which could have been the ultimate for every scientist and researcher working in the field of medicine.

2.2.1 Applying Evidence Base to Ayurvedic Clinical Practice

Why do we need an evidence base to Ayurvedic practice? Do we really require an evidence search for a health-care practice which is in vogue since ages? This often made argument from core Ayurveda fraternity needs to be analyzed in terms of extended benefits of putting an evidence basis to the practice of Ayurveda, primarily for a prospectively better and dependable health care and secondarily for the prospective growth of Ayurveda as a contemporary science. An evidence basis is required to be adopted at every level of health-care practice from diagnostics to the therapeutic decision making. Ayurveda requires a thorough work to bring out an evidence basis to its diagnostics primarily to support its fundamentals and to create a sound scientific and logical basis upon which a decision of therapeutic intervention can be made [7–9].

In addition, it also requires evidences to support its interventions in various clinical conditions to the extent that it may justify their application in a given condition. Evidence basis, in its essence, is proposed to be beneficial for the benchmarking of any medical practice. This is meant for maximization of predictable benefits to any clinical intervention besides minimization of any untoward effect through looking into and utilizing the documented evidences to reach at a clinical decision. In contemporary Ayurvedic clinical practice, subjective inferences often loom larger than the objective evidences. Therefore, an evidence-based approach seems to be the most appropriate one in bringing uniformity initially to the practice style and standards and subsequently to the responses obtained. An illustration of *prakriti* analysis in contemporary Ayurvedic practice holds a good example in case. Despite of its sound fundamental basis and clinical importance, it is often diagnosed with huge intra- and interrater variability. Absence of an unambiguous, reproducible, and uniform tool to analyze *prakriti* in Ayurvedic clinical practice not only limits its application as a help to Ayurvedic diagnostics and therapeutics but also questions the decisions taken on behalf of its analyses which remains challengeable [10–13].

Ayurveda fundamentally appreciates the evidence-based decision making. It appreciates the evidences generated through clinical observations (*pratyksha*), speculation (*anumana*), experimentation (*yukti*), and documentation (*apta*). Classical texts of Ayurveda stand in favor of a comprehensive utilization of these evidences in decision making in Ayurvedic practice.

Ayurveda has been in practice for thousands of years now and has gathered a huge sum of personal experiences regarding its benefits in many clinical conditions. Unfortunately, for a larger part of its historical succession, Ayurveda did not adopt a method of documentation or record keeping, and therefore these personal experiences by and large could not be utilized for their mass applications by growing Ayurvedic physicians in the post-independence period. Moreover, bringing documentary evidence to support a clinical decision is the utmost thing which makes the concerned physician accountable for their acts.

We can see evidence-based practice as largely applicable to Ayurveda within its purview and by essentially utilizing its own tools of evidence generation. Application of the stringent methods of evidence generation may not appear essential to Ayurvedic practice initially, but this is of utmost importance that their own tools of disease diagnosis and progress indicators should be utilized efficiently.

2.2.2 *Applying Evidence Base to Ayurvedic Clinical Practice: What Are the Tools?*

To apply the evidence base as a help to decision making in practice of Ayurveda, we need to search, assemble, and systematically reappraise the evidences available. Seeing the paucity of researches and thereby evidences generated in Ayurveda, the issue of adopting EBA is significantly different than that of EBM. For EBA, we not only need to appraise the researches done in field of Ayurveda but also need to reappraise various researches done in contemporary science with a different objective but which may hold a close resemblance to the principles and practice of Ayurveda. This is a simple adoption of what is already available and accessible in science for making a better understanding and applicability of our own science. Simultaneous to this, we need to systematically reappraise whatever meager researches are available to Ayurveda through various sources, and finally, we need to generate more evidences and their documentation in order to have a better applicability of Ayurveda into clinical practice.

2.2.2.1 Searching the Evidences from Contemporary Science

In effort to bring an evidence base awareness to the basic science of Ayurveda and its clinical application, the first thing which can and which should be done is the thorough exploration of contemporary science to reappraise various pieces of information from research done primarily with a different objective but which may find a substantial relevance and applicability to Ayurveda.

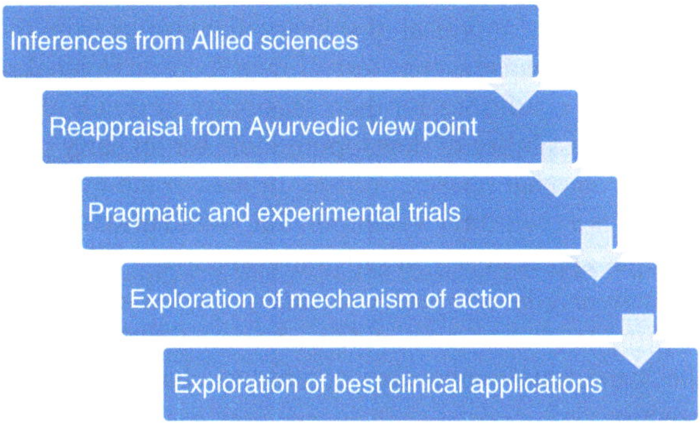

Fig. 2.1 Generating evidences through researches in allied sciences

We all agree that the phenomenal growth of biomedicine in past few decades was not primarily because of the work done in the field of medicine but because of the work done in the field of allied sciences and through their application to the field of medicine.

Looking into available information from science, with a view to find their relevance and applicability in Ayurveda, could prove to be a simple yet powerful exercise to make a foundation to more specific and innovative exercises which are required to be planned in future. This exploration and reappraisal of contemporary science could be done in a random or a systematic manner. This could also be done with a view to find information with a clinical relevance as well as those with fundamental or pharmaceutical importance (Fig. 2.1).

2.2.2.2 Reappraising the Information Helping in Diagnostic Decision Making

We recently have come across the concept of biomarkers which are proposed to be the specific biological substances arriving early in the process of a pathogenesis and whose identification can bring an early identification of a disease process. The pioneering work done by David Wong brought a paradigm shift in the field of salivary diagnostics [14]. Salivary diagnostics was further proposed to be a *point-of-care* (POC) diagnostics, where a limited amount of resource was to be used to handle a larger patient load for diagnosing diseases reciprocally [15]. A noninvasive, well-tolerated oral sample of saliva is used here to identify biomarkers, diagnostic to various diseases during the patient's periodic or initial dental visits.

Making an extension to the salivary diagnostics, Indian Council of Medical Research (ICMR), as an effort to provide a handy, inexpensive, and screening tool to diagnose and monitor diabetes, is proposing its screening test through saliva. This test would be a less expensive and noninvasive tool to enable a mass screening and monitoring of huge diabetic population in India [16]. Interestingly, Ayurveda identifies *asya madhurya* (sweet taste in mouth) as a prodromal symptom to *prameha*, an entity having a good resemblance to what we understand as diabetes [17].

Now, this reappraisal of salivary diagnostics from the point of view of Ayurveda gives us a strong reason to test all Ayurvedic prodromal sign and symptoms described in various conditions for their feasibility of quick identification clinically and also for any possibility of developing tools for an early diagnosis of the disease during their prodromal phases. Adding further to the quest, just to approve sweetness of mouth as a prodromal symptom, this would also be of interest to know if an increase in sugar appears early in saliva in comparison to blood. It is therefore, taking a clue from Ayurveda, any such evidence provided to diagnostics would not only be able to provide a substantial evidence base to the clinical description of Ayurveda but at the same time would also be able to change the face of contemporary medical practice.

Prakriti, as a fundamental construct of Ayurveda, forms the genetic and epigenetic basis to the human morphological and biological specifications. As per the genetic specifications determined at the time of conception and further under the influence of immediate environment, an individual is made distinct in terms of its appearance, behavior, and physiology. We have come across many studies which have approved a genetic basis to *prakriti* constructs.

As independent researches, we also have come across few recent studies and publications of Oxford University, Medical Research Council of Britain, Concordia University, British Journal of Psychology, and Bath University who are linking certain morphological features of human body to some specific psychological attributes. Among them, most interesting ones are those who link the shape and size of fingers to some special psychological abilities [18]. Reappraising these independent works in reference to Ayurveda, we can easily point that morphological attribute of an individual are primarily the reflection of a differential distribution of *dosha* in every individual determined in early phases of intrauterine life. Psychological attributes are also essentially the reflections of these *dosha* distributions only. It is therefore obvious to find a link between morphological and psychological features in individuals in reference to their *dosha* preponderance. Understanding such associations between morphology and psychology can make remarkable changes in the field of preventive and curative medicine. Moreover, this can also possibly offer a great help to counselors who suggest a career opinion in reference to the aptitudes of an individual.

A reappraisal of exogenous researches, however, may not prove to be helpful always. The example in case is the findings obtained through the identification of genetic correlates of longevity and selected age-related phenotypes. In a genome-wide association, Framingham study identified a relationship between walking speed and longevity [19]. In the study, it was found that those who walk faster have a better probability to live longer than those who walk slow. This inference, however, is in contrast to the perception of Ayurveda. People with *vata* predominance are proposed to have a faster walking speed, but at the same time, these people are presumed to have less happy and shorter life in comparison to *kapha* people who are marked with a slow walking speed yet a happy and long life.

An intricate relationship between gut and joint pathologies has long been proposed in Ayurveda. *Ama*, an outcome of incomplete digestion, has been proposed as the principal incriminator to many joint pathologies marked by pain and stiffness [18]. We have come across many such researches who are proposing a gut pathology in terms of increased permeability, mucosal denudation, and increased influx of complex macromolecular antigen to the gut periphery and also to the systemic circulation [20]. As a result, an immune aberrance is proposed to occur which may finally give rise to systemic presentations like arthritis [21–23]. This observation gives us a unique opportunity to understand *ama* in light of qualitative and quantitative observation of in-fluxed antigen and their corresponding antibodies. Needless to emphasize, this can also give us a unique opportunity of objectively quantifying *ama* for its application in making the judgments about clinical and therapeutic evaluation in reference to an *ama*-related disease.

2.2.2.3 Reappraising the Information Relating to Ayurvedic Pharmaceutics and Therapeutics

Ayurvedic pharmaceutics is composed of certain unique propositions of drug delivery system which largely are based upon Ayurvedic methods of drug preparations. An arbitrary classification of Ayurvedic pharmaceutical preparations as those of *guru* (strong) and *laghu* (mild) is in recognition to their rapidity of delivering the active molecules and thereby bringing them into action.

Nanomedicine argues for small nano-sized drug particles to enable them for some target-oriented functions where size of the particle matters. This is especially true for target-oriented intracellular activities where drug particles are required to be engulfed intracellularly to initiate a cellular response. Many independent researchers have established the role of particle size in initiation of a drug response [24]. Ayurvedic preparations containing metal are processed through a controlled incineration method (*puta*) where heat is offered to disintegrate metal into smaller particles. *Puta* as a traditional measure to the intensity and duration of heat offered in the process relates inversely to the particle size, i.e., the larger the *puta* number and size, the smaller would be the particle size [25]. Any correlational study to compare a drug response in a defined clinical condition through use of drugs which are prepared variously through utilization of different *puta*, and thereby offering different particle size, can establish the fact of particle size and its clinical effect as is perceived in Ayurveda. A pharmacodynamic and kinetic study may further follow to confirm the mechanism behind these assumptions. This simple study can have a substantial effect upon bringing an evidence-based logic to the selection of drugs in clinical practice of Ayurveda.

Bronchial asthma has been among few most frequently occurring illnesses which affect the quality of life of the sufferer significantly. Ayurveda approaches toward it variously but with less significant responses. Identification of bitter taste receptors of airway smooth muscles (ASM) [26], however, may change the Ayurvedic management protocol in bronchial asthma. Bitter taste receptors (TAS 2 Rs) on the tongue were presumed to be evolved as protective mechanism to protect individual from accidental intake of plant substances containing bitter taste. Identification of these receptors on ASM was also thought to be an extension of the earlier phenomena. In view of this, this was hypothesized that an inhalation containing bitter tastants would lead to an ASM contraction. Paradoxically, experimentation done to test this hypothesis proved it on the contrary. A bitter tastant inhalation caused a significant relaxation of the ASM. It further has decreased the airway obstruction in a mouse model of asthma. These observations can give a strong impetus to Ayurvedic *dhumapana* (fume inhalation) method of drug delivery recommended to asthmatics. *Dhumapana* is traditionally recommended to all asthmatics who undergo a purificatory *vamana* (emesis) therapy. A dried hollow stick made of paste of certain herbs is dipped at one end in ghee (clarified butter) and is then ignited to produce fumes. This fume is inhaled from the rear end of the stick. This is noteworthy that most herbs recommended for *dhumapana* in asthmatics are bitter in taste. After receiving a scientific understanding to why bitter are recommended to asthmatics, we can now propose for its improved delivery system where the quantity and quality of fume produced and inhaled can be monitored to produce dependable responses every time. Alternatively, a steam inhalation where steam is impregnated with bitter tastants can also be tried. In either way, this would be providing a sound evidence base to Ayurvedic recommendations for bronchial asthma therapy.

2.3 Generating Evidences: What Are the Needs of Ayurvedic Research?

Ayurveda is often being criticized by scientific fraternity for its ambiguity and paucity of evidences required to bring a strong scientific footing to its belief. On the contrary, hard-core Ayurvedic physicians are often found emphasizing the inadequacy of scientific tools in evaluating the intricate subjective details of human biology as are perceived in Ayurveda.

What do we primarily require to initiate a research? For a scientifically tuned mind, the answer is easy to find. It is the research question around which we plan our whole research. This is therefore important to understand that the methods are only secondary and are the means to reach at the desired objective. A method should therefore follow the primary research question and not the contrary as is happening to many of current researches in Ayurveda.

When we try to honestly define the research questions in Ayurveda, we would be surprised to see that there are millions of questions unanswered and which can be approached by simple research methods available around us. For few more complicated issues, we may possibly require more sophisticated research models which may be developed de novo or through required modifications into the existing models.

What we need in Ayurveda is to develop a spirit of scientific inquiry for the search of truth. Whatever methods are found adequate, unbiased, and helpful in taking us to the ultimate objective would be the most appropriate method of research in Ayurveda.

The guiding dictum should be to identify such appropriate tools and methods of research in Ayurveda which may be capable to respect equally the desired rigor of science as well as the original holistic nature of Ayurveda. We discuss here a few research methodologies which seem most appropriate for bringing evidence base to contemporary Ayurveda.

2.3.1 Reporting Single Cases and Case Series

Ayurvedic clinical practice is overwhelmingly marked by huge sum of anecdotal claims which are not substantiated through thorough scientific screening of a cause and effect relationship between the changed status of patient and the intervention given. This is however largely realized that until we develop a culture to generate stronger evidences, it is worthy to begin with nurturing a culture to report more and more cases where some noticeable changes have occurred. This adoption of case-reporting culture would possibly help initially to develop an aptitude of scientific scrutiny to each and every point we presume important in case management, and secondly, this will provide us a huge raw data upon which a magnitude of future research can be erected. Many biomedical breakthroughs have had a modest beginning in the form of an isolated case report without a presumption that what could be the future impact of this report. We have observed many case reports from Ayurveda in recent past claiming for substantial changes among clinical status where the intervention was made. These conditions are as diverse as mono-ocular vision loss [27], cerebellar ataxia [28], insomnia [29], PAOD [30], migraine [31], rhinosinusitis [32], osteoarthritis, [33] and many more. Number of case reports published in literature in reference to Ayurveda, however, are limited. Creating an awareness among primary care physicians besides those who are maintaining a specialty practice might have a lasting impact in producing more case reports as a definitive help to the ultimate evidence generation.

Information generated through several similar cases may constitute a case series. It has been considered as a strong pre-evidence which can conclude in more dependable evidences if the signals generated through the case series are trapped and evaluated further. Seeing the overwhelming claims of complementary and alternative medicine (CAM) in various terminal and incurable illness, National Institute of Health (NIH) has taken a novel initiative. Through its program of best case series launched at National Cancer Institute (NCI), it aimed at filtering the CAM interventions where the claims of clinical improvements are substantiated through radiological and biochemical evidences. It further emphasizes the importance of a good documentation both in pre- and post-treatment phases as an essential preclude to evidence generation. NCI proposes a detailed and thorough experimentation with the interventions where an improvement is substantiated through proper documentation [34]. Despite of their considerable importance as a curtain raiser to future evidences, single cases and subsequent series find a little attention in Ayurvedic fraternity which is evident through their poor availability at

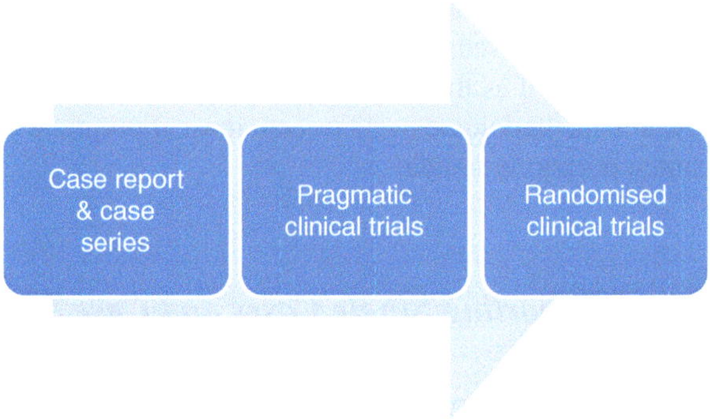

Fig. 2.2 Generating evidences through case reporting

the searchable databases [35]. We need to find ways for an optimal utilization of this so far underutilized tool to generate clinical evidences per se (Fig. 2.2). An encouragement to clinical research in practice settings is required to be done in this purview.

2.3.2 Evidences from Classical Ayurveda

Figure 2.3 explicitly explains how the classical knowledge of Ayurveda can be changed into dependable contemporary evidences just by exposing it to some objectively defined research models. Every single statement made in Ayurvedic classics may thereby, as per their clinical and therapeutic importance, be brought into scientific scrutiny, and as a result, what we get is a pure, dependable, and applicable knowledge which may help the optimization of Ayurvedic interventions in any given condition.

Various new research experiments may also be proposed referring to evidence generation in Ayurveda. Examples in case are the augmentation in level of glutathione and Cyt P450 enzyme levels in reference to *panchakarma* procedures of Ayurveda. Various enzyme systems that are responsible for inactivation and elimination of toxins and xenobiotics get activated in response to intake of herbal compounds. This enzyme activation can be a potential mechanism behind detoxification which is said to be obtained through *panchakarma* [36]. Lele has proposed four plausible mechanisms to understand action of Ayurvedic drugs. A pleiotropic nature of Ayurvedic drugs is largely attributed to sharing of their molecular targets by many cell systems and cell membrane components [37, 38].

Bioavailability of Ayurvedic herbal drugs has not been given the importance in research so far which it deserves to be. Inverted intestine loop model is used to study the bioavailability of *Terminalia arjuna* extracts and is proved as a valid model to study the bioavailability of various Ayurvedic herbs [39]. Many more such models and experiments can be proposed to validate various Ayurvedic postulates for their better applicability into clinical practice.

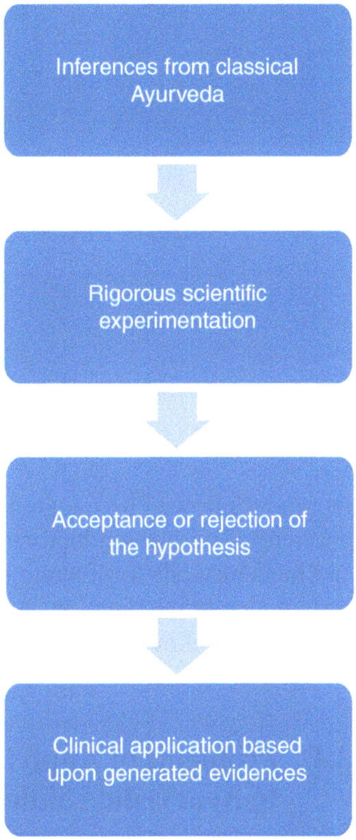

Fig. 2.3 Evidence generation from classical Ayurveda

2.3.3 Evidences from Contemporary Ayurvedic Research

Ayurvedic researches conducted in past few decades have not really been rewarding [40]. Poor research methodology and their equally poor presentation have lead to a substantial unacceptability of Ayurvedic research papers through many peer reviewed and indexed journals. This is how we find a huge bulk of Ayurvedic researches that remain unpublished [41]. Many Ayurvedic publications are also referred unavailable because of inaccessibility to their editions through digital media. This is how the researches done so far in Ayurveda could neither be made available for their wider analysis nor could be utilized for any future work. A paucity of research literature in Ayurveda, therefore, has helped skepticism to grow about its principles and interventions. The conditions, however, currently are found improving by seeing a boom of journals both indexed and peer reviewed solely dedicated to the cause of Ayurveda. This has given an opportunity to less privileged researchers to have published their researches and thereby exposing them to a larger screening through a peer readership [42].

Converting published and unpublished literature into an evidence requires a conventional approach. It is composed of an assemblage and systematic sorting of

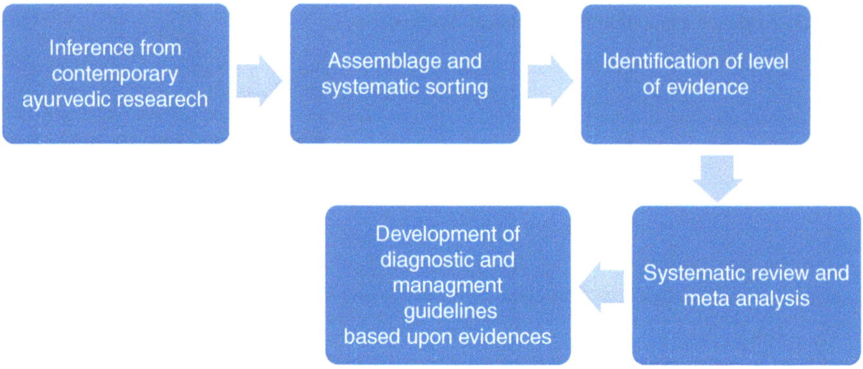

Fig. 2.4 Evidence generation from contemporary Ayurvedic research

literature followed by assigning a level of evidence to them as per their research protocols. These assembled researches then can be exposed to systematic review and meta-analysis to generate strength to evidences either favoring or disfavoring certain idea or intervention. A development of diagnostic and management protocols and guidelines may follow these basic exercises (Fig. 2.4).

2.4 Problems of Applying Effective Evidence Base to Ayurvedic Clinical Practice

Application of evidence basis to Ayurvedic practice is adhered with plenty of inherent problems. Comparing to the modern medical practice, where evidence-based practice is concerned about effective and handy utilization of continuously emerging pool of evidences subsequent to mass influx of clinical and experimental researches, Ayurvedic clinical practice suffers with a paucity of documented evidences. Besides this paucity, the meager existing evidences in Ayurveda are also not readily retrievable for lack of a single and accessible database accessible to its clinicians.

Lack of objective screening and standardization of various Ayurvedic tools utilized in diagnostic and therapeutic decision making is another limitation which makes bringing transparency in Ayurvedic clinical practice rather difficult.

The problems in bringing evidence basis to Ayurvedic practice can be enumerated as under:

1. Suboptimal perception of the importance of bringing evidence basis to Ayurvedic clinical practice among peers. This is leading to a lack of thought status among most of our Ayurvedic peers. A recently conducted survey in Maharashtra, UP, and Bihar identified the acceptance of ignorance about newly emerging safety and practice issue among over 80% respondents who were institutionally qualified Ayurvedic physicians.

2. Un-updated literature pertaining to the clinical specialties. Current Ayurvedic clinical practice largely relies upon classical texts like *Charaka*, *Sushruta*, and *Vagbhatta*. Unfortunately, many of the classical formulations described in these texts are unavailable or obsolete. The production and use of classical Ayurvedic formulations have shrunken greatly in recent years, and the new proprietary formulations which have now flooded the market seriously lack theoretical logic as well as scientific evidence besides big dosage-form crisis. Minimal approaches have been made to update these classical texts to the contemporary requirements or to develop an acceptable treatment protocol for clinical conditions approaching in Ayurvedic clinics.
3. Poor diagnostic framework. Ayurveda has its own set of understanding a disease, and its treatment pattern is in accordance to its own understanding. Various key fundamentals like *prakriti*, *tridosha*, and *srotus* are involved in making a pathogenic and subsequent diagnostic and management approach of Ayurveda. Unfortunately, most of these fundamentals have not been brought into the critical scientific screening for their utilization in clinical practice in a more objective and reproducible manner. In lack of objectivity, these fundamentals and hence their utilization in practice are subject to individual judgments and variations leading to incomprehensibility in practice.
4. Inadequate sharing of experiences and inadequate documentation are another pitfall which limits the application of evidence-based practice in Ayurveda. Ayurvedic physicians, in general, are not aware and not adequately trained in documentation of the clinical records. In lack of these records, a substantial intervention in a clinical condition may remain unnoticed for its thorough exploration to be utilized further.
5. Inaccessibility to recent advances in Ayurveda or modern medicine. Ayurvedic physicians are poorly acquainted with accessibility to resources to make them updated about the recent advances occurring in the field. Researches done at various institutes of Ayurveda in India are only manually accessible and hence cannot be utilized by the people practicing away from those places.
6. Unavailability of meta-analysis studies about Ayurvedic interventions in various clinical conditions.

2.4.1 Solutions: Creating an Effective Evidence Resource and Ensuring Its Utilization

Keeping in view of an immediate need of bringing evidence base to Ayurvedic clinical practice to ensure transparency and uniformity in practice initially and to the overall clinical benefits subsequently, we may need the following as the way out to reach at a modest beginning of an evidence-based practice in Ayurveda. Having a careful look at the existing problems is supposed to help framing an effective and need-based strategy for the ultimate cause:

- Creating a strong, accessible, and free electronic database pertaining to the researches done in Ayurveda. This database, however, needs to be vigilant before putting any information for its source, reliability, and authenticity.
- Promotion of documentation in Ayurvedic clinical practice. Documentation has been the key factor ensuring a transparency in practice and its adherence to protocols. Ayurvedic physicians are required to be made aware of importance of documentation and should be promoted for scientific writing.
- Case report documentation should be promoted at all the clinical forums, and journals should develop a liberal and flexible approach to consider writings from new professionals.
- Promotion of in-house clinical and scientific journal publication from Ayurvedic institutes involved in research.
- Introduction of Ayurvedic tools of diagnostics and therapeutic decision making into strict scientific scrutiny, to bring out their uniform, applicable, and standard forms which can unambiguously be applied into clinical practice.

2.5 Conclusions

Singh [7] in his guest editorial to a recent issue of IJAR explains how the classical frame of evidence from Ayurveda can be utilized to a contemporary tune. While talking of searching and applying evidence base to Ayurveda, we need to understand that in conventional sense, the term "*evidence*" is primarily coined to help clinical decision making in light of best among overwhelmingly available inferences within modern medicine [1]. Conventional modus operandi of applying evidence base to medical practice, therefore, is limited to screening of best evidences helping a decision making. Thereby, defining the best evidence and finding them pragmatically in a clinical setting are the only real challenges.

Referring to Ayurveda, however, the issue of applying evidence base needs to be redefined in reference to its unique propositions. There is a ubiquitous agreement upon the traditional evidences of Ayurveda of which experience, long-term use, and textual classical references form a large sum. This substantial primary evidence base of Ayurveda is not static; rather, it is vitally "dynamic" because the practitioners use the principles contained in the *shastra* and tradition in their day-to-day practice dynamically. Still, this primary evidence needs secondarily to be supported by new science evidence. A primary evidence base of Ayurveda, therefore, is required to be brought in a format which can become retrievable to help decision making in a clinical dilemma. A thorough documentation, therefore, comes as the foundation of evidence-based practice, and it warrants an unfailing and untiring documentation of every evidence from Ayurveda, conventional or unconventional [8]. Besides, this is also important to address the issue of human biology as is observed from Ayurvedic or conventional perspective. If we are deferring from conventional theories and their experimental designs, we need to innovate our own methods to understand a biological process and also the ways through which this understanding can help a decision making [39]. Needless to emphasize, these methods are essentially required to be flawless, dependable, reproducible, and acceptable. Designing these methods require a rigorous brainstorming initially about what is available and what is required, and subsequently the ground research by designing suitable models which can solve the dilemma of understanding the Ayurvedic biology [10–12].

The issue of evidence base in Ayurveda, therefore, requires to be dealt at various levels like documentation of existing evidences, designing diagnostic and clinical parameters which can act as evidence to help a decision making, and generating more evidences in reference to the safety and efficacy pertinent to Ayurvedic practice. This is the time when we need to understand that bringing evidence base to the practice of Ayurveda is mandatory if it is thought to be raised as a medical system where predictability and dependability are featured as key components. An evidence-based search and development of the materials and methods to promote such practice in Ayurveda would go long in benefitting the human being. "Ayurveda for future" therefore is the most appropriate direction which should be focused with utmost zeal and care [43–45].

References

1. Sackett DL, Rosenberg WMC (1995) The need for evidence-based medicine. J R Soc Med 88:620–624
2. Roberts C, Torgerson D (1998) Randomisation methods in controlled trials. Br Med J 317:1301
3. Kang M, Ragan BG, Park JH (2008) Issues in outcome research: an overview of randomization technique for clinical trials. J Athl Train 43:215–221
4. Besley J (2009) What is evidence-based medicine? Hayward Medical Communication, downloaded from http://www.whatisseries.co.uk/. Accessed on 23 Nov 2010
5. Bennet KJ, Sackett DL, Hayness RB, Neufield VR (1987) A controlled trial of teaching critical appraisal of the clinical literature to medical students. JAMA 257:2451–2454
6. Shin JH, Hayness RB, Johnston ME (1993) Effect of problem based, self directed undergraduate education on lifelong learning. Can Med Assoc J 148:969–976
7. Singh RH (2010) Exploring larger evidence-base for contemporary Ayurveda. Int J Ayurveda Res 1:65–66
8. Rastogi S (2010) Bringing evidence basis to Ayurvedic clinical practice: applicability, problems and solutions. NETRUM News Lett 3:7–10
9. Rastogi S (2010) Exploring larger evidence-base for contemporary Ayurveda. Int J Ayurveda Res 1:195–196
10. Rastogi S, Chiappelli F (2010) Bringing evidence basis to decision making in complementary and alternative medicine (CAM): prakriti (constitution) analysis in Ayurveda. In: Chiappelli F et al (eds) Evidence-based practice towards optimizing clinical outcomes. Springer, Berlin/Heidelberg, pp 91–106
11. Singh RH (2003) The holistic principles of Ayurvedic medicine. Chaukhamba Surbharati, Varanasi
12. Valiathan MS (2003) Towards Ayurvedic biology. Decadal document. National Academy of Science, New Delhi
13. Tripathi PK, Patwardhan K, Singh G (2011) The basic cardiovascular responses to postural changes, exercise and cold pressure test: do they vary in accordance with the dual constitution

types of Ayurveda. Evid Based Complement Altern Med 2011:2. doi:10.1155/2011/328380, Article ID 251850
14. Bauer JG (2010) Foreword. In: Chiappelli F, Brant XMC, Neagos N, Oluwadara OO, Ramchandani MH (eds) Evidence–based practice: towards optimising clinical outcomes. Springer, Berlin/Heidelberg, pp v–vii
15. Malamud D (2006) Salivary diagnostics: the future is now. J Am Dent Assoc 137:284–286
16. Cassiday L (2009) Nothing to spit at: the salivary proteome of type 2 diabetes. J Proteome Res 8:3
17. Sharma PV (1986) Charaka Samhita English translation and commentary. Chaukhamba Orientalia, Varanasi
18. Stenstrom E, Saad G, Nepomuceno MV, Mendenhall Z (2010) Testosterone and domain-specific risk: digit ratios (2D:4D and rel2) as predictors of recreational, financial, and social risk-taking behaviors. Pers Individ Differ. doi:10.1016/j.paid.2010.07.003
19. Lunetta KL, Agostino RBD, Karasik D, Benjamin E, Guo CY, Govindaraju R, Kiel DP, Hayes MK, Massaro JM, Pencina MJ, Seshadri S, Murabito JM (2007) Genetic correlates of longevity and selected age related phenotypes: a genome-wide association study in the Framingham study. BMC Med Genet 8(suppl 1):S13
20. Rastogi S (2012) Gut and joint interconnections: a reappraisal to Ayurvedic understanding of joint diseases. In: Rastogi S, Chiappelli F, Ramchandani MH, Singh RH (eds) Evidence-based practice in complementary and alternative medicine: protocols, pitfalls and potential in Ayurveda. Springer, Berlin/Heidelberg (In press)
21. Soderholm JD, Perdue MH (2001) Stress and the gastrointestinal tract II. Stress and intestinal barrier function. Am J Physiol Gastrointest Liver Physiol 280:G7–G13
22. Cordain L, Toohey L, Smith MJ, Hickey MS (2000) Modulation of immune function by dietary lectins in rheumatoid arthritis. Br J Nutr 83:207–217
23. Hvatum M, Kanerud L, Hallgren R, Brandtzaeg P (2006) The gut joint axis: cross reactive food antibodies in rheumatoid arthritis. Gut 55:1240–1247
24. Mukharjee P, Bhattacharya R, Bone N, Lee YK, Patra CR, Wang S et al (2007) Potential therapeutic application of gold nanoparticles in B-chronic lymphocytic leukaemia (BCLL): enhancing apoptosis. J Nanobiotechnol 5:4
25. Sarkar PK, Chaudhari AK (2010) Ayurvedic bhasma: the most ancient application of nanomedicine. J Sci Ind Res 69:901–905
26. Deshpande DA, Wang WCH, Mcllmoyle EL, Robinett KS, Schillinger RM, An SS, Sham JSK, Liggett SB (2010) Bitter taste receptor on airway smooth muscle bronchodilation by localized calcium signaling and reverse obstruction. Nat Med 16:1299–1304
27. Rastogi S, Chawla S, Singh RK (2009) Ayurvedic management of unilateral loss of vision following a blunt injury to eye: a case report. Complement Health Pract Rev 14:84–92
28. Sriranjini SJ, Pal PK, Devidas KV, Ganpathy S (2009) Improvement of balance in progressive degenerative cerebellar ataxias after *Ayurvedic* therapy: a preliminary report. Neurol India 57:166–171
29. Vinjamury SP (2007) Ayurvedic shirodhara treatment for insomnia: a case study. Presented in The 135th APHA annual meeting and exposition of APHA, 2007, California
30. Rastogi S (2008) CAM management of peripheral arterial occlusive disease (PAOD): a case report. Complement Health Pract Rev 13:198–203
31. Vaidya PB, Vaidya BS, Vaidya SK (2010) Response to Ayurvedic therapy in the treatment of migraine without aura. Int J Ayurveda Res 1:30–36
32. Rastogi S, Ranjana RR (2007) Jala neti application in acute rhino sinusitis. Indian J Tradit Knowl 6:328–333
33. Sarmukaddam S, Chopra A, Tillu G (2010) Efficacy and safety of Ayurvedic medicines: recommending equivalence trial design and proposing safety index. Int J Ayurveda Res 1:175–180
34. NCI Best case series program (2010). Available at http://cancer.gov/cam/. Accessed on 25 Nov 2010

35. Rastogi S (2009) Poor quality and improper use: a review of common reasons of possible adversity in Ayurvedic practice. Int J Risk Saf Med 21:121–130
36. Waterschoot RAB, Rooswinkel RW, Wagenaar E, Kruijssen CMM, Herwaarden AE, Schinkel AH (2009) Intestinal cytochrome P450 3A plays an important role in the regulation of detoxifying systems in the liver. FASEB J 23:224–231
37. Lele RD (2010) Four new approaches for validation of Ayurvedic herbal drugs. Int J Ayurveda Res 1:136–137
38. Lele RD (2008) Clinical science and clinical research, 2nd edn. National Book Depot, Mumbai
39. Rastogi S (2010) Building bridges between Ayurveda and modern science. Int J Ayurveda Res 1:41–46
40. Singh RH (2010) Exploring issues in the development of Ayurvedic research methodology. J Ayurveda Integr Med 1:91–95
41. Baghel MS (2010) Issues in publication of Ayurvedic research work, -National and International scenario-Shortcomings and Solutions, downloaded from http://www.servedeva.org/documents/msbaghel.pdf/. Accessed on 20 Nov 2010
42. Narahari SR, Ryan TJ, Aggithaya MG, Bose KS, Prasanna KS (2008) Evidence–based approaches for the Ayurvedic traditional herbal formulations: towards an Ayurvedic CONSORT model. J Altern Complement Med 14:769–776
43. Mashelkar RA (2008) Second world Ayurveda congress (theme: Ayurveda for the future)—inaugural address: part I. Evid Based Complement Altern Med 5:129–131. doi:10.1093/ecam/nen014
44. Mashelkar RA (2008) Second world Ayurveda congress (theme: Ayurveda for the future)—inaugural address: part II. Evid Based Complement Altern Med 5:243–245. doi:10.1093/ecam/nen014
45. Mashelkar RA (2008) Second world Ayurveda congress (theme: Ayurveda for the future)—inaugural address: part III. Evid Based Complement Altern Med 5:367–369

Chapter 3
Diet and Nutrition Concepts in Ayurveda: Gleaming into Opportunities for Evidence-Based Applications in Health Care

Devesh Rastogi, Shalini Gupta, Ranjana Rastogi, and Rajiv Rastogi

3.1 Introduction

Evidence-based medicine is the conscientious, explicit and judicious use of current best evidence in making decisions about the care of individual patients. The practice of evidence-based medicine means integrating individual clinical expertise with the best external clinical evidence available through systematic research. It is, however, important to note that external clinical evidence can inform, but can never replace, individual clinical expertise, and it is this expertise that decides whether the external evidence applies to the individual patient at all and, if so, how it should be integrated into a clinical decision [1]. This aspect of evidence-based practice looks more apt to Ayurveda where a therapeutic individualisation in light of subjective variations plays a key role towards ultimate decision-making.

Ayurveda *(Ayu + Veda)* as science of life deals with almost every aspect of life to ensure a sustainable health. Its methods involve lifestyle improvements and dietary recommendations and also the therapeutic interventions aiming to promote harmony between spiritual, physical and material needs of a human contextual with the environment. Ayurveda proposes human health as an outcome of a harmonic balance between an individual and their environment [2].

D. Rastogi (✉)
Indulgence Food Pvt. Ltd., Nagpur, India
e-mail: rastogi.devesh@gmail.com

S. Gupta
Department of Physiology, C.S.M. Medical University, Lucknow, India

R. Rastogi
Department of Obstetrics and Gynaecology, Vatsala Hospital, Lucknow, Uttar Pradesh, India
e-mail: rastogiranjana2010@rediffmail.com

R. Rastogi
Department of Ayush, Central Council of Research in Yoga and Naturopathy, MOH&FW, New Delhi, India

S. Rastogi (ed.), *Evidence-Based Practice in Complementary and Alternative Medicine*,
DOI 10.1007/978-3-642-24565-7_3,

Individualisation in Ayurveda begins with the idea of individual body types (*prakriti*) and subtypes based on predominance of certain factors (*dosha*) presumed responsible in determining individual physical, physiological and mental aptitudes. *Prakriti* based upon *dosha* therefore forms the fundamental basis of Ayurvedic therapeutics, upon which its decisions are largely based.

As *dosha* are set to drive a specific kind of physiology, it has a differential aptitude to deal with different substrates. This is how, to make a balance of *dosha*, every one may have its own set of preferred food, which may not be shared equally by people of the same age or sex.

Ayurvedic concepts of food and nutrition are holistic and in harmony with the individual as well as with environment. On the contrary, modern understanding of food is elemental, generalised and symptomatic.

3.2 Food and Nutrition: Contemporary and Classical Viewpoints

3.2.1 Food Classification

Modern classification of food comprises of nutrients which help normal functioning of the body. Six major kind of nutrients identified are carbohydrates, fats, proteins, vitamins, minerals and water.

Carbohydrates are the main source of energy, meeting about 70% of the energy requirements. Excess carbohydrates are converted into fat and glycogen and accumulate in the body in the form of adipose tissue.

Fats or lipids are the concentrated form of energy in the food. Comparing to carbohydrates, lipids yield more energy on oxidation. About 30% of energy requirements are met by lipids. Excess of fats and lipids are stored as adipose tissue.

Proteins are structural constituents to cell membranes. The quality of protein depends upon the content of the amino acids, from which it is made up of. Proteins can be used as an alternative source of energy if other sources are insufficient.

Vitamins and minerals are accessory nutrients. Vitamins together with minerals regulate the biological processes. As constituents of enzymes, they catalyse biological reactions.

Water is an ideal vehicle for transporting dissolved nutrients and waste from the body. Apart from the direct intake of water, body needs of water are also met through the consumed food [3].

The Centers for Disease Control and Prevention (CDC) advocates knowledge of food groups in order to generate healthy eating plan. A healthy eating plan (balanced diet) helps in identifying calorie needs, quantity of each food group to be taken and to make healthy choices (Table 3.1) [4].

In Ayurveda, food is classified into 12 groups: grains, pulses, meat, vegetables, fruits, salads, wines, water, milk and milk products, sugar cane products, cooked

Table 3.1 CDC classification of food groups

Food groups	Examples
Grains	Whole wheat bread and rolls, whole wheat pasta, English muffin, pita bread, bagel, cereals, grits, oat meal, brown rice, unsalted pretzels and popcorn
Fruits	Apples, apricots, bananas, dates, grapes, oranges, grapefruit, grapefruit juice, mangoes, melons, peaches, pine apples, raisins, strawberries, tangerines and 100% fruit juice
Vegetables	Broccoli, carrots, collards, green beans, green peas, kale, lima beans, potatoes, spinach, squash, sweet potatoes and tomatoes
Fat-free or low-fat milk and milk products	Fat-free (skim) or low-fat (1%) milk or butter milk, fat-free or low-fat or reduced-fat cheese, fat-free or low-fat regular or frozen yogurt
Lean meats, poultry and fish	Beef, poultry, pork, game meats, fish, shellfish, select only lean; trim away visible fats; broil, roast or poach; remove skin from poultry
Nuts, seeds and legumes	Almonds, hazelnuts, mixed nuts, peanuts, walnuts, sunflower seeds, peanut butter, kidney beans, lentils and split peas

foods and accessory foods (e.g. oils and spices). It is noticeable that Ayurvedic classification of food group is wider in range and envelops all the possible food combinations [5].

Modern medicine and Ayurveda both recommend that food choices should be met as per individual needs and chosen from available variety. Modern science refers to this as individual calorie requirement, whereas Ayurveda refers to it as per individual *prakriti* and digestive capability [2, 4].

3.2.2 Understanding the Digestion Process

Ayurveda teaches that poor digestion is the primary cause of most diseases. *Ama* (toxin generated from undigested food in the stomach) is root to many of the gastro-intestinal disorders. *Ama* can be created because of inappropriate combination of food, food contamination, excess food intake or a hypo-digestive state. If the digestive tract inadequately processes the intake loads, *ama* generates. *Ama* subsequently leaks into the system and settles at vulnerable places. Such weakened places are called *khavaigunya* (weak or defective spaces in the organs or tissues where *dosha* begin to settle and initiate subsequent pathologies). *Khavaigunya* can be created in many ways including physical or emotional injury, inherited disorders or unhealthy lifestyle choices. This weakening concept is akin to weak immune system in the modern science. It is a common knowledge that every individual has inherent capability of immune system and hence posses different sensitivity to weather and food.

The strength of digestive fire, called *agni* (biological energy to metabolise nutrients in the body for absorption and complete assimilation without generating much waste), determines an individual's appetite. Adequate digestive fire promotes better appetite. *Agni* regulates digestion, absorption and metabolism of nutrients to transform them into cellular structures. The subtle energy of *agni* transforms the molecules of food into the substrates of the cell. If the *agni* is improper, the digestion, absorption and metabolism of nutrients will be improper, leading to poor nourishment and *ama* generation. *Ama* eventually coats cells, creates cellular confusion and causes dull, inadequate and lethargic feeling.

Modern science does recognise poor digestion process due to poor release of digestive juices but does not relate it with any body type indications like BMI etc. for individual appreciation. Though it specifically defines digestive metabolism of proteins, carbohydrates and fats clearly, their effect on a combined diet is not so particular.

3.2.3 Eating Principles

Ayurveda identifies individual body constitution as the factor determinant to the appropriateness of a particular diet for a person. This emphasises the fact that one single diet cannot suit every individual. The United States Department of Agriculture (USDA) has also taken cognisance of the fact that one size does not fit all. *My Pyramid* program (now named Choose My Plate) offers personalised eating plans and interactive tools to help an individual planning one's food choices based on specific dietary guidelines [6].

Ayurveda also has defined its dietary guidelines as follows.

3.2.3.1 Appropriate Quantity

Ayurveda stresses substantially for a differential approach towards quantity (*matra*) determination of food in individual cases. Contrary to the generic quantity measurement system based upon calorie requirements in defined age and sex groups, Ayurveda defines it more clearly in terms of individual metabolic status. Ayurveda presumes that a quantitatively appropriate diet is essential for health and that quantity is determined by the *agni* (*Charaka Samhita Sutra Sthana* 5/3) [7]. Quantitative determination of diet in Ayurveda is primarily based upon a sensory specific satiety (SSS) regulation system where one transiently looses the liking for a specific food after consuming it to the satiety level.

In contemporary context, we know that there are many factors which actually drive the food quantity determination, applying on a case-to-case merit. In reference to obesity, we have seen that distorted meal portions and size have eluded the perception of normal food size in general context (variable size of bread, spoons and bowls) which eventually leads to overeating without getting noticed [8].

A quantity may exceed the SSS limits here in presumption that one has not eaten well. Very interestingly, sensory-specific desire (SSD) also plays a role in quantitative determination of food. Foods in a definitive food group share the sensory attribute and thereby act cumulatively on SSS index. This explains how reaching to satiety with one food stops the desire of having the food from the same group again. SSD operates differently among adults and children. Among adults, this is found to be group specific, whereas among children, this is more food specific. This is how children may suffer with overeating more often than adults [9].

This is evident that to avoid food quantity related troubles, we need to have a cognisance of SSS unaffected by other factors which may alter the consumed food quantity. Ayurveda recognises this cognisance as *anuphatya* (the quantity of food which does not cause a trouble in physical and physiological functions).

A food quantity determination also has a qualitative bearing. The food which is simple and easy to get digested may be taken in quantities bigger than the food which is complex to get digested. Ayurveda thereby proposes a *guru* (complex) and *laghu* (simple) classification of food. Contemporary knowledge of food elaborates about the differential quantities of food required in reference to various food groups. The idea is to supplement adequate amount of components from each group as per its requirement in the body to arrive at a complete food. At no point in time, however, does it talk about an intra-group quantification of foods as per their digestibility.

Within every major food group like carbohydrate, protein and fat, there are variable items which vary on account of their digestibility. Starch, for example, can be categorised into three basic groups: rapidly digestible starch (RDS), slowly digestible starch (SDS) and resistant starch (RS) [10].

Slowly digestible starches are found to blunt the postprandial increase and subsequent decline of plasma glucose and insulin concentrations, leading to prolonged energy availability and satiety, compared to more rapidly digestible starch. Sandsa et al. [11] examined the postprandial metabolic and appetitive responses of a slow-digestible starch (wax maize, WM) and compared it with rapidly digestible carbohydrate, a maltodextrin-sucrose mixture (MS).The result supported that WM provides sustained glucose availability in young, insulin-sensitive adults [11].

For their long yet slow release properties, slowly digestible substances are recommended in lesser quantity when compared to rapidly digestible substances required to meet the immediate requirements of energy. Similar distinctions are also made among the protein category where amino acid composition and digestibility are found to affect critically the net nutritional value of a protein. Contrary to the rapid amino acid release as is observed in rapidly digestible protein, slowly digestible proteins are recommended less on account of amino acid losses post-ileum. Amino acids passing beyond ileum are largely consumed by faecal microorganisms and therefore become unavailable to human metabolism [12].

Ayurvedic perspective of *guru* and *laghu* food may have special implications among various target groups while designing an ideal food combination. For example, in debility where a rapid replenishment is required, a large quantity of *laghu* food with a rapid digestibility and subsequent metabolism may be more suitable comparing to a well-fed obese where a filling and satiating *guru* food may be more apt to suppress the hunger urge for longer time comparing to other foods.

Interestingly, Ayurveda describes an elaborate list of foods which are classified either as *laghu* or *guru*. They, however, are required to be cross-checked through controlled enzymatic hydrolysis and protein digestibility corrected amino acid score (PDCAAS) to generate evidences for their rational clinical applications.

3.2.3.2 Avoidable Food and Food Recommended for Occasional and Regular Use

Preserved foods, for their nutritional deficits or antinutrient properties, are not recommended for regular consumption in Ayurveda. Pork, beef, fish, curd, *yava* (barley) and *mash* (black bean) are also accounted among the foods which are not recommended for regular use. On the contrary, some special varieties of rice (*sasti, sali*), cow's milk, goose berry (*amla*), rock salt (*saindhava lavana*), clarified butter (*ghee*) and cow pea (*munga*) are recommended for their regular use. We are not yet fully aware of the health promotive and restorative properties of many among such regular components of Ayurvedic foods. Their exploration and subsequent application therefore in Ayurvedic clinical practice may have larger health care implications than are presently perceived. A regular selection of diet is also a matter of personal selection as Ayurveda perceives. The food which does not generate such diseases, which are yet unborn (*ajatanam vikaranam anutpattikara*) and which maintains health (*swasthyam ye nanuvartate*) is considered ideal and should be consumed regularly. This is clear that this choice allows us to be variable as per our liking and susceptibility towards a particular food group. A food individualisation besides a generalisation among categories of frequently recommended foods (FRF), occasionally recommended food (ORF) and not recommended food (NRF) seems to have formed the basis of Ayurvedic food science.

3.2.3.3 Food in Reference to Seasons

India, the birthplace of Ayurveda, has been blessed with a variety of seasons comprising mainly of winter, summer and rain. Ayurveda interestingly links the climatic variations of these seasonal groups with corresponding changes in human physiology. Seasons, therefore, are linked with the dominance of corresponding *dosha* activity marking the flaring up of season-specific pathologies. To prevent such seasonal pathologies, Ayurveda advises a definitive code of food intake besides many other instructions to keep one healthy. Seasonal variability among the disease epidemiologies is a well-observed fact [13]; however, little work has been done to identify these epidemiological variations in reference to the corresponding changes in the human physiology. A seasonal variation in reproductive, physiological and immunological behaviour in mammal is an observed fact [14, 15].

Pajman [13] noticed that the respiratory tract infection–related sepsis is significantly more common in winter compared to their incidence in fall. This clearly gives us an inference of reduced immunity during extreme weather compared to more cosy weather. Ayurveda beautifully charts a seasonal scaling up and down of body resistance and innate immunity in reference to summer and winter. In reference to innate immunity, the seasons are classified as *adana* (the period of scaling down) and *visarga* (the period of scaling up), where the former is composed of late winter to summer and the latter of rain till early winter. Changes in physiological and immune functions are well defined in reference to a change in weather.

An appearance or disappearance of pathogens, environmental changes and host behaviour are considered responsible for seasonal epidemiological changes. Besides seasonal variables like temperature, humidity and food availability, photoperiod or a light-dark cycle has also been proposed to play a role in seasonal variability of host responses [16].

Ayurvedic seasonal food preferences typically address to the seasonal compromises in order to rebalance them, favouring a sustainable health maintenance. A lot of work, however, would be required to bring this hypothesis of '*seasonal disease prevention through an effective dietary modification*' into an evidence-based reality.

Incidentally, Ayurveda has given enough flexibility to its dietary concepts by accepting that dietary substances are adaptable if they are regularly used (*oaksatmya*). Similarly, it also advocates a tapering method to allow changes into an existing dietary schedule with new ones. A *padanshik* (change in fractions and phases) order is beautifully elaborated in Ayurveda to enable such changes during the transition of seasons without causing an unwarranted illness because of a dietary transition.

3.3 Ayurvedic Diet: Classical Viewpoint

Ayurveda identifies that the physical body and the food are both composed of same five basic elements: earth, water, fire, air and space. If prepared and taken in correct proportion of their taste, food creates a natural balance between these essential elements within the body. The six tastes, sweet, salty, sour, pungent, astringent and bitter, are said to have unique elemental compositions, rendering them *dosha* specific.

3.3.1 Considerations to Decide Food Suitability

Ayurveda defines eight qualities while determining the best use of food to a particular person:

(a) *Natural quality of food* – Every food has its natural quality which affects the digestion process, and it is more nutritive in its natural form. Some foods like pulses are heavy, having complex molecular structure (take longer time in digestion), while others, like fruits, are light, having simple molecular structure (easily digestible).
(b) *Processing of food* – Processing changes the natural shape and form of the food and renders it safe and palatable. Processing includes steps like cooking, steaming, roasting, baking, etc. Food processing requires a sense of discrimination in the blending of flavours, as well as of textures, colours and shapes. Sprouting, fermentation and combining different foods in a meal are ways to get the maximum nutritive value from some of our foods. Preservation of its maximum nutritive value should remain the principle behind any food processing.

Table 3.2 Effect of cooking on foods

Cooking
Improves the flavour and palatability of the foods
Makes the food more digestible
Enhances the availability of some nutrients, for example, trypsin inhibitors present in protein foods is destroyed by cooking, which makes the trypsin freely available in the body
Destroys bacteria, thus making the food safe for consumption. This also improves the keeping quality of the food

Appropriate cooking has definite advantages, as mentioned in Table 3.2 [17]. Ayurveda explicitly explains food processing by defining the amount of heat and water required to make a particular food. By changing a processing method, the ultimate qualities of prepared food can also get changed.

(c) *Combination of food* – Certain foods, when combined together, increase their nutritive value. Various food products are combined or supplemented to enhance the nutritive value of the total offering. However, it should be a proper combination so that it does not cause any complication during digestion, absorption and metabolism of nutrients and not further lead to metabolic disorder [18]. Ayurveda further explains various foods which may have a deleterious effect if combined together. These foods are called *viruddha-ahara* (incompatible diet) and are said to be avoided for their disease-causing potential. Food compatibility may further be defined in reference to individual susceptibility also. A food which is suitable to one individual may not be equally suiting to some other having a different *prakriti*.

(d) *Habitat and climate of food* – Food should be natural to the climate and habitat where it is being eaten. The foods that naturally appear in winter normally have warm properties. Likewise, the natural summer foods contain good amount of water to keep the body cool. One of the biggest reasons why one should opt for seasonal foods is because they are full of antioxidants that are so good for health. Antioxidants fight free radicals and prevent various disorders [18].

(e) *Time and disease state during food intake* – Time of food intake and the state of mind and body during intake are also very important. The food intake should be based on the favouring food products (*pathya*) which may offer tranquillity to mind and body in normal state and pathogenic dissociation in disease state. This consideration essentially includes the food required to be avoided (*apathya*) in certain specific conditions. Time (duration between each meal in a day) is based upon the number of frequency per meal in a day, probably based on the physiological condition.

This holistic concept does not find an overbearing reference in modern science.

(f) *Rules of Use* – Eating order should be guided by digestive sequence of food to offer a better digestion. (One can draw reference to three-course meal culture, popular in Western world. A typical three-course meal starts with a starter, followed by a main course, and ends with dessert.) Simply put, first in the eating sequence is light food which promotes *agni*, so that by the time one eats the main course, his *agni* is in full flame to digest the complex protein and fat structures. *Dipana* in Ayurveda are like the starters which ignite the *agni*. This is followed by *pachana* which can subsequently help in digestion.

(g) *User* – Ayurveda puts a great emphasis upon user for maximisation of beneficial effects of diet. A food therefore is required to be individualised. If the food layout and aroma does not generate a neuro-humoral response, *agni* will remain low and hence digestion will remain poor [2].

3.3.2 Balanced Diet: Classical and Contemporary Views

In Ayurveda, the concept of balanced diet, is a harmonious combination of six food qualities and six food tastes with due consideration of five elements. It is proposed that a person who includes all the six tastes in his food enjoys good health.

Ayurvedic dietary principles do not limit the quantity or variety of food that can be eaten. As a result, such a diet is not likely to be deficient in any nutrients, assuming that the person is eating enough calories through selection of a wide variety of foods [4].

The *My Pyramid* education framework provides specific recommendations for making food choices that will improve the quality of an average diet. These recommendations are interrelated and should be used together. Taken together, they will result in the following changes from a typical diet [19]:

- Increased intake of vitamins, minerals, dietary fibre and other essential nutrients, especially of those that are often low in typical diet
- Lowered intake of saturated fats, trans fats and cholesterol and increased intake of fruits, vegetables and whole grains to decrease risk from some chronic diseases
- Calorie intake balanced with energy needs to prevent weight gain and/or to promote a healthy weight

The recommendation in this education framework falls under four overarching themes:

- Variety – eat foods from all food groups and subgroups
- Proportionality – eat more of some foods (fruits, vegetables, whole grains, fat-free or low-fat milk products) and less of others (foods high in saturated and trans fats, added sugars, cholesterol, salt and alcohol)
- Moderation – choose forms of food that limit intake of saturated and transfats, added sugars, cholesterol, salt and alcohol
- Activity – be physically active every day

There is a commonality in approach for variety of intake, but healthy diet in modern science is more exclusive rather than inclusive, as in Ayurveda.

In contemporary science, there is no reference of balancing of tastes altogether [19].

3.4 Special Diets

Both modern science and Ayurveda recognise the need of special food for immunologically compromised people. Ayurveda supplements to these thoughts by adding concepts of *pathya* and *apathya*.

3.4.1 Concept of Pathya–Apathya

A food which is beneficial for our body is *pathya*. The contrary is *apathya*. It is further pointed out that there is no rule of thumb to decide upon *pathya* or *apathya*. It depends upon many factors like time, place, season and individual suitability. *Charaka* outlines six factors to decide upon *pathya* and *apathya*. They are quantity (*matra*), time (*kaal*), mode of preparation (*kriya*), habitat (country/place), body constitution (*deh*) and physiological status (*dosh*) [2]. These concepts have been explained above.

Food as a medicine can literally be supplemented with the fact that certain foods contain chemicals which have proven disease-preventing history [20]. Disease-preventing phytochemicals, present in plant food, are shown in Table 3.3 [21]. Properties of functional foods are shared by several phytochemicals present in plant foods [22]. It is interesting to note that several nutrients like vitamin E (tocopherol), provitamin A (β-carotene), ascorbic acid and selenium also have disease-preventing and health-promoting potential, just like phytochemicals. Evidences are piling up for greater possibilities of using food as medicine in many intractable conditions where medicine alone does not suffice to help. Expanding upon the Ayurvedic concept of *pathya-apathya*, a type 2 diabetes reversal is claimed recently by Lim et al. [23].Using a dietary intervention alone, this study claimed normalisation of beta cell function in association with decreased pancreas and liver triacylglycerol [23]. This study gives similar inferences to those the author observed in a pilot study upon five patients [24]. There are more compelling evidences showing preventive as well as remedial role of diet in obesity and type 2 diabetes [25]. Many dietary ingredients to the Indian conventional diet have been identified for their beneficial roles in various diseases, particularly to diabetes. *Momordica charantia* (*karvellaka*), a highly acclaimed *pathya* for *prameha*, (Ayurvedic synonym for diabetes) is found to contain an insulin-like peptide called foetidin, momordicin or charantin (polypeptide p-insulin). It is postulated that this mimics or improves insulin action at the cellular level or even exhibits extra-pancreatic action [26].Various mechanisms involved behind its antidiabetic action are proposed as enhanced insulin secretion by pancreas, reduced glycogenesis in liver tissue, enhanced peripheral glucose utilisation and increased serum protein levels [27]. *Piper nigrum* (*marica*) seeds, a common ingredient in Indian kitchen, are also found to have a hypoglycaemic effect. This is also found effective against complications arising due to glycation and glycooxidation of proteins and membranes [28]. *Ocimum sanctum* (*tulasi*) is a house hold name in India. Besides its medicinal usage, it is conventionally used as daily religious offerings and also as flavouring agent to Indian milk tea. Tulasi leaves are

Table 3.3 Disease-preventing phytochemicals in plant food

Specific food groups	Main health-promoting chemical	Useful in prevention of
Whole cereal, grains	Dietary fibre, tocopherols	Cancer, diabetes, cardiovascular disease, hypercholesterolaemia
Vegetables, fat	α-linoleic acid, linoleic acid, tocopherols[a]	Cancer, diabetes, cardiovascular disease, hypercholesterolaemia
Palm oil	Tocopherols, tocotrienols[a], carotenoids	Cancer, heart diseases, atherosclerosis, cataract, pulmonary diseases, muscle injury
Yellow or green leafy vegetables, yellow fruits	Carotenes[a], ascorbic acid[a], dietary fibre, omega-3 fatty acids	Cancer, heart diseases, atherosclerosis, cataract, pulmonary diseases, muscle injury
Rice bran oil	Sterols, PUFA	Hypercholesterolaemia, diabetes, cardiovascular disease
Linseed oil, fish oil, flax seed oil	Omega-3 fatty acids	Hypercholesterolaemia, diabetes, cardiovascular disease
Spices, fenugreek seeds	Gums, curcumin, eugenol, capsaicin	Cancer, cardiovascular disease, detoxification of drugs and toxins

[a]Anti oxidants

found to stimulate insulin secretion from the â cells via physiological pathways [29].Curcumin, the yellow phenolic curcuminoid present in turmeric, is reported to have a wide range of biological activities. It delays galactose-induced cataract in rats [30] and also exhibits very high lipid-soluble antioxidant action and may be helpful in diabetes [31]. *Curcuma longa* root also contains Rumarin, used for its antipruritic activity and may be helpful in reducing itching sensations in those with hyperglycaemia [32, 33]. *Trikatu* is a phytocombination (*Piper longum*, *Piper nigrum* and *Zingiber officinale*) that increases bioavailability by promoting rapid absorption from the gastrointestinal tract, or preventing metabolism/oxidation during first passage through the liver after being absorbed, or a combination of these mechanisms, helping improve most drugs' therapeutic activity [34].Their bioenhancing role has recently been proposed for combining them with various known pharmacological molecules to increase the bioavailability of the latter and hence reducing their dose requirements to produce desired therapeutic effects [35].

The concept of '*diet in disease*', however, still needs a thorough probing to bring these scattered observations and inferences on a larger scale to establish their applicability in various disease conditions on a practically adaptable model.

3.4.2 Body Acclimatisation as a Food Recipient

Detoxification of the body or acclimatisation of the body as a food recipient has been practised in ancient and modern world. A weakened body (weakened by virtue of age or disease or digestive power) is always acclimatised to normalcy through a ritual from simple (easy to digest) to complex (difficult to digest) foods. Panchkarma is a very popular Ayurvedic ritual for detoxification of the body. After performing the panch-karma, the subject is kept on a specific dietary regimen (*samsarjana*) consisting of rice preparations first, from *peya* preparations (almost liquid preparations) to *anna* (semi solid preparations) to *vilepi* (solid preparations). The ritual is from easy to complex food to adapt and improve the body's digestive powers slowly but systematically.

After the rice preparation, the subject is given pulse preparations called *yush*. Again, the first one to be adopted here is *akrit yush* (*dal* without frying) followed by *krit yush* (dal with frying).

Once these two courses are over, only then is the subject exposed to *mans rasa* (animal protein). The *mans rasa* can again be in *akrit* and *krit* sequence. After sequencing the food in the given order, the person may finally be allowed to take full meal consisting of wheat.

We can find these adaptation examples in baby foods, which are the most acknowledged type of feeding mechanism for newborn infants. They are first kept on mother's milk as natural recipients and then on infant food followed by weaning food. Rice-based weaning food are always recommend for infants first, up to a certain age, followed by wheat-based weaning foods. The logic is the same – from simple to complex food in terms of digestibility and in terms of strengthening of the digestive system to deal with more complex foodstuffs.

3.4.3 Food, Age and Lifestyle

Traditional wisdom has always guided different food combinations and processing techniques to enhance the nutritive value of food. In modern science, food fortification is used for maintaining and enhancing the nutritional status of foods. Food fortification or supplementation is also used as a tool to provide essential nutrients to people with compromised metabolic conditions or to people with specific nutritional requirements. For example, high-protein foods are not given to old-age people as their ability to digest complex food gets slower with time. Sportspersons would require protein-rich diet. A rich diet (high in calorie, protein, fat, calcium, iron) is recommended for pregnant and lactating women. Impacts of adequate diet during pregnancy are obvious and evident. They not only reduce the pregnancy-related complications but also add to the health of newborn in the form of their improved weight [22]. In disease condition, dietary modifications not only control the disease condition but also help in recovery of the patient.

Modern science acknowledges that lifestyle is one substantial reason for diseases. Lifestyle diseases include metabolic syndrome and cancer. There are considerable epidemiological evidences suggesting that adequate lifestyle including exercise and dietary modification would lower the risk for these diseases [36]. Diabetes is the best-described lifestyle disease. In 2005, 17 million people were diagnosed with diabetes in the USA, while another one third remained undiagnosed. By 2050, the USA alone will have around 48 million people with diabetes. In 2004, India had an estimated 37.76 million diabetics – 21.4 million in urban areas and 16.36 million in rural areas [37, 38].

Indian habitual diets are predominantly based on plant and animal foods like cereals, pulses, green vegetables and fats. They generally are good sources of bio-active phytochemicals, particularly dietary fibre, vitamin E, omega-3 fatty acids, carotenoids and phenolic compounds. Studies carried out during the past two to three decades have shown that these phytochemicals have an important role in preventing chronic diseases like cancer, diabetes, coronary heart disease and hyper-lipidaemia. Table 3.3 shows a list of disease-preventing phytochemicals in plant foods [21].

3.5 Pitfalls and Opportunities

While Ayurveda essentially scores over modern science for being more inclusive, there is a clear complexity in the nature of defining it. Few of the examples are:

(a) There are seven types of *prakriti* that can have infinite combinations based on the proportion of each *dosha* present. Again, *vikriti* factors also should be taken into account. What may be nurturing to one may be harmful to another. This complexity would mean literally an individual food pyramid (akin to My Pyramid program by USDA) for each person.
(b) Within the subgroups of food lists, preferences have not been provided for seasonality and conditions of growing.
(c) Quantity is not based on calories but on the power of digestion and fullness of stomach [5].

Clearly, it generates probing thoughts like:

(a) How will a common man decipher his *prakriti*? With every person having a *tridoshic* complexity, it seems impossible until met with a trained doctor on a regular basis.
(b) Every aspect related with food has been given consideration. However, their relative importance has not been defined.
(c) Dietary quantification in relation with *prakriti* is lacking in specificity.
(d) How do we define mental state of a person who is eating or who is preparing food?

3.6 Opportunities for Creating Evidence Basis

From the complexity lies the opportunity for investigation and creation of evidence basis. We have observed that Ayurvedic viewpoints, when tested against modern scientific knowledge, stand the testimony as a better and inclusive source of knowledge. At some places, this correlation has strong evidence basis and at other places, found logical [39–41]. However, in general, we find them more at the abstract level without enough guidelines for their applications onto individuals.

Clearly, there are opportunities for further data collection and analysis to establish the evidence basis to achieve the following at the least:

1. Bringing objectivity to the methods of observation with the help of modern diagnostic tools to create definitive determinants for *prakriti* identification
2. Establishing quantitative relationship in between factors affecting *prakriti* and diet of a person using population survey techniques
3. Creating a season-*prakriti*-diet matrix, based on the common knowledge of food groups
4. Methods of raw material selection and their preparation with the current knowledge of active ingredients present in them which have curing properties, etc.

These studies would help create evidence basis to achieve some of the desired objectives as follows:

1. Decide on relevancy of the ancient text vis-à-vis modern practices and make it more contemporary
2. Decide upon preparations since a lot of raw materials have changed their character, owing to soil erosion, global warming and gene modifications for better yield desires
3. Make it more user-friendly and result-oriented
4. Make it more safe with respect to risk of heavy metals, chemical fertiliser and pesticides

There is an urgent need to bring relevance to such a scripture for the new-age human being and his contemporary lifestyles. This fact has recently been recognised by a leading Indian agency, The National Institute of Nutrition (NIN). NIN has come out with its new 'Dietary Guidelines for Indians – A Manual', and the 'Guideline No. 9' is considered the most important for the changing lifestyle of Indians. When NIN came out with its first manual in 1998, it had several guidelines except this one. The economic transition has changed the lifestyles of people. It was taken for granted people would anyway give their body some physical exercise 15 years ago. This, however, is not happening, was a glooming observation made by NIN scientists [42]. Interestingly, besides a wholesome nutrition, physical exercise has also been given due importance in Ayurveda for the purpose of a composite health.

Clearly, there are lots of such probing thoughts in Ayurvedic understanding of food and nutrition and their contemporary relevance in modern context, which need to be considered for objective evaluation, to bring their benefit into the clinical reality. This work is a small step towards this direction.

References

1. Sackett LD, Rosenberg W, Muir Grey JA et al (1996) Evidence-based medicine: what it is and what it isn't. BMJ 312:71
2. Singh RH (2007) Kaya chikitsa. Chaukhamba Sanskrit Pratishthana, Delhi

3. Shakuntala M (2006) Food: facts and principles. New Age International, New Delhi
4. Nutrition for every one (2011); Centers for Disease Control and Prevention. Downloaded from http://www.cdc.gov/nutrition/everyone/ Accessed on 09 Jan 2011
5. Patel MR (2010) Applying the knowledge of Ayurveda to appraise the US nutritional paradigm. Dissertation, California College of Ayurveda, Nevada
6. Choose my plate (2011); United States Department of Agriculture. Downloaded from http://www.choosemyplate.gov/ Accessed on 17 July 2011
7. Tripathi BN (ed) (2008) Charaka Samhita. Chaukhambha Publication, Varanasi
8. Smith JM, Ditschun TL (2009) Controlling satiety: how environmental factors influence food intake. Trends Food Sci Technol 20:271–277
9. Olsen A, Ritz C, Hartvig DL, Moller P (2011) Comparison of sensory specific satiety and sensory specific desires to eat in children and adults. Appetite 57:6–13
10. Englyst HN, Kingman SM, Cummings JH (1992) Classification and measurement of nutritionally important starch fractions. Eur J Clin Nutr 46(Suppl 2):33–50
11. Sandsa AL, Leidyb HJ, Hamakercd BR, Maguiree P, Campbellad WW (2009) Consumption of the slow-digesting waxy maize starch leads to blunted plasma glucose and insulin response but does not influence energy expenditure or appetite in humans. Nutr Res 29:383–390
12. Schaafsma G (2000) The protein digestibility–corrected amino acid score. J Nutr 130: 1865S–1867S
13. Pajman AD, Sinha S, Moss M, Haber MJ, Martin GS (2007) Seasonal variation in the epidemiology of sepsis. Crit Care Med 35:410–415. doi:10.1097/01.CCM.0000253405.17038.43
14. Rojansky N, Brzezinski A, Schenker J (1992) Seasonality in human reproduction: an update. Hum Reprod 7:735–745
15. Wehr T, Moul D, Barbato G, Giesen HA, Seidel JA, Barker C et al (1993) Conservation of photoperiod-responsive mechanisms in humans. Am J Physiol 265:R846–R857
16. Dowell SF (2001) Seasonal variation in host susceptibility and cycles of certain infectious diseases. Emerg Infect Dis 7:369–374
17. Moorthy G (2001) Food & nutrition. Arya Publishing House, New Delhi
18. Food combining diet. Downloaded from http://www.free-fad-diets.com/food-combining.html/ Accessed on 10 Sept 2010
19. United States Department Of Agriculture, My pyramid food guidance system education frame work. Downloaded from http://www.choosemyplate.gov/downloads/MyPyramid_education_framework.pdf/ Accessed on 17 July 2011
20. Srilakshmi B (2003) Dietetics. New Age International, New Delhi
21. Narsingarao BS (2003) Bioactive phytochemicals in Indian foods and their potential in health promotion and disease prevention. Asia Pac Jr Clin Nutr 12:9–22
22. Rastogi S, Rastogi R, Rastogi D, Rastogi R, Singh G, Chiappelli F (2010) Evaluating the impact of a pragmatic nutrition awareness program for expectant mothers upon birth weight of the newborn. Evid Based Complement Alternat Med. doi:10.1093/ecam/neq034, Advance Access published on 28 April 2010
23. Lim EL, Hollingsworth KG, Aribisala BS, Chen MJ, Mathers JC, Taylor R (2011) Reversal of type 2 diabetes: normalization of beta cell function in association with decreased pancreas and liver triacylglycerol. Diabetologia. doi:10.1007/s00125-011-2204-7
24. Rastogi D, Rastogi S et al (2011) Impact of a nutritionally engineered processed and packed food regime on Type II diabetes – a preliminary study. Light on Ayurveda Journal (accepted for publication, Nov 2011)
25. Astrup A (2001) Healthy lifestyles in Europe: prevention of obesity and type II diabetes by diet and physical activity. Public Health Nutr 4:499–515. doi:10.1079/PHN2001136
26. Ojewole JA, Adewole SO, Olayiwola G (2006) Hypoglycaemic and hypotensive effects of *Momordica charantia Linn* (*Cucurbitaceae*) whole-plant aqueous extract in rats. Cardiovasc J S Afr 17:227–232

27. Shanmugasundaram KR, Panneerselvam C, Samudram P, Shanmugasundaram ER (1983) Enzyme changes and glucose utilisation in diabetic rabbits: the effect of *Gymnema sylvestre*, R.Br. J Ethnopharmacol 7:205–234
28. Kaleem M, Sheema SH, Bano B (2005) Protective effects of *Piper nigrum* and *Vinca Rosea* in alloxan induced diabetic rats. Indian J Physiol Pharmacol 49:65–71
29. Hannan JM, Marenah L, Ali L, Rokeya B, Flatt PR, Abdel-Wahab YH (2006) Ocimum sanctum leaf extracts stimulate insulin secretion from perfused pancreas, isolated islets and clonal pancreatic-cells. J Endocrinol 189:127–136
30. Suryanarayana P, Saraswat M, Mrudula T, Krishna TP, Krishnaswamy K, Reddy GB (2005) Curcumin and turmeric delay streptozotocin-induced diabetic cataract in rats. Invest Ophthalmol Vis Sci 46:2092–2099
31. Itokawa H, Shi Q, Akiyama T, Morris-Natschke SL, Lee KH (2008) Recent advances in the investigation of curcuminoids. Chin Med 3:1–13
32. Yoganarasimhan SN (2000) Medicinal Plants of India, Vol II, Tamil Nadu; Interline Publishing House, Bangalore, 1st edn. 2:471
33. Modak M, Dixit P, Londhe J, Ghaskadbi S, Paul A, Devasagayam T (2007) Indian herbs and herbal drugs used for the treatment of diabetes. J Clin Biochem Nutr 40:163–173
34. Atal CK, Zutshi U, Rao PG (1981) Scientific evidence on the role of Ayurvedic herbals on bioavailability of drugs. J Ethnopharmacol 4:229–232
35. Atal N, Bedi KL (2010) Bioenhancers: a revolutionary concept to market. J Ayurveda Integr Med 1:96–99
36. Segasothy M (1999) Vegetarian diet: panacea for modern life style diseases? Q J Med 92:531–544
37. IDF (2007) Diabetes atlas, 3rd edn. International Diabetes Federation, Brussels
38. ICMR (2006) Assessment of burden of NCDs. New Delhi, Indian council of Medical Research
39. Rastogi S (2010) Building bridges between Ayurveda and modern science. Int J Ayurveda Res 1:41–46
40. Valiathan MS, Thatte U (2010) Ayurveda: the time to experiment. Int J Ayurveda Res 1:3
41. Vaidya AB, Raut AA (2006) Evidences based Ayurveda sorting fact from fantasy. In: Ayurveda and its scientific aspects – opportunities for globalisation. Department of AYUSH and C. S. I. R, New Delhi, pp 1–39
42. NIN's new diet guidelines. Downloaded from http://articles.timesofindia.indiatimes.com/2011-07-05/hyderabad/29738444_1_food-supplements-microwave-oven-nin/ Accessed on 10 July 2011

Chapter 4
Clinical Evidence in the Tradition of Ayurveda

P. Ram Manohar

4.1 The Evolutionary Dynamics of Ayurveda

Ayurveda is a medical tradition indigenous to the Indian subcontinent with a remarkable evolutionary history that spans several thousands of years. This unbroken continuity of tradition is perhaps unparalleled, given the fact that Ayurveda has survived vicissitudes of great intensity including foreign invasions, political subjugation, and epistemological challenges from other knowledge systems.

The earliest textbooks of Ayurveda that have been preserved for posterity also reflect the dynamism in the tradition of Ayurveda. The works of *Charaka* and *Sushruta*, for example, date from several centuries before the Common Era and have undergone editorial revisions for several hundreds of years, if not a millennium. These texts have been edited [1] for scribal errors [*pathasuddhi*], appended [2] with missing information [*sampurana*],[1] and updated [2] with contemporary knowledge [*samskarana*].[2]

Agnivesha, based on the teachings of his preceptor *Atreya*, originally composed the *Charaka Samhita* several centuries before the Common Era, and historians have been unable to arrive at a consensus regarding the dating of these texts. This text got its present name after *Caraka* redacted the work before the Common Era. *Dridhabala* later appended missing portions in the early centuries of the Common Era [1]. In a

[1]The colophon in the *Charaka Samhita—ityagniveshakrte tantre charakapratisamskrte/prapte drdhabalasampurite*—itself summarizes the revisions made on the text [2].

[2]This verse from the *Charaka Samhita* describes the process of editing and updating a classical text—*samskarta kurute tantram puranam cha punarnavam* [2].

P.R. Manohar
The Ayurvedic Trust,
Coimbatore, Tamil Nadu, India
e-mail: rammanoharp@gmail.com

S. Rastogi (ed.), *Evidence-Based Practice in Complementary and Alternative Medicine*,
DOI 10.1007/978-3-642-24565-7_4, © Springer-Verlag Berlin Heidelberg 2012

similar manner, the *Sushruta Samhita* was first composed by *Sushruta* based on the teachings of *Divodasa*, the King of *Kashi*, and this work was edited and revised by *Nagarjuna* and also critically edited by *Chandrata* in the tenth century CE [1].

Hundreds of thousands of manuscripts are preserved on palm leaves or other writing materials like birch bark in a number of private and public repositories. These documents testify the elaborate documentation, revision, and validation that Ayurvedic knowledge has undergone over thousands of years. At the first historical reference point, we encounter Ayurveda as a codified and organized system of medicine that has already diversified into eight clinical specialties developed well-defined epistemological and ontological premises, with well-structured formats for technical writing and protocols for engaging in scientific discussions as well as research methodologies for generating and validating knowledge.

In other words, acquaintance with the classical writings of Ayurveda gives us the impression of a tradition that laid the foundation for a rational and scientific development of medical knowledge in India.

4.2 Ayurveda in the Global Health-Care Scenario

In the backdrop of the renewed worldwide interest in complementary and alternative medicine [CAM], traditional systems of health care like Ayurveda are gaining in popularity on one hand and are also being subjected to scientific scrutiny as well as legislative regulations by various countries in the world on the other.

CAM includes a wide range of modalities including complete medical systems, stand-alone interventions as well as herbal recipes, mind-body techniques, and the like.

The CAM modalities of healing are classified in different ways. According to National Institutes of Health, USA, there are broad categories like natural products, mind-body medicine, manipulative and body-based practices, and other CAM practices. Ayurveda is considered as a whole medical system under other CAM practices [15]. It is a fact that Ayurveda, though mentioned by name, does not figure prominently among the CAM range of healing approaches in the developed nations. The WHO looks at Ayurveda as traditional medicine [TM] as it is practiced widely in its country of origin rather than as complementary or alternative medicine in other countries [4].

4.3 The Demand for Evidence of Safety and Efficacy of Ayurvedic Interventions

In spite of being understood generally as an independent system of medicine, there is great skepticism when it comes to acceptance of its credibility as a scientifically valid approach to health care. In the UK, for instance, the *House of Lords Select Committee on Science and Technology's Report on Complementary and Alternative*

Medicine [HMSO, 2000] classified Ayurveda as the third group of CAM modalities that were considered to have no evidence base for clinical effectiveness. After a strong protest and representation by the Ayurvedic community, Ayurveda has been included as a subgroup of herbal medicine. Group I, which represents the most organized CAM therapies, includes osteopathy, acupuncture, herbal medicine, chiropractic, and homeopathy [5].

Visibility for Ayurveda in international databases like the PubMed is poor. Query with Ayurveda as search word returns about 2,000 results, whereas Chinese medicine fetches more than 50,000 results.[3]

The Agency for Healthcare Research and Quality attempted to generate evidence report of published literature on use of Ayurvedic therapies for treatment of health conditions. It was found that there are currently few RCTs and CCTs in the literature, and this becomes an impediment in the assessment of safety and efficacy of Ayurvedic interventions from a scientific point of view [6].

An evidence-based approach is being emphasized as imperative to adopt if Ayurveda is to gain credibility and acceptance at a global level in the spectrum of CAM interventions or as an independent system in its own right for that matter.

In the current scenario, there is indeed dearth of published research and documentation in a format that would be acceptable to scientific and regulatory authorities. However, it is also important to realize that this does not mean that Ayurveda does not have an evidence-based approach traditionally. It is just that the documentation is not available in a form that is accessible or will make sense to the modern scientific community.

4.4 Clinical Evidence in the Tradition of Ayurveda

This chapter is an attempt to discuss the methodologies that evolved in the classical tradition of Ayurveda to generate clinical evidence that can assure the safety and efficacy of its medicines and interventions.

Even as we address the challenge of generating updated evidence on the safety and efficacy of Ayurveda with the help of modern research tools and methodologies, it is essential that the traditional perspective on evidence is also adequately explored and investigated in detail.

At the outset, it has to be emphasized that Ayurveda has the characteristics of a knowledge system. It has a well-defined epistemology and ontology [14]. Experience had to be validated before it could be accepted as knowledge. Direct perception, perception-aided inference, and testimonials of authorities [2] in the field were accepted as sources of reliable knowledge.[4] There is ground to suppose that some

[3]PubMed search with keywords Ayurveda and Chinese medicine on www.pubmed.com

[4]The *Charaka Samhita* lists the tools for validating knowledge—*trividhe tvasmin jnanasamudaye purvamaptopadesajjnanam, tatah pratyakshanumanabhyam parikshopapadyate* [2].

kind of clinical experimentation was also advocated to formulate and devise clinical intervention protocols[5] [2]. A careful study of classical Ayurvedic literature gives ample evidence in support of the position that Ayurveda is a knowledge system rather than a belief system [8].

Ayurvedic texts emphasize the need to be open to new information as well as the importance of constant updating of knowledge[6] [2]. A valid source of knowledge is not against the spirit of systematic acquisition of knowledge, has been expounded by people who have investigated into the truth of the matter, is accepted by peers in the field, has beneficial applications for the world, and is presented in a rational and scientific manner[7] [2].

It is, therefore, not surprising to find that the most authentic textbooks of Ayurveda have advocated evidence-based approach to clinical practice.

4.5 Stringent Criteria for Incorporating Drugs into the Pharmacopeia

Making a sweeping statement that there is no substance in the world that cannot be potentially used as medicine[8] [9], the classical texts issue a warning against the use of substances that have not been adequately understood. Any plant, animal, or mineral substance could be incorporated into the Ayurvedic pharmacopeia only if it has been adequately understood in terms of nomenclature, identity, properties, and applications[9] [2]. The texts also warn against abuse of well-known medicines, emphasizing the point that even poison becomes medicine when used appropriately, whereas the best medicine can turn out to be harmful if used improperly[10] [2]. Out of nearly 10,000 plants used for medicinal purposes in the Indian subcontinent, only 1,200–1,500 plants got incorporated into the Ayurvedic pharmacopeia officially over a period of more than 3,000 years. Every plant is to be studied thoroughly before it becomes a part of Ayurvedic pharmacopeia.

---

[5]Chakrapani's comments on *Charaka Samhita* explaining the logic of combining herbs and individualizing formulations—*yuktih yojana bheshajasya dehadoshadyapekshaya* [2].

[6]*Charaka Samhita* emphasizes the need for continuous learning in Ayurveda—*na chaiva hyasti sutaramayurvedasya param, tasmadapramattah sasvadabhiyogamasmin gacchet* [2].

[7]*Charaka Samhita* lays down the criteria for acceptance of new knowledge—*yaschanyopi kashcidvedarthadaviparitah parikshakaih pranitah sishtanumato lokanugrahapravrttah sastravadah* [2].

[8]The *Astanga Hrdayam* declares that there is no substance in the world without medicinal property—*jagatyevamanaushadham, na kincit vidyate dravayam* [9].

[9]The *Charaka Samhita* stresses the danger in using unknown substances and abuse of known substances—*aushadham hyanabhijnatam namarupagunaistribhih, vijnatam chapi duryuktam anarthayopapadyate* [2].

[10]*Charaka Samhita* explains how poison can also be used as medicine by adjusting the dosage—*yogadapi visham tikshnamuttamam bheshajam bhavet, bheshajam chapi duryuktam tikshnam sampadyate visham* [2].

Great importance was given in the tradition of Ayurveda to assess safety and efficacy of a medicinal substance in a realistic manner. It was recognized that there is no substance that is absolutely safe. Any potential medicine also possessed undesirable qualities, and hence, there was a need to assess the risk-benefit ratio[11] [2].

It is very interesting to note that the *Charaka Samhita* has documented what is perhaps one of the earliest public warnings issued against the unethical use of spurious medicines. The text alerts the intelligent laity to refuse medications prescribed irrationally by a physician for the sake of their own health and life[12] [2].

Toxicity of drugs and foods was to be determined by exposing animals to these substances[13] [9], and clues were also obtained from animals on efficacy of drug sources by a process of observation that is akin to what is known today as zoopharmacognosy[14] [10].

4.6 Chance Effect Versus Real Effect of a Clinical Intervention

The need to distinguish between chance effect and real effect of a medicine or clinical intervention for that matter has been stated in unequivocal terms. The physician who can provide relief from an ailment is one who administers a medicine with clear knowledge of its indications and outcomes. One whose success depends on accidental or chance effect of a medicine or clinical intervention cannot be considered as a physician. If such a quack finds success in clinical practice, then it is mere coincidence, just like the accidental creation of letter patterns by insects on a manuscript[15] [2].

The chance effect of an intervention was known as *Yadrcchiki Siddhi* and the real effect as *Pratiniyamiki Siddhi*[16] [2]. *Pratiniyamiki Siddhi* means a predictable and repeatable effect of an intervention, which has been experimentally tested and proven by authorities in the field. The Sanskrit equivalent for efficacy is the term *Siddhi*, and an efficacious medicine was known as *Siddhabheshaja*. However, it is important to point out that efficacy and safety was evaluated in terms of an

[11]The *Charaka Samhita* points out that one must assess the risk-benefit ratio—*na tu kinchidadoshanirgunam gunabhuyastvamato vichintyate* [2].

[12]The *Charaka Samhita* issues a public warning against physicians who prescribe medicines irrationally—*tasmanna bhishaja yuktam yuktibahyena bheshajam, dhimata kinchidadeyam jivitarogyakankshina* [2].

[13]The *Ashtanga Hrdayam* recommends testing of toxicity by administering substances to animals—*mryante makshikah prasya kakah kshamasvaro bhavet.....* [9].

[14]*Atharva Veda* refers to zoopharmacognosy for identification of medicinal plants—*varaho veda virudham nakulo veda bheshajam, sarpa gandharva ya viduh ta asma avase huve* [10].

[15]Chakrapani comments on *Charaka Samhita*, explaining the chance effect of clinical intervention—*yadrcchikasiddhau hi vaidyo na rogapramokshe karanam, kintu ghunaksharanyayena daivagato bheshajasya samyagyoga iti* [2].

[16]In his comments on *Charaka Samhita*, Chakrapani coins a term for real effect of clinical intervention—*siddhirakhyatiti ukta pratiniyamiki siddhih na yadrchhiki* [2].

intervention, which is specific to a particular clinical condition of the patient. The same medicine, which is safe and efficacious in one context, can become dangerous in another context. Such a complete intervention was known as *Prayoga*[17] [2].

An evidence-based intervention was known as a *Siddhaprayoga*. Ayurveda is thus a tradition of evidence-based clinical interventions [*Siddhaprayogas*] rather than evidence-based medicines [*Siddhabheshajas*].

When formulations are listed in the context of a particular disease, the texts often emphasize the fact that most efficacious [*Siddhatama*][18] [2] recipes have been chosen, implying the fact that those particular recipes which demonstrated superior efficacy were chosen after a lot of experimentation and observation of their clinical outcomes.

Safety is also evaluated in a similar vein with respect to the intervention rather than a medicine. Contending that there is no medicine that is absolutely safe, the texts point out that the clinical intervention that provides relief to a particular disease without provoking the manifestation of new diseases is pure and safe. Technically, a safe intervention is known as a *Shuddhaprayoga*[19][2].

Adverse events are known as *Vyapats*, and strategies for management of adverse events were prescribed in anticipation [*Vyapat Siddhi*][20] [2]. Thus, the Ayurvedic approach to safe medicine included both risk assessment and safety measures. Ayurvedic texts also alert the physician about the possibility of iatrogenic diseases [*Mithyopacarajanyavyadhi*][21] [2].

The *Charaka Samhita* blatantly states that claims of successful clinical outcomes will be dismissed as chance effect if these are not substantiated with evidence and rationale[22] [2]. The ancient proponents of Ayurveda were very well aware of the difference between chance effect and real effect of a medicine or clinical intervention. The texts have documented debates on the relevance of clinical intervention. Students,[23] [9] as well as skeptics[24] [2], are seen questioning the role of clinical intervention in giving relief from diseases on the ground that patients who do not get

[17]*Charaka Samhita* explains that a complete and wholesome intervention becomes successful—*samyakprayogam sarvesham siddhirakhyati karmanam* [2].

[18]*Charaka Samhita* lists the most efficacious formulations—*atah siddhataman yogan srnunmada-vinasanan* [2].

[19]*Charaka Samhita* defines a safe intervention—*thus prayogah samayedvyadhim yonyamanya-mudirayet, nasau visuddhah suddhastu samayedyanna kopayet* [2].

[20]*Charaka Samhita* on strategies for anticipating adverse events and planning their management—*samyakprayogam chaushadhanam, vyapannanam cha vyapatsadhanani siddhishuttarakalam* [2].

[21]*Chakarapani's comments on Charaka Samhita refer to iatrogenic diseases—mithyopachara iti asamyakkaranamasamyagupacharascha* [2].

[22]*Charaka Samhita* emphasizes the need to support claims of cure with evidence and rationale—*vina tarkena ya siddhih yadrcchasiddhireva sa* [2].

[23]Students question the role of clinical intervention in the *Ashtanga Hridaya—bhedadinam sam-mato bhaktinamrah papracchedam samsayanognivesah* [9].

[24]The arguments put forth by skeptics in *Charaka Samhita* to prove the futility of clinical intervention—*yatascha pratikurvan sidhyati, pratikurvan mryate, apratikurvan siddhyati, apratikurvan mryate, tataschintyate bheshajamabheshajenavisishtamiti* [2].

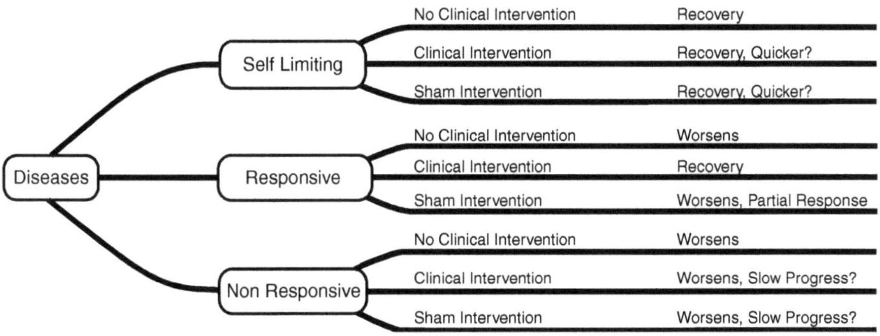

Fig. 4.1 Ayurveda classifies diseases into three categories based on prognosis: (a) self-limiting disease, (b) diseases that respond to treatment, and (c) diseases that do not respond to treatment. Legitimate claims of efficacy can be made only with regard to diseases that respond to treatment

treated are observed to recover, while those that receive treatment are seen to succumb to the disease. At a very early stage of its evolutionary history, Ayurveda has addressed the question of the reliability of clinical intervention and the predictability of clinical outcomes.

4.7 Natural Course of Diseases and Claims of Efficacy

Ayurveda was perhaps the earliest medical system to describe self-limiting diseases, which were referred to as *Anupaya-Sadhya* in the *Charaka Samhita*[25][2]. This is also referred to in other texts like the *Ashtanga Hrdayam*[26] [9]. The limitation of medicine was also recognized and acknowledged by accepting the fact that many diseases do not respond to treatment [*Upaya-Asadhya*] [2]. The physician has a role only in the management of diseases that respond to treatment [*Upaya-Sadhya*] [2]. The debates on the significance of medical intervention in managing diseases conclude with the statement that medicine is unfailing in diseases that are responsive to treatment and the skillful physician should distinguish between self-limiting, curable, and incurable diseases. He cannot make a claim in having cured a self-limiting disease and cannot be held responsible for his inability to cure an incurable disease. If equipped with the proper knowledge, a well-trained physician can effectively manage diseases that are amenable to treatment[27] [2] (Fig. 4.1).

---

[25] The arguments in support of the role of clinical intervention proposed by the *Charaka Samhita—na hi sarve vyadhayo bhavantyupayasadhyah, na chopayasadhyanam vyadhinamanupayena siddhirasti, na chasadhyanam vyadhinam bheshajasamudayoyamasti* [2].

[26] *Ashtanga Hridya* refers to self-limiting diseases—*vinapi kriyaya svasthyam gacchatam shodasamsaya* [9].

[27] *Charaka Samhita* on diseases that respond to treatment—*sadhyasadhyavibhagajno jnanapurvam chikitsakah, kale charabhate karma yattat sadhayati dhruvam* [2].

Apart from self-limiting diseases, it appears that the masters of Ayurveda were also aware of the placebo effect, though it was not employed in clinical research. It was well known that by influencing the mind, people could get better. When the mind is favorably disposed, the immunity and response of the body is enhanced, leading to decrease in severity of disease[28] [2]. The so-called placebo effect was used as a therapeutic tool to induce a healing response from the patient.

There are also references to what can today be understood as spontaneous remission. Certain diseases are understood to remain dormant for years without clinical manifestations, and chronic diseases may resolve unexpectedly under favorable circumstances[29] [2].

To put it in a nutshell, the ancient exponents of Ayurveda knew about the natural course of a disease. They have described the possible courses that a disease may take in the absence of medical intervention as well as in response to medical intervention. Claims of efficacy have been carefully established in the tradition of Ayurveda by ruling out chance effect and with due consideration of the natural course of a disease.

4.8 Methodology for Generating Clinical Evidence

These discussions lead us to very important questions. Did the tradition of Ayurveda employ a well-defined methodology of research to generate evidence on safety and efficacy of its clinical interventions? If so, how rigorous and reliable was it? We know today that evidence can be generated at different levels, and the reliability depends on the rigor of the methodology that has been used to establish causal relationships.

It was clearly understood in Ayurveda that both health and disease are events dependent on cause and effect relationships, and in order to cure disease and establish health, it was essential to understand the complex ways in which the chain of cause and effect unfolds to create the outcomes of health and disease[30] [2].

The goal of the medical system was to create the knowledge of cause and effect relationships in the context of both pathology and therapeutics. The text is explicit when it states that the disease disappears when the cause and effect reactions are eliminated. The ancient researchers who painstakingly compiled the knowledge of Ayurveda were aware of the challenge of understanding the intricate causal

---

[28] *Charaka Samhita* explains how the mind can influence treatment outcomes favorably—*manasorthanukulyaddhi tushtirurjabalodayah, sukhopabhogata cha syad vyadheschato balaksayah* [2].

[29] *Charaka Samhita* discusses how favourable factors can induce remission in diseases—*iha khalu nidanadoshadushyaviseshebhyo vikaravighatabhavabhavaprativiseshah bhavanti* [2].

[30] *Charaka Samhita* emphasizes that all biological events are based on cause and effect relationships—*vikarah prakrtischaiva dvayam sarvam samasatah, tadhetuvasagam hetorabhavannanuvartate—Charaka Samhita* [2].

relationships that lead to manifestation of diseases. They were quite wary of the possibility of erroneous observations and judgments without the deployment of a rigorous methodology.

4.9 Levels of Evidence and Controlled Studies

Mere coincidence [*Sahacarya*] does not imply causation [*Hetu*]. If cause and effect are seen associated together repeatedly, then a coincidence is suspected. This is known as *Sahacarya*, which means to be together. When the coincidence becomes established as a norm [*Sahacarya Niyama*], it is understood as a correlation [*Vyapti*][31] [3]. Deducting a correlation was not considered sufficient to establish causation. The correlation had to be tested using controls, i.e., positive and negative controls. This was known as *Pakshadharmata* and was considered as the final test for confirming a cause and effect relationship[32] [3]. This process consisted of examining the plausibility of causation in three contexts—the context where causation is probable and suspected known as *Paksha*, the context where causation is established known as *Sapaksha*, and the context where causation has been ruled out known as *Vipaksha*[33] [3]. This is achieved by studying the relationship between variables, which was known as *lingaparamarsha*.

From the above discussion, it appears that evidence for causation was considered at three levels that correspond to anecdotal evidence, observational studies, and controlled experiments. It is interesting to note that the concept of controlled clinical trials finds a parallel in the concept of *Pakshadharmata*. *Paksha* corresponds to the trial drug; *Sapaksha*, to the positive control; and *Vipaksha*, to the negative control.

It can be safely presumed that clinical evidence was generated in the tradition of Ayurveda by using quite a rigorous method of observation and analysis.

4.10 Meticulous Study of Independent and Dependent Variables

It is also interesting to find that a statistical approach was adopted to test the significance of the relationship between two variables, the dependent [*lingi*] and the independent [*linga*], considering both positive and negative correlations[34] [3]. It is not

[31]The *Tarkasangraha* explains the concept of correlation—*yatra yatra dhumastatra tatra vahniriti sahacaryaniyamo vyaptih* [3].

[32]The *Tarkasangraha* on establishing causation—*vyaptivisishtapaksadharmatajnanam paramarsah* [3].

[33]The *Tarkasangraha* explains the method to confirm causation with the help of controls—*sandigdhasadhyavan pakshah, nischitasadhyavan sapakshah, nischitasadhyabhavavan vipakshah* [3].

[34]The *Tarkasangraha* explains negative and positive correlations between variables—*lingam trividham, anvayavyatireki, kevalanvayi, kevalavyatireki ceti* [3].

possible to study causation without the study of variables or *lingaparamarsha*[35] [3]. Three tests are used in the tradition for this purpose. The first is the test of specificity. The dependent variable should have a specific correlation with the independent variable, and vice versa. When the independent variable is present, the presence of the dependent variable is implied without fail. In other words, one independent variable should not be associated with two or more dependent variables. This is known as *Avyabhicaritva* and implies that an independent variable is specific to a dependent correlate. Rise in body temperature implies fever and nothing else. The fact that fever might imply something else is another question altogether.

Next is the test of sensitivity. The independent variable should have a continuous association with the dependent variable, and vice versa. This is known as *Avinabhavasambandha*. Rise in body temperature always means active fever. One cannot be febrile without a rise in temperature.

The third one is the test of integrity. When the independent variable is absent, the dependent variable is also absent, and vice versa. If there is no fever, then there is no rise in temperature, and if the temperature is not raised, then there is no fever. This is known as *Ayutasiddhatva*[36] [11].

Studying the relationship between the independent and dependent variables in a very rigorous manner helped to arrive at diagnosis of disease. Very specific and reliable criteria were formulated to ensure a clear diagnosis to the extent possible. Clinical outcomes were also analyzed rigorously on the basis of the abovementioned tests of significance.

Suffice to say, Ayurveda, being a knowledge system, developed and evolved as evidence-based approach to health care over several thousands of years. There have been breaks in this process and in the last few hundred years; the Ayurvedic community has not been able to effectively continue this activity or present the evidence in a form that is acceptable to modern scientists and researchers.

4.11 Creating a Matrix of Evidence: Integrating Text, Tradition, and Modern Research

Blind adoption of modern methods of research will not serve the purpose of understanding the strengths of Ayurveda as a comprehensive approach to health care. Personalization of the clinical intervention underpins the rationale behind the Ayurvedic approach of prevention and management of diseases. Multiple formulations and multiple modalities of therapies make up a typical clinical intervention that is tailored to suit the specific requirements of a particular individual. Ayurveda defines a pharmaceutical formulation as that which is formulated with specific reference to the requirements of a disease condition and body constitution. Suitable

[35]The *Tarkasangraha* on how to establish causation by study of variables—*svarthanumitiparartha-numityoh lingaparamarsa eva karanam, tasmat lingaparamarsonumanam* [3].

[36]*Padartha Vijnana* discusses these concepts in detail [11].

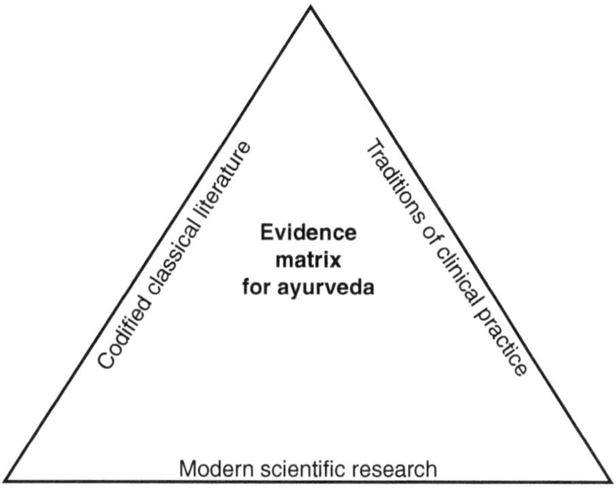

Fig. 4.2 The triangular evidence matrix for Ayurveda and traditional medicine draws evidence from three streams: classical literature preserved in the tradition, current practices, and modern research. Such a matrix will give a comprehensive view of available evidence to validate Ayurveda

methods of research will have to be envisaged to generate evidence of safety and efficacy of Ayurvedic clinical interventions.

Review of clinical research done on Ayurveda reveals that majority of the studies, which are experimental and with controls, focus on single herbs, a single formulation, or a single therapy. Ayurveda has rarely been studied in a complete way and in the manner in which it is actually practiced [7]. On the other hand, reports on whole system interventions often lack rigor in the study design and hence do not provide compelling evidence.

The challenge before us is to generate rigorous evidence that is built upon the foundations of the tradition of Ayurveda and at the same time incorporating modern methodologies and approaches without compromising the rigor of science or the holism of Ayurveda. Such an approach will be able to make the best use of knowledge that has been carefully compiled and preserved over the millennia as well as the latest advancements in scientific research.

The National Institutes of Health funded a pilot study for evaluating the efficacy of personalized outpatient Ayurvedic clinical intervention against standard allopathic treatment in rheumatoid arthritis. This study was able to demonstrate that randomized, double-blind, placebo-controlled design could be used to study personalized Ayurvedic clinical interventions. A short communication about the study design and the success of blinding has been published in the Annals of Rheumatic Diseases [12]. The outcomes of the study have also been presented at the Annual Meeting of the American College of Rheumatology [13] and demonstrate that modern science and the tradition of Ayurveda can be integrated to generate evidence of the highest level. Encouragingly, the full outcome paper is being favorably considered by peer-reviewed rheumatology journals in the USA (Fig. 4.2).

The meaningful way forward seems to be an approach to evidence building in clinical research that draws from classical literature, current clinical practice, and modern research in an integrative manner, which will help us to create a comprehensive evidence matrix for Ayurveda and traditional medicine.

References

1. Meulenbeld GJ (1999) A history of Indian medical literature [Ia and Ib]. Egbert Forsten, Groningen
2. Yadavji T (ed) (1992) Caraka Samhita. Munshilal Manoharlal Publishers Pvt. Ltd, New Delhi
3. Annambhatta (1876) Tarkasangraha. Nirnayasagara Press, Bombay
4. WHO (2002) WHO traditional medicine strategy 2002–2005. WHO, Geneva
5. Herbal Regulatory Group of UK (2003) Recommendations on the regulation of herbal, practitioners in the UK. The Prince of Wales's Foundation for Integrated Health, UK
6. Hardy M, Coulter I, Venuturupalli S, Roth EA, Favreau J, Morton SC, Shekelle P (2001) Evidence report/technology assessment, number 41, Ayurvedic interventions for diabetes mellitus: a systematic review, AHRQ Publication No. 01-E040
7. Hardy M (2001) Research in Ayurveda: where do we go from here? Altern Ther Health Med 7:34–35
8. Balasubramanian AV, Nirmala Devi TD (eds) (2006) Traditional knowledge systems of India and Sri Lanka. CIKS, Chennai
9. Sastri H (ed) (2002) Ashtanga Hridayam. Chaukhambha Orientalia, Varanasi
10. Anonymous (2003) Atharvaveda Samhita. Nag Publishers, Bombay
11. Mishra YC (2005) Padartha Vijnana. Chaukhambha Sanskrit Bhawan, Varanasi
12. Furst DE, Booth-LaForce C, Kumar PRK, Krishnaswamy BG, Mahapatra A, McGann M, Ram Manohar P, Sarin R, Venkatraman M (2011) Well controlled, double-blind, placebo-controlled trials of classical Ayurvedic treatment are possible in rheumatoid arthritis. Ann Rheum Dis 70:392–393
13. Furst DE, Booth-LaForce C, Gopinath J, Kumar PRK, Khanna D, Krishnaswamy BG, Mahapatra A, McGann M, Ram Manohar P, Raveendran KG, Sarin R, Venkatraman M (2010) Double-blind, randomized, controlled, placebo-included, pilot study comparing classical Ayurvedic medicine, methotrexate, and their combination in RA. Arthritis Rheum 62:S463
14. Kapoor K, Singh AK (eds) (2005) Indian knowledge systems, vol 1. Indian Institute of Advanced Study, New Delhi
15. NCCAM (2011) NCCAM third strategic plan, exploring the science of complementary and alternative medicine, NIH Publication No. 11–7643 D458

Chapter 5
Evidence-Based Traditional Persian Medicine

Mahsa Dousti, Manisha Harish Ramchandani, Andre Barkhordarian, Sohrab Danaei, and Francesco Chiappelli

5.1 History of Persian Traditional Medicine

5.1.1 Introduction

Medicine has always played a significant role in Iranian culture and civilization. Archeological discoveries such as a skull found at the site of the "*Torched City*" *suggest a* surgical operation performed on a 13-year-old girl suffering from hydrocephalus some 4,850 years ago. The name "*Iran*" derives from "*Aryan*" and has a history stretching over 7,000 years. Only a bit larger than the state of Alaska, Iran is among the most geographically diverse countries in the world. This ancient nation can be divided into 12 separate geographic environments and boasts five major climates. Iran's geographic diversity allows for more than 7,500 species of plants, of which nearly 1,800 of which are used in medicine. Many of Iran's most precious herbal treasures are plants found nowhere else in the world. This astounding environmental diversity has led to numerous natural herbal remedies.

Iran's traditional medicine (ITM) has its roots in Persian, Greek, Indian, and Egyptian medicine. Over long years, the ITM secured a firm foothold not only in Iran but also in the vast part of Europe and India subcontinent proving crucial in promotion of medicine as a whole. After Islam, significant efforts of Iranian scientists like Rhazes (a.k.a. *Muhammad ibn Zakariya al-Razi*, 865–925 AD), Avicenna (a.k.a. *Abū 'Alī al-Husayn ibn 'Abd Allāh ibn Sīnā*, 980–1037 AD), Birouni (a.k.a. *Alberonius*, *Abū Rayhān al-Bīrūnī*, 973–1048 AD), and Jorjani (a.k.a. *Abd al-Qahir al-Jurjani*, ca. 1007–1078 AD), the writers of immortal textbooks on traditional medicines respectively entitled Al-Havi, Canon, Al-Seydaneh, and Zakhireh, are

M. Dousti (✉) • M.H. Ramchandani • A. Barkhordarian • S. Danaei • F. Chiappelli
Division of Oral Biology and Medicine, UCLA School of Dentistry, Los Angeles, CA, USA
e-mail: mahsa.dousti@yahoo.com; rmanisha@ucla.edu; andreucsb@hotmail.com; sohrab.danaei@yahoo.com; fchiappelli@dentistry.ucla.edu

S. Rastogi (ed.), *Evidence-Based Practice in Complementary and Alternative Medicine*,
DOI 10.1007/978-3-642-24565-7_5, © Springer-Verlag Berlin Heidelberg 2012

clear throughout the history of medicine. They were not only responsible for accumulating all the existing information on medicine of the time, but adding to this knowledge by their own astute observations, experimentation, and skills.

5.1.2 Principles of Persian (Iranian) Traditional Medicine (ITM)

ITM looks at patients and diseases through an angle different from that of modern medicine. Modern medicine has an abstract supervision on the work of organs, tissues, and genes, considering the disease as the driving force behind an imbalance in body performance. It does its utmost to strike a balance in organ, tissue, or gene performance to cure the disease. ITM, however, views man as one entity. From the perspective of ITM, a disease shows that the whole body is imbalanced. So, it tries to strike an overall balance. One among the most prominent of Iranian physicians, Avicenna, stated "Medicine is the science by which we learn the various states of the human body in health and when not in health, and the means by which health is likely to be lost and, when lost, is likely to be restored back to health. In other words, it is the art whereby health is conserved and the art whereby it is restored after being lost."

5.2 The Role of Avicenna in Persian (Iranian) Traditional Medicine

5.2.1 The Canon of Medicine

Avicenna was a brilliant physician of the late 900s and early 1000s who systematized medicine in Persia. He is known as the "*Prince of Physicians*" for the introduction of clinical trials, evidence-based medicine, the experimental use and testing of drugs, and a precise guide for practical experimentation in the process of discovering and proving the effectiveness of medical substances in his medical encyclopedia, *The Canon (or Laws) of Medicine (Al-Qanoon fi al-Tibb)*.

The Canon of Medicine was the first book dealing with experimental medicine, evidence-based medicine, randomized controlled trials [1, 2], and efficacy tests [3, 4], which still form the basis of clinical pharmacology [4] and modern clinical trials [5]. It was used for centuries as a major medical reference in the world, particularly in Europe [6]. A quick glance at *the Canon of Medicine* shows that Avicenna relied heavily on history, physical examination, diet and lifestyle, environmental factors, individual temperament of the patient and visual observation in the diagnosis, treatment, and prevention of diseases. Volume 3, Sects. 6, 7, and 8, of Avicenna's *Canon of Medicine* deal with the description of anatomy and diseases of the oral structures including tongue, teeth, gingiva, and their treatments. It consists of three main sections:

- Mouth and tongue
- Tooth
- Gingiva and lip

Many of these are still common issues in modern communities, and their diagnosis and treatment are routine and even might be challenging for today's dentistry. Examples are ankyloglossia (tongue-tie), ranula, tooth wear, supraeruption, and also infectious diseases such as periodontal diseases and differentiating it from odontogenic problems, halitosis, and even bruxism and tooth discoloration. Avicenna introduced a broad spectrum of herbal and traditional medicines for treatments of oral diseases. His emphasis on having special diets for improving dental health and describing a wide spectrum of oral diseases shows his knowledge and deep concepts regarding today's dentistry.

5.2.2 *Temperaments, Elements, and Humors in Avicenna's Medicine*

Avicenna extended the theory of temperaments in *The Canon of Medicine* to encompass "emotional aspects, mental capacity, moral attitudes, self-awareness, movements and dreams" [7].

- Temperaments arise from the interaction of the elements and the humors. Temperaments determine the way in which the soul functions. Each organ of the body has its own temperament.
- Elements represent the primary constituents, the *primary qualities,* of the human body, and are four:
  - Earth
  - Air
  - Fire
  - Water
- The elements are dynamic and have direction, as they point to each other—attract and are attracted reciprocally. Health comes when the strength of the *primary qualities* are in balance.
- When one quality predominates, stress and ill health can result:
  - Slow and heavy movement signifies a predominance of cold and dryness (earth).
  - Fearfulness and sluggishness suggests excess of cold and wet (water).
  - Cheerfulness indicates heat and wetness (air).
  - Anger, aggressiveness, and violence indicate heat and dryness (fire).

- The humors are the primary fluids of the body, which move within it. Food and drink are transformed into heat through the digestive process. The humors arise in the liver during the second stage of digestion. The four humors sustain and nourish the body as they move through their channels:
  - Sanguineous (blood)
  - Serous (phlegm)
  - Bilious (choler, yellow bile)
  - Atrabilious (melancholy, black bile)
- These channels correspond to air, water, fire, and earth. In a state of health, the humors are assimilated by the organs and completely integrated into the tissues. In a state of the absence of health—disease—some material is unable to be assimilated and must be eliminated by the body.

Avicenna further summarized the relationship among the four humors and the temperaments as follows [8]:

- ***Choleric*** (yellow bile) corresponds to hot and dry, yellow, and bitter. It corresponds to the fluid of yellow bile, the season of summer, and the element of air. A person who is choleric is easily angered or bad tempered. This humor prevents the body from becoming heavy, sleepy, and dull. In over abundance, a person described as "choleric" would be mean-spirited, suspicious, and angry.
- ***Melancholic*** (atrabilious) refers to earthy, thick, black, and sour. This humor feeds the bones, the spleen, and other parts of the body, which are "*melancholy*" in nature. It tempers the two hot humors (sanguineous and bilious). When the atrabilious humor is in too much abundance, melancholia, characterized by aversion to food, despondency, sleeplessness, irritability, restlessness, and depression could result. It is now generally believed that melancholia is the same phenomenon as clinical depression.
- ***Phlegmatic*** (serous) is watery, cold, moist, and white. It moderates the strength, heat, and thickness of blood, nourishes the brain, and moistens such parts of the body that are involved with motion. A phlegmatic person is calm and unemotional.
- ***Sanguine*** (blood) pertains to the blood and is hot and moist. It imparts strength and color to the body. The characteristics of a *sanguine* temperament are courage, hopefulness, and amorousness.

5.2.3 Avicenna's Materia Medica

Following Avicenna's teaching, Iran's traditional medicine (ITM) brings together natural sciences, anatomy, diagnosis, therapeutic, and materia medica and is based in the following principles [8]:

- The universe is a single orderly unit.
- All components of the universe act in coordination with one another and are subject to certain rules.

- Temperature causes expansion. So if bodies are closer to their origin, they are warmer and have more motion. If bodies are far from their origin, they will be more and more motionless. As a result of this, they become contracted, which in turn makes them more fragile and stiff.
- The earth is the lowest-ranking body in the universe.
- Warmness, coldness, wetness, and dryness are the basic components of the universe. Warmness and coldness are the primary natures while wetness and dryness are dubbed as secondary natures.

The principle then states that adding up these natures will create features for bodies and elements. In a first-ever encounter, man viewed things as purely physical. Later, after mulling them over, he came up with the following classification:

1. The solid represented by soil
2. The liquid represented by water
3. The gas or steam represented by air
4. The force represented by fire and light

The more we move from "the force" toward "the solid," the less warmth we will have. In other words, the solid and soil are the lowest while light and fire are the highest in nature.

- All beings are complex in the nature. The above features are more or less present in all creatures. However, some features are hidden in some creatures, while they are more apparent in others.
- Among other features of the beings is "constant transition from one stage to another." Transition and metamorphosis are ever-present features of the world. Nothing goes waste in the world.
- Rules and regulations apply to both the little world (particles) and the great world (universe). Both which are also known as microcosm and macrocosm and are subject to fixed regulations.
- Every "body" goes through three stages:
  - Spirit—afterlife (*solid spirit, vegetal spirit, animal spirit, human spirit*).
  - Soul (life)—life
  - Body (corpse)—world. There are four different kinds of spirits.

  In addition to the features already mentioned for the above spirit, human spirit has free will that enables man to obtain other human feature such as "knowledge, skill, and creativity" to move toward evolution.
- All beings in the world (solids, plants, animals, and humans) affect each other.
- There are certain rules governing the relations between components of the world. Some of them are clear-cut and evident at certain times. The others, which outnumber the first group, are invisible. The two groups surely interact. As science advances, the number of known and evident rules increases. This will surely decrease the number of the unknown.
- Elements, which make up world beings, were created by the revolution of heavens. In a first stage, warmness, coldness, wetness, and dryness came into being. In the second stage, these four elements joined forces to create fire, air, water,

and soil. The third stage saw the creation of compound beings. In a later stage, plants and animals came into being. In the latest revolution stage, humans were created. The number of natural elements, which are the cornerstone of life, stands at seven.

5.3 Traditional Persian Herbal Medicine

5.3.1 Herbal Remedies in Medicine

Iran's traditional medicine has long been respected and utilized as the main source of remedy for many in rural communities. Traditional medicine consists of health cares and medicine related to specific cultures and customs and has been practiced before the introduction of Western scientific medicine. This indigenous local traditional medicine relies on practice and observations that have been passed down generations. Thus, ITM can be understood as an amalgam of knowledge and recognition of medical science, inherited and practical experiences, and cultural beliefs that have emerged and expanded in the course of its history.

Local medicine originated from biological and social needs of the people and is a part of a culture. However, in each society, people profit by manners of treatment regarding to customs, mores, beliefs, skills, and techniques. In the last years, as a consequence of multitude factors, including dissatisfaction with sophisticated medical health care systems, alternative medicine has become increasingly popular. Furthermore, conventional medicine has not fully been able to treat complex chronic conditions (arthritis, allergies, pain, hypertension, cancer, depression, digestive problems, etc.), and more people have decided to take control of their own health care. This clearly begs the question whether or not a given herbal remedy is more effective in treating said conditions. It is best answered through randomized clinical trials. Where such evidence exists, it is often contradictory. In this situation, the best evidence is provided by a systematic review or meta-analysis, i.e., an evaluation of the totality of the available data on a specific topic. With this approach, although problems may still exist, selection bias and random error are minimized.

5.3.2 Implications for Dentistry

Alternative dentistry is defined as the process of using alternative medicine such as herbal supplements to treat dental problems. Recently, the use of alternative dentistry in treating teeth has been fast growing and gaining popularity. Here are some of the major factors that attract people to alternative dentistry.

5.3.2.1 The Holistic Approach

In alternative dentistry, dentists view the body as one whole system. This means that what happens to one body part may be caused by a malfunction in another body part. If there is a problem with your teeth, holistic dentistry views this as something that is due to a possible malfunctioning of one of your organs. Therefore, through this kind of dentistry, the physicians are able to find and treat two or more diseases at once.

Because alternative dentistry focuses on the natural healing properties of plants and vegetables, the natural resources are certified to be healthy for the patient. In addition to this, there is a possibility that the patient may not need to undergo a life-threatening dental operation because a holistic treatment may heal both issues, internal and dental.

Alternative dentistry is far cheaper than modern medicine because the brand of medicines that dentists use comes from natural sources. Therefore, the patient would not need to pay as much as going to a modern dental office. Alternative dentistry is centered around the entire body system rather than the current paradigm which is the oral cavity. There are fewer side effects in alternative dentistry because everything is naturally compounded. The medicine that the patient would take comes from nature itself and has fewer chemicals than synthetic medicine.

5.3.2.2 Traditional Persian Herbal Medicine—Implications for Dentistry

Holistic dentists promote the use of alternative methods to diagnose, treat, prevent, and cure a wide range of disorders that traditional medicine cannot yet cure. The herbs aloe vera, bloodroot, calendula, echinacea, goldenseal, and grapefruit seed extract are useful for treating periodontal problems, while clove oil, garlic, lemon balm, licorice, and propolis are helpful for fighting toothaches. Alfalfa, dandelion, horsetail, and plankton can help reduce tooth decay, and yohimbe increases salivation in some patients. Herbal components such as chamomile, clove oil, echinacea, eucalyptus, fennel, ginger, licorice root, tincture of myrrh, nettle leaves, tea tree oil, witch hazel, and watercress are included in herbal dental products [9].

Common natural resources used in oral health care include:

- **Alfalfa** (*Medicago sativa*) has been used as an herbal medicine for over 1,500 years. The Roman writer Palladius referred to alfalfa as "*medica*." The ancient Greeks and Romans believed that the alfalfa plant came from the Medes land, which is modern day Iran. Its leaves, petals, flowers, and sprouts are believed to be beneficial for people suffering from arthritis, water retention, and blood disorders. One of the richest sources of trace minerals and an antioxidant, alfalfa is also used for hemorrhaging and fungal infections.
- **Aloe** (*Aloe vera*) juice is commonly used internally to relieve digestive discomfort. It is also used for soothing wounds, radiodermatitis, sunburn psoriasis, fungal

infection, and ulcers [10]. The resinous yellow aloin from wounding the a*loe* plant is used externally to relieve skin discomforts. This plant extract has the ability to protect the skin against sunburn. Some modern research suggests Aloe vera can also protect the skin from gamma rays due to radiotherapy. Aloe accelerates healing and reduces pain associated with canker sores, lichen planus, and gingivitis. The gel's effect is nearly immediate; it can also be applied over wounds due to its antibacterial effects.

- **Althadin**, used as a mouth and throat anti-inflammatory medicine, is formulated from marshmallow plant (*Althaea officinalis*), licorice (*Glycyrrhiza glabra*), and essential oil of peppermint (*Mentha piperita*). Althadin mucilage and other substances with similar properties are effective lubricants that reduce irritation and inflammation of the lining of the mouth and throat by creating a physical barrier membrane.
- **Bee pollen** (bee bread) is used in naturopathic medicine as a nutritional supplement. It was utilized by Avicenna for dyspnea (possibly for treating hay fever). Bee pollen has an antimicrobial effect. Moreover, it is effective for combating fatigue, depression, and colon disorders.
- **Burdock** (*Arctium lappa*) roots contain a variety of chemicals and nutrients. Its oil extract, called bur oil, is popular as a scalp treatment. Its seeds are a known antibiotic. Folk herbalists consider dried burdock to be a diuretic, diaphoretic, and a blood-purifying agent. Burdock poultices are excellent for the relief of muscle tension and headaches associated with temporomandibular joint disorders (TMJDs).
- **Catnip** (*Nepeta cataria*) leaves are excellent for calming the nervous system and controlling irritability. Catnip also has antimicrobial and repellent activities [11]. Drinking catnip tea or taking in capsules helps to relax patients before dental treatment.
- **Chamomile** (*Matricaria chamomilla*) has been used as a treatment for different disorders, particularly inflammatory and infectious diseases [12, 13]. Preliminary research suggests chamomile is an effective therapy for anxiety. It is commonly used as a nerve tonic, sleep aid, and digestive aid. It is used as a poultice for pain and swelling and also as a mouthwash to soothe inflamed, irritated gums.
- **Cloves** (*Syzygium aromaticum*) have been used in dentistry for a long time, where the essential oil is used as an anodyne (painkiller) for dental emergencies. Tellimagrandin II is an ellagitannin found in *S. aromaticum* with antiherpesvirus properties [14]. The buds also have antioxidant properties. Western studies have supported the use of cloves and clove oil for dental pain. Clove oil can be applied to a cavity in a decayed tooth. It also helps to decrease infection in the teeth due to its antiseptic properties. When applied on sore gums, it eases pain. Chewing whole cloves helps to diminish bad breath.
- **Comfrey** (*Symphytum officinale*) leaves and roots have traditionally been used for treating bronchial problems, broken bones, sprains, arthritis, gastric and varicose ulcers, severe burns, acne, and other skin conditions. It is believed to have bone and teeth building properties in children and have value in treating "many female disorders." Modern science confirms that comfrey can influence the

course of bone ailments [15]. Comfrey tea is used as a compression to ease jaw tension and relieve the pain of jaw and tooth fractures or adjustments to braces.

- **Dandelion** (*Taraxacum officinale*) contains a wide number of pharmacologically active compounds [16]. In Persian, it is called "*qasedak*," meaning the "small postman"—so-called because of the belief that this flower brings good news. Rhazes (around 900 AD) wrote "*The Tarashaquq is like Chicory*." Avicenna (around 1000 AD) wrote a book chapter on *Taraxacum*. Culturally, it was used to treat infections, bile and liver problems, as well as cancers and used as a diuretic. There is evidence to suggest it may have anti-inflammatory effects and assists with urinary tract infections in women. Dandelion is helpful for treating abscesses in the oral cavity.
- **Dragonhead** (*Dracocephalum kotschyi*), grown in the central regions of Iran, was historically used for fever and rheumatism. It was also used as an antihyperlipidemic, antinociceptive, analgesic, antipyretic, and anti-inflammatory [17].
- **Eastern purple coneflower** (*Echinacea*) was used historically against syphilis and gonorrhea and was believed to purify ones blood. Its roots and leaves contain many enzymes, fatty acids, and polysaccharides, which are recognized as stimulators of the immune system. Echinacea has antibiotic, antiviral, and anti-inflammatory properties. Hence, it is excellent for the treatment of abscesses in the mouth.
- **Fennel** (*Foeniculum vulgare*) is a highly aromatic and flavorful herb with culinary and medicinal uses. Along with the similar-tasting anise, it is one of the primary ingredients of absinthe. An anti-inflammatory herb, fennel is commonly used in tea form to soothe the gums. Fennel is also used as a flavoring in some natural toothpaste [9]. Chewing fennel seeds is helpful to eliminate halitosis.
- **Garlic** (*Allium sativum*) has been used for centuries to prevent and treat a variety of illnesses and to ensure longevity. *Allium sativum* has been found to reduce platelet aggregation and hyperlipidemia [18]. Garlic is also claimed to help prevent heart disease and cancer. Garlic cloves are used as a remedy for infections, digestive disorders, and fungal infections such as thrush. Garlic can be used as a disinfectant because of its bacteriostatic and bactericidal properties. More recently, it has been found from a clinical trial that a mouthwash containing 2.5% fresh garlic shows good antimicrobial activity [19].
- **Goldenseal** (*Hydrastis canadensis*) is used as a mucous membrane tonic. Goldenseal increases the secretion of the mucous membranes. At the same time, goldenseal contains astringent factors, which counter excessive flow. Thus it was referred to as a mucous membrane "*alterative*," increasing deficient flow but decreasing excessive flow. Topically, they are used to help relieve open sores, inflammations, and rashes. Herbalists today consider goldenseal an anti-inflammatory, antibacterial, anticatarrhal, antiseptic, astringent, and muscular stimulant. When used as a toothpaste or mouthwash, goldenseal is excellent for soothing inflamed gums.
- **Guava** (*Psidium guajava*) has been a subject for diverse research in order to identify their chemical constituents and pharmacological properties. From preliminary medical research, extracts from guava leaves and bark are implicated in

therapeutic mechanisms against cancer, bacterial infections, inflammation, and pain. It can be used as an antiseptic and mouthwash to disinfect oral cavities from oral infections such as gum infections. It can also be used to treat tooth decay. Aside from its antiseptic property, *guava* is also loaded with a high concentration of vitamin C. Guava bark may be used as a substitute for a toothbrush. This is a very effective alternative to a standard toothbrush. In fact, in the Middle East, guava bark is manufactured and even packaged into individual blister packs and is inexpensive.

- **Gum tree** (*Eucalyptus*) yields a powerful antiseptic essential oil that has long been used medicinally [20]. *Eucalyptus* has been used as a means of reducing malaria. Its leaves have been commonly used to lower fevers, which gave it the name "*fever tree*." Eucalyptus oil is used on sore and inflamed gums for temporary relief.
- **Horsetail plant** (*Equisetum telmateia*) has a long history of medicinal uses. This plant is rich in healing silica and is commonly used for its antipyretic effects. It also has anti-inflammatory properties. It is used as a mouthwash to relieve mouth and gum infections.
- **Kelp** (algae) was used to treat goiter, ulcers, and obesity and to protect people against the effects of radiation. Alginate, a kelp-derived carbohydrate, is used to thicken products such as toothpaste. Alginate powder is also used frequently in general dentistry and orthodontics for making impressions of the upper and lower arches. One of the richest sources of vitamins, minerals, and trace elements, kelp helps ensure healthy gums and bones.
- **Lavender** (*Lavandula angustifolia*) is used extensively with herbal medication and aromatherapy. According to folk wisdom, lavender has many uses; lavender leaves help treat inflammation, cough, and spasm. Essential oil of lavender has antiseptic and anti-inflammatory properties [21]. Lavender seeds and flowers are widely used as relaxants. Its extract is also used as an analgesic, neuroprotective, and anesthetic [17].
- **Lemon balm** (*Melissa officinalis*) is claimed to have antibacterial and antiviral properties [17]. It is also used as an anxiolytic and mild sedative. Lemon balm extract was identified as a potent inhibitor of GABA transaminase. The major compound responsible for GABA transaminase inhibition activity in lemon balm is rosmarinic acid [22]. Lemon balm also has shown to improve mood and mental performance. Positive results were achieved in a small clinical trial involving Alzheimer patients [23]. The extract of lemon balm is also found to have exceptionally high antioxidant activity [24]. Lemon balm is used in some variations of an herbal toothpaste for its soothing and aromatic properties.
- **Licorice root** (*Glycyrrhiza glabra*), often called "the grandfather of herbs," has been used medicinally for thousands of years. In herbalism, licorice acts as an "adaptogen" to help regulate the hypothalamic-pituitary-adrenal axis. It can also be used for autoimmune conditions including lupus, scleroderma, and rheumatoid arthritis. Its antibiotic properties are reportedly effective in the treatment of ulcers. Licorice may be useful in conventional and naturopathic medicine for both mouth and peptic ulcers [25, 26] and also may be used as a topical antiviral

agent for shingles, ophthalmic, oral, and genital herpes. There is further evidence that glycyrrhizin, the active ingredient in licorice, inhibits plaque growth by acting against *Streptococcus mutans*, the bacteria associated with tooth cavity development. As a sweet or flavorful, licorice is often added to toothpaste and mouthwash.

- **Miswak** (*siwak*) is a teeth-cleaning twig made of the stem of the *Salvadora persica* tree. It has a long, well-documented history and is reputed for its medicinal benefits. It also features prominently in Islamic hygienic jurisprudence. In addition to strengthening the gums, preventing tooth decay and eliminating toothaches, the *miswak* is also said to halt further increase in decay that has already set in. Benzyl isothiocyanate, which is extracted from roots of miswak, has inhibitory effect on growth of *Streptococcus mutans* and has antiviral effect against herpes simplex virus type 1. Furthermore, miswak creates a fragrance in the mouth, eliminates bad breath (i.e., halitosis), improves the sense of taste, and causes the teeth to glow and shine. Studies indicate that *Salvadora persica* extract is somewhat comparable to other oral disinfectants and antiplaque agents like triclosan and chlorhexidine gluconate if used at a very high concentration [27, 28].
- **Marigold** (*Tagetes*) is commonly used as a homeopathic remedy (Calendula, called "the homeopathic antiseptic"). Marigold flowers have been used internally as a diuretic, a stimulant, and an antispasmodic. Externally, they are used in the treatment of burns, wounds, and impetigo of the scalp. As a mouthwash, it helps relieve ulcers, wounds, and inflamed areas and helps to relax muscles tension in the temporomandibular joint and pressure from braces.
- **Myrrh** (*Commiphora myrrha*) is a powerful antiseptic that is said to have special efficacy on the heart, liver, and spleen meridians. It is recommended for rheumatic, arthritic, and circulatory problems and for amenorrhea, dysmenorrhea, menopause, and uterine tumors. Myrrh is used as an antiseptic in mouthwashes, gargles, and toothpastes for treatment of gum disease. Myrrh has also been recommended as an analgesic for toothaches and can be used in liniment for bruises, aches, and sprains. Washing the mouth with myrrh tea and brushing with its powder is useful when gum disease exists. It is widely used to eliminate bad breath [9].
- **Myrtle** (*Myrtus*) has antibacterial, antifungal, anti-inflammatory, and analgesic properties [17]. In addition, a recent systematic review of herbal medicines has proven a positive effect of myrtle compounds for treatment of sinusitis. An ointment containing the essential oil myrtle is also effective against herpes simplex virus (HSV-1) infection, and an extract of the berries of *Myrtus communis* has significant ulcer-protective effects [29].
- **Oregano** (*Origanum vulgare*) is commonly used as an antiseptic as well as a cure and relief for toothache, headache, anxiety, rheumatism, vermifuge, asthma, spasm, and gastrodynia [8, 17]. Oregano is high in antioxidant activity due to a high content of phenolic acids and flavonoids [30]. It also has shown antimicrobial activity against some strains of the food-borne pathogens [30].
- **Otostegia persica** (*Labiatae*) is used as analgesic and antioxidant [31]. It is used for minor pains especially for relieving toothaches [17, 32].

- **Peppermint** (*Mentha piperita*) is a very popular herb, which is largely used in local medicine. The chemical composition of peppermint has been the subject of many investigations. The essential oil of peppermint is used as an antiseptic agent. It is also effective in alleviating body aches including toothaches. It has been shown that peppermint acts through a specific anti-pain channel called TRPM8 to reduce pain-sensing fibers. The aroma of peppermint has been found to enhance memory [33]. It is also has antimycobacterial, antifungal, antiallergic, antiviral, and antioxidant properties [17]. Peppermint has promising radioprotective effects for patients undergoing cancer treatment [34]. *Mentha* also reduces aphtha severity and relapse frequency.
- **Plantain** (*Plantago*) leaves are usually used as an anti-inflammatory and analgesic [17]. It is a potent coagulant; because of this unique quality, plantains were used as wound dressings for the injured on the battlefield (it was also called "soldier's herb"). *Plantago* is used as a replacement for hepatotoxic comfrey in herbal preparations. Current studies show that it can be used as a mouthwash to prevent chemotherapy-induced mucositis.
- **Rosemary** (*Rosmarinus officinalis*) has a reputation for improving memory [35] and has been used as a symbol for remembrance. Rosemary contains a number of biologically active compounds, including antioxidants. Carnosol, found in rosemary, is also a promising anticancer agent. Rosemary increases the production of bile and raises blood pressure. It also has antioxidant, antinociceptive, diuretic, antiulcerogenic, hyperglycemic, and relaxant properties [17, 36, 37]. Rosemary is used as mouthwash for the treatment of gum disease and bad breath.
- ***Satureja khuzistanica*** is an endemic plant in the southern parts of Iran. It is widely recommended for relieving inflammation, toothache, and the common cold. It also has antiseptic, analgesic, antihyperlipidemic, antidiabetic, and antioxidant properties [17, 38].
- **Sage** (*Salvia officinalis*) had a high reputation throughout the Middle Ages, with many sayings referring to its healing properties and value. Today, the leaves are used to treat laryngitis, tonsillitis, and sore throats. Modern evidence shows possible uses as an antibiotic, antifungal, astringent, antispasmodic, estrogenic, and hypoglycemic. In a double-blind, randomized, and placebo-controlled trial, sage was found to be effective in the management of Alzheimer's disease [39]. As a mild antiseptic, sage was said to heal bleeding gums and mouth ulcers (cold sores). Drinking a cup of hot sage and chamomile tea eases apprehension before dental treatments.
- **Shepherd's purse** (*Capsella bursa-pastoris*), also known as St. John's wort, has astringent, diuretic, and stimulant properties. The herb is widely used to treat infectious diseases such as syphilis, tuberculosis, dysentery, and whooping cough [17]. The fresh tops of Shepherd's purse may be used to stop bleeding after tooth extraction.
- **Tea tree oil** (*Melaleuca* oil), extracted from the leaves of *Melaleuca alternifolia*, is a highly effective topical antibacterial and antifungal agent. It is used in several commercial products including mouthwash and toothpaste [9]. It is highly antiseptic and used for cuts and abrasions. As a mouthwash, it relieves oral inflammation.

- **Thyme** (*Thymus vulgaris*) medicinally is used for respiratory infections in the form of a tincture, salve, syrup, or by steam inhalation. The essential oil of common thyme (*Thymus vulgaris*) is made up of thymol. Thymol, an antiseptic, is the main active ingredient in Listerine mouthwash. Before the advent of modern antibiotics, it was used to medicate bandages. It has also been shown to be effective against the fungus that commonly infects toenails. Thyme helps relieve and ease fever and toothache [17]. Many studies have explained and described its anti-inflammatory and antifungal properties [17, 40].
- **Yarrow** (*Achillea millefolium*) is among plants whose anti-inflammatory properties have proven effective. The most medicinally active part of the plant is the flowering top. Today, yarrow is valued mainly for its effects on colds and influenza and also for its effects on the circulatory, digestive, excretory, and urinary systems. It also has analgesic, antiphlogistic, and anti-inflammatory properties [41]. Yarrow mouthwash promotes healing of oral injuries due to surgery, teeth cleaning, and braces.

5.4 Conclusion

5.4.1 Empowering the Patient by Raising Health Literacy

Some individuals who take alternative medicines are afraid the dental team will not respect their decision to take an herbal medication and will subsequently tell them to stop taking those medications [9]. However, as herbal medications become more popular, many clinicians are beginning to use them in their practices. Patients are likely to feel an herbal supplement is beneficial to their health and well-being, making it difficult to give guidance without interfering with the patient's ideas or beliefs.

The dental aspects of herbal supplementation are not as diverse as those faced by the medical community. However, plant extracts affecting inflammation and bleeding are of significant interest to the dental professional. If the patient inquires about the effects of a particular herb, it is essential that the facts about herbal supplements be presented as objectively as possible to allow the patient to make an informed decision. However, the dental professional is also obliged to supply professional judgment.

Children under the age of 15 and elderly patients seem to be more prone to the possible adverse effects and should avoid taking herbal medications. Pregnant women should not take any herbal supplements because of the potential of teratogenic toxicity. Breast-feeding women should also avoid herbal supplements [9].

5.4.2 Decision-Making for Dental Practice

Clinical decision-making is defined as "explicit use of information to quantify probabilities and outcomes to analyze decisions under conditions of uncertainty." For dentists, like other physicians, it is a part of the daily routine in their practice.

Decision-making in dental practice involves use of information in order to assess the probabilities and outcomes of each possible decision and also to analyze decisions that best suits the patient [42]. Clinical decision-making includes a chain of processes to be performed in order: The first is a diagnosis or detection phase, the second is the decision about intervention, and the third is selection of suitable treatment among alternatives [43]. Clinical decision-making is therefore referred to as a social process in which the dentist, the patient, and the other bodies such as the insurer each contribute a crucial role [44, 45].

Based on the source of the evidence on which clinical experts establish their decision- making, two principal models for clinical decision-making are intuitive (traditional) and analytical (evidence-based). In the traditional model, clinical experts (dentists) apply knowledge logically based on their education and expertise in order to decide about the appropriate care for each patient. The source of such information is dentists' undergraduate training, personal experience, activity in continuing education, and consultation with colleagues [46]. In this traditional model of decision-making, the evidence may be influenced by the context of practice, practice behavior, and biases of the dentist, which originates from dentists' intuitive knowledge and experience [45, 47].

In regards to the large volume of information in the scientific literature, a new process for evaluating scientific evidence has emerged in medicine and other health fields to help clinicians with the best care options. In this model, known as evidence-based medicine, evidence comes from a consensus of current research, filtered by precise evaluation of the existing literature [48]. The best evidence, however, does not replace dentists' clinical skills, judgment, or experience but provides another tool to help dentists in the process of decision-making [49]. "Best evidence" refers to information obtained, according to the results from studies, such as the systematic reviews and meta-analyses examined by randomized controlled clinical trials, nonrandomized controlled clinical trials, cohort studies, case-control studies, crossover studies, cross-sectional studies, case studies, or the consensus opinion of experts in appropriate fields of research or clinical practice [45, 50].

5.4.3 Current Situation of Traditional Persian Medicine in Today's Iran

The practice of traditional medicine is deeply rooted in the cultural heritage of Iran and constitutes an integral part of the culture of the people of this country. Different forms of traditional medicines have been used in this country as an essential means of treatment of diseases and management of various health problems from time immemorial. The practice of traditional medicine in this country has flourished tremendously in the recent years along with that of modern medicine. As a result, even cutting edge technology of allopathic medicine, a large majority of the population of this country, particularly in the rural and semi-urban areas, still prefer to use traditional medicine in the treatment of most of their diseases even though modern medical facilities may be available in the neighborhood. The concept, practice, type, and method of application of traditional medicine vary widely among the different ethnic groups living in different parts of the country according to their culture, living standard, economic status, religious belief, and level of education. Traditional medicine practice in Iran includes both the most primitive forms of folk medicine as well as the highly modernized systems.

According to WHO, more than three-quarters of the world population rely upon traditional remedies (mainly herbs) for the care of different ailments. This is due to the fact that traditional medicine is accessible, affordable, culturally and socially acceptable, and most people prefer it to the "exorbitantly priced" conventional Western medicine. There are some differences and similarities between ancient and modern medicine. But in fact, modern medicine has been inspired by ancient medicine in many ways. Morphine, digoxin, quinine, atropine, reserpine, physostigmine, pilocarpine, vincristine, vinblastine, artimesinin, and taxol are a few examples of what medicinal plants have given us in the past. Despite these facts, there are enormous contributions of traditional practices in the modern medicine; practitioners of the two systems still keep distance. Most physicians of the allopathic medicine believe that only pure compounds can be used in modern medicine. Herbalists, on the other hand, are reluctant to use the pure compounds, even isolated from plants, as they believe that the plant-derived pure compound loses their identity and is no longer natural or represents the crude plant drug, but rather it is like any synthetic chemical. To further clarify the pros and cons of using each form of healing for our body, here is a list of the advantages and disadvantages of using herbal medicine vs. conventional drugs.

Competent scientific researchers have tested conventional drugs or synthetic medicine before releasing them into the market. These drugs have been formulated after a multitude of experimentation and testing. Intake of conventional drugs can be controlled. According to the prescription, the patient can control the dosage of the medicine. There is less potential of drug overdose [9].

Conventional drugs may have unwanted side effects. Although these conventional drugs have been tested scientifically, there still may be some aspect of the drug that may affect the health of the patient. Even with prescription drugs, there is still a tendency for the patient to overdose without supervision, for example, medications like antidepressants. The patient may be tempted to take more than he/she should specially when he/she feels depressed and just wants to relax. The same goes for sleeping pills. Some drugs have harmful effects on the body even though directions were on the prescription. The body may react differently depending on what class of drug administered to the patient. A good example would be narcotics.

Herbal medications are all natural; the ingredients and components are made from natural resources. This ensures the efficacy and healing capabilities of the medicine. It is less costly than synthetic drugs. It usually does not have any side effects.

There are some disadvantages to herbal medicine, and it extends from delicate treatment of Avicenna and Rhazes to superstitious beliefs. The efficacy of herbal medication is not concrete. It indeed has little scientific basis, and how effective it can be is usually questionable. Another problem is that there are many species that are used locally by indigenous people in different parts of Iran, and there is little information or documented references about their uses.

With all the information, if we attempt to compare and adjust the modern medical findings to the traditional medicine, then we would achieve an interesting and noticeable understanding. This leads us to present a clear explanation in relation to etiologies of the diseases, and in this way we will be able to suggest many effective and efficient measures in the field of prevention and treatment of diseases.

Acknowledgments We gratefully acknowledge all scientists who openly share their data in public repositories and publish their research findings in the open access literature. MD would like to express her sincere thanks to Mona Dousti for her advice and support from the early stage of the preparation of this manuscript, and Edmond J. Samadi and Scott Roberston for their assistance.

References

1. Eldredge JD (2003) The randomised controlled trial design: unrecognized opportunities for health sciences librarianship. Health Info Libr J 20:34–44
2. Bloom BS, Retbi A, Dahan S, Jonsson E (2000) Evaluation of randomized controlled trials on complementary and alternative medicine. Int J Technol Assess Health Care 16:13–21
3. Daly WJ, Brater DC (2000) Medieval contributions to the search for truth in clinical medicine. Perspect Biol Med 43:530–540
4. Brater DC, Daly WJ (2000) Clinical pharmacology in the middle ages: principles that presage the 21st century. Clin Pharmacol Ther 67:447–450
5. Tschanz DW (2003) Arab roots of European medicine. J Gulf Heart Assoc 4:69–81
6. Siraisi NG (1987) Avicenna in Renaissance Italy: the Canon and medical teaching in Italian universities after 1500. Princeton University Press, Princeton, pp 77–124
7. Lutz Peter L (2002) The rise of experimental biology: an illustrated history. Humana Press, Totowa, p 60
8. Avicenna (1989) The canon of medicine, vol 2, 4th edn. (trans: Sharfakandy A). Sorush Publication, Tehran
9. Kaweckyj N (2010) Eastern medicine meets dentistry: the use of herbal supplements in dentistry today. Continuing education course at dental care. Revised December 9, 2010, pp 15–17
10. Kokai J (1989) Anti -inflammatory and wound healing topical skin preparations containing aloe extract and allergenic acid. Jpn J Pharmacol 1:231–408
11. Peterson CJ, Nemetz LT, Jones LM, Coat JR (2002) Behavioral activity of catnip (Lamiaceae) essential oil components to the German cockroach (Blattodea:Blattellidae). J Econ Entomol 95:377–380
12. Luppold E (1989) Maticaria chamomilla—old and new medicinal plants. Pharm Unsrer Zeit 13:65–70
13. Tubaro A, Zilli C, Redaelli C, Della Loggia R (1984) Evaluation of anti-inflammatory activity of chamomile extracts topical application. Planta Med 50:359–363
14. Kurokawa M (1998) Purification and characterization of Eugenin as an anti-herpesvirus compound from geum Japonicum and Syzygium aromaticum. JPET 284:728–735
15. Grube B, Grünwald J, Krug L, Staiger C (2007) Efficacy of a comfrey root (symphyti office Radix) extract ointment in the treatment of patients with painful osteoarthritis of the knee: results of a double-blind, randomised, bicenter, placebo-controlled trial. Phytomedicine 14:2–10
16. Schutz K, Carle R, Schieber A (2006) Taraxacum—a review on its phytochemical and pharmacological profile. J Ethnopharmacol 107:313–323

17. Naghibi F, Mosaddegh M, Mohammadi Motamed S, Ghorbani A (2005) Labiatae family in folk medicine in Iran: from ethnobotany to pharmacology. Iran J Pharm Research 2:63–79
18. Steiner M, Lin RS (1998) Changes in platelet function and susceptibility of lipoproteins to oxidation associated with administration of aged garlic extract. J Cardiovasc Pharmacol 31:904–908
19. Groppo F, Ramacciato J, Motta R, Ferraresi P, Sartoratto A (2007) Antimicrobial activity of garlic against oral streptococci. Int J Dent Hyg 5:109–115
20. Vigo E, Cepeda A, Gualillo O, Perez-Fernandez R (2004) In vitro anti-inflammatory effect of eucalyptus globulus and thymus vulgaris: nitric oxide inhibition in J774A.1 Murine macrophages. J Pharm Pharmacol 56:257–263
21. Hajhashemi V, Ghannadi A, Sharif B (2003) Anti- inflammatory and analgesic properties of the leaf extracts and essential oil of Lavandula angustifolia mill. J Ethnopharmacol 89:67–71
22. Awad R, Muhammad A, Durst T, Trudeau VL, Arnason JT (2009) Bioassay-guided fractionation of lemon balm (Melissa officinalis L.) using an in vitro measure of GABA transaminase activity. Phytother Res 23:1075–1081
23. Akhondzadeh S (2003) Melissa officinalis extract in the treatment of patients with mild to moderate Alzheimer's disease: a double blind, randomised, placebo controlled trial. J Neurol Neurosurg Psychiatry 74:863–866
24. Dastmalchi K, Damiendorman H, Oinonen P, Darwis Y, Laakso I, Hiltunen R (2008) Chemical composition and in vitro antioxidative activity of a lemon balm (Melissa officinalis L.) extract. LWT - Food Sci Technol 41:391–400
25. Das SK, Das V, Gulati AK, Singh VP (1989) Deglycyrrhizinated liquorice in aphthous ulcers. J Assoc Physicians India 37:647
26. Krausse R, Bielenberg J, Blaschek W, Ullmann U (2004) In vitro anti-helicobacter pylori activity of Extractum liquiritiae, glycyrrhizin and its metabolites. J Antimicrob Chemother 54:243–246
27. Almas K (2002) The effect of salvadora persica extract (miswak) and chlorhexidine gluconate on human dentin. J Contemp Dent Pract 3:27–35
28. Almas K, Skaug N, Ahmad I (2005) An in vitro antimicrobial comparison of miswak extract with commercially available non-alcohol mouth rinses. Int J Dent Hyg 3:18–24
29. Zolfaghari ME, Salamian P, Riazi A, Khaksa A (1997) Clinical trial of efficacy of myrtle oil in the treatment of herpes simplex. Iran J Med Sci 22:134–137
30. Faleiro L (2005) Antibacterial and antioxidant activities of essential oils isolated from *Thymbra capitata* L. (Cav.) and *Origanum vulgare* L. J Agric Food Chem 53:8162–8168
31. Shaiq Ali M, Saleem M, Ali Z, Ahmad V (2000) Chemistry of zataria multiflora (Lamiaceae). Phytochem 55:933–936
32. Sharififar F, Yassa N, Shafiee A (2003) Antioxidant activity of Otostegia persica (Labiatae) and its constituents. Iran J Pharm Res 2:235–239
33. Moss M, Hewitt S, Moss L, Wesnes K (2008) Modulation of cognitive performance and mood by aromas of peppermint and ylang-ylang. Int J Neurosci 118:59–77
34. Samarth RM, Goyal PK, Kumar A (2004) Protection of Swiss albino mice against whole-body gamma irradiation by Mentha piperita Linn. Phytother Res 18:546–550
35. Moss M, Cook J, Wesnes K, Duckett P (2003) Aromas of rosemary and lavender essentials oils differentially affect cognition and mood in healthy adults. Int J Neurosci 113:15–38
36. Al-Hader AA, Hasan ZA, Aqel MB (1994) Hyperglycemic and insulin release inhibitory effects of osmarinus officinalis. J Ethnopharmacol 43:217–221
37. Dias PC, Foglio MA, Possenti A, de Carvalho JE (2000) Antiulcerogenic activity of crude hydro-alcoholic extract of Rosmarinus officinalis L. J Ethnopharmacol 69:57–62
38. Abdollahi M, Salehni A, Mortazavi SHR, Ebrahimi M, Shafie A, Fouladian F, Keshavarz K, Sorouri S, Khorasani R, Kazemi A (2003) Antioxidant, antidiabetic, antihyperlipidemic, reproduction stimulatory properties and safety of essential oil of Satureja Khuzestanica in rat in vivo: a toxicopharmacological study. Med Sci Monit 9:331–335
39. Akhondzadeh S, Noroozian M, Mohammadi M, Ohadinia S, Jamshidi AH, Khani M (2003) Salvia officinalis extract in the treatment of patients with mild to moderate Alzheimer's disease: a double blind, randomized and placebo-controlled trial. J Clin Pharm Ther 28:53–59

40. Pina-Vaz C, Goncalves RA, Pinto E, Costa-de-Oliveira S, Tavares C, Salgueiro L, Cavaleiro C, Goncalves MJ, Martinez-de-Oliveira J (2004) Antifungal activity of thymus oils and their major compounds. J Eur Acad Dermatol Venereol 18:873–879
41. Lewis DA (1989) Anti-inflammatory drugs from plant and morine source. Birkhauser Reriag Baser, Berlin, pp 121–147
42. White BA, Maupomé G (2001) Clinical decision- making for dental caries management. J Dent Educ 65:1121–1125
43. Bader JD, Shugars DA (1995) Variation in dentists' clinical decisions. J Public Health Dent 55:181–188
44. Grembowski D, Milgrom P, Fiset L (1998) Factors influencing dental decision-making. J Public Health Dent 48:159–167
45. Ghasemi H (2008) Preventive orientation and caries management by Iranian dentists. Academic dissertation, Department of Oral public health, Institute of Dentistry, Faculty of medicine, University of Helsinki. Yliopistopaino, Finland, p 24–27. ISBN: 978-952-10-4707-7
46. Anderson JD (2000) Need for evidence-based practice in prosthodontics. J Prosthet Dent 83:58–65
47. Bauer J, Spackman S, Chiappelli F, Prolo P, Stevenson R (2006) Evidence-based dentistry: a clinician's perspective. J Calif Dent Assoc 34:511–517
48. Sackett DL, Rosenberg WM, Gray JA, Haynes RB, Richardson WS (1996) Evidence based medicine: what it is and what it isn't. BMJ 312:71–72
49. Forrest JL, Miller SA (2002) Evidence-based decision making in action: part 1-finding the best clinical evidence. J Contemp Dent Pract 3:10–26
50. Bruce M (1999) Evidence-based learning in general dental practice. Evid Based Dent 1:20–21

Part III
Substantiating Ayurvedic Theory and Practice Toward Evidence-Base

Chapter 6
Prakriti Analysis in Ayurveda: Envisaging the Need of Better Diagnostic Tools

Sanjeev Rastogi

6.1 Introduction

Recent resurgence of traditional medicine (TM) has resulted in a renewed ubiquitous curiosity toward their fundamental constructs. Their clearer understanding and subsequent applications based upon evidences are the primary motive of this global curiosity. Ayurveda has responded well to these emerging global demands from TM by making a paradigm shift into its research priorities which now focuses more upon basic research besides the clinical ones [1].

Ayurveda as a major stakeholder among global TM practices proposes its unique pronature biophysical basis toward the understanding of health and disease. It identifies four *purusharthas* (spiritual, economical, sensual, and renounceable) as the primary objectives of a human life and foresees the enabling health as an essential mean to achieve those. Interestingly, despite of its appearance as a subjective science, Ayurveda stands to be a truly logical, systematic, and comprehensive health science encompassing the wider perspectives of an individual. *Charaka Samhita* defines Ayurveda as a science dealing with quality of life within philanthropic, misanthropic, pleasurable, and miserable modes of living (*Charaka Samhita Su.*1/41). Ayurveda deals explicitly with the materials and methods to intervene into the state of disease and health. A disease in Ayurveda is proposed to be an outcome of imbalance among the body constituents, viz., *dosha, dhatu*, and *mala*. This imbalance is depicted clinically through altered body functions. Disease management in Ayurveda, therefore, is intended to restore the balance of the inner milieu by regulating diet, lifestyle, and supplementation of naturally occurring compounds. A medical prescription from Ayurveda uniquely considers finer details of the patient and the disease to bring out a typical prescription suiting to individual requirements.

S. Rastogi
PG Department of Kaya Chikitsa, State Ayurvedic College, Lucknow University, Lucknow, Uttar Pradesh, India
e-mail: rastogisanjeev@rediffmail.com

S. Rastogi (ed.), *Evidence-Based Practice in Complementary and Alternative Medicine*, DOI 10.1007/978-3-642-24565-7_6, © Springer-Verlag Berlin Heidelberg 2012

Despite of its textual novelty, for want of objectively applicable tools, the fundamental constructs in Ayurveda could not be adequately utilized to raise a dependable and predictable health care. Recent global upsurge of TM, at this juncture, opens up the widening opportunities of critically evaluating Ayurvedic fundamentals for their dependability and reproducibility in health care for meeting the expectations of science [2–4]. Eventual to the global expectations, a few key fundamentals from Ayurveda, viz., *prakriti* and *tridosha* have come to a critical reappraisal for their better appreciation and subsequent utilization in health care [5–7].

Prakriti in Ayurveda is defined as an individual quality quantified in terms of *dosha* and determined by various innate variables expressing that *dosha*. *Dosha*, as progenitor to the idea of *prakriti*, describes physiological system specificity which regulates the physiological and in turn the anatomical expressions specific to human body. Dosha are categorized as *vata, pitta*, and *kapha* as per their principal activities and subsequently named together as *tridosha*. An individual *prakriti*, in turn, is a realization of predominant *dosha* activity in a person leading to its physical, physiological, and mental identity [6, 7].

For their omnipresence in principles and practice of Ayurveda, *prakriti* and *tridosha* come forward as central dogma in Ayurveda. Conceptually, the duo propose a greater understanding to disease etiology, presentation, and management and eventually offer help in evidence-based decision-making for personalized treatments [5]. Translating this concept into a dependable evidence for decision-making, however, still requires much work. Dahanukar and Thatte [8] have correlated therapeutic outcomes in certain conditions to the *prakriti* specifications of an individual [8]. Construct of *prakriti* has recently been correlated HLA alleles [9]. The same is also furthered by biochemical correlates and whole genome expression referring to the various *prakriti* types [10].

Irrespective to these recent scientific appraisals, a fair utilization of *prakriti* into the clinical practice still require a dependable, reproducible, and objective method to determine it. We, therefore, need to have a standard tool to determine *prakriti* unequivocally for its use in clinical practice.

6.2 Examining *Prakriti*: Are We Properly Equipped?

Adoption of unambiguous, reproducible, and universally applicable tools to generate evidence is a prerequisite to evidence-based decision-making [11]. *Prakriti*, for its conceptual and clinical importance to Ayurvedic health care, deserves a detailed yet determinant examination for its possible usage in clinical practice. In Ayurvedic practice, *prakriti* is examined in connotation to the *dosha*-related features available to an individual. This feature examination aiming at *prakriti* diagnosis is usually done through an interaction between patient and physician. To help the interview process and also to bring objectivity to the results obtained through such process, a symptom-based checklist (questionnaire) model is adopted. Most published Ayurvedic researches including many recent ones, requiring a *prakriti* examination,

Table 6.1 Conventionally used triple choice questionnaire model to make a *prakriti* diagnosis

Features	*Vata*	*Pitta*	*Kapha*
Skin	Dry	Less oily	Oily
Appearance	Nonpleasing	Less pleasing	Pleasing
Color of skin	Black	Copper	White
Hair	Less, dry, rough	Less, soft, white	Soft
Veins and tendons	More and superficially visible	Average and not visible	Not visible
Joints	Loose with crepitus	Loose with no crepitus	Compact with no crepitus
Walking speed	Fast	Average	Slow
Speech	Fast	Average	Slow
Sleep	Less, easily arousable	Average	Deep sleep

From PG Dept. of Sharir, State Ayurvedic College, Tulsi Das Marg, Lucknow
Only a few features are represented here in the table. The actual questionnaire contains 13 anatomical, 16 physiological, and 12 psychological features

adopted a similar *prakriti* examination approach to reach at its diagnosis. Ironically, a validation to any such method aiming at *prakriti* diagnosis has never been attempted in these studies. It is because of this reason, a *prakriti* diagnosis made through conventional methods is found to have substantial interrater variability in terms of quantitative estimation of *dosha* referring to ultimate *prakriti* diagnosis. Biostatistical quantification of *tridosha* [12], classification of human population on basis of HLA gene polymorphism and linking it to *prakriti* [9], and whole genome expression and biochemical correlates of extreme *prakriti* types [10] are few among recent studies aiming to explore the scientific basis of *prakriti*. Among these, Joshi [12] adopted a semiobjective questionnaire method utilizing a comprehensive list of 28 features referring to different *dosha* [12]. The study identified feature classes as important traits with variable expressions as per the *dosha* influence in an individual. Three possible expressions to every feature class were proposed referring to three major *dosha* classes: *vata*, *pitta*, and *kapha*. This *prakriti* analysis model, therefore, was a triple choice questionnaire model where each question represented a feature class and each choice represented a *dosha* category (Table 6.1). The ultimate *prakriti* diagnosis in this model is reached through an active–passive interaction between patient and physician to choose the most appropriate expression against selected feature classes. Numbers of expressions favoring individual *dosha* are then counted, and a proportionate *prakriti* is inferred by identifying the *dosha* which is most commonly expressed. Irrespective of its ease of application, this method, however, fails to recognize "*the phenomenon of absolute or differential expression of dosha*," a key characteristic of *prakriti* understanding in Ayurveda. It is important to understand that independent *dosha* may have an absolute expression of their own in a feature class which is not shared by other *dosha* or may have a differential expression by sharing the same feature class by other *dosha* too. *Dosha* are thereby expressed through a few shared and yet few exclusive features which are phenotypical expressions of their inherent properties or *guna* (Table 6.2). A compulsive search of expression for some *dosha* against some trait as is done in triple response model may therefore lead to an erroneous result. The argument of absolute or differential

Table 6.2 Cross and independent distribution of features among different *dosha prakriti*

Feature class	*Kapha*	*Pitta*	*Vata*
Face features	Yes	No	No
Skin features	Yes	Yes	Yes
Color of skin	Yes	Yes	No
Nutritional status of body	Yes	No	Yes
Appetite	Yes	Yes	No
Thirst	Yes	Yes	No
Bowel movements	No	Yes	No
Involuntary movements	No	No	Yes
Intolerance to heat or cold	Yes	Yes	Yes

"Yes" represents the features represented in individual dosha class
"No" represents the features not represented in individual dosha class

expression of *dosha* becomes more explicit when we reanalyze Table 6.1 for its application in *prakriti* diagnosis. In reference to the skin appearance, the first trait, an expression of dry, less oily, and oily skin is considered representative to *vata*, *pitta*, and *kapha*, respectively. Similarly for second trait, an expression of unpleasing, less pleasing, and pleasing appearance is considered representative to *vata*, *pitta*, and *kapha*, respectively. This is important to note that these feature classes are primarily expressed by *vata* and *kapha*, respectively, and any moderate expression of features is wrongly attributed to *pitta*, where these traits are actually not expressed. Ignorance to this important observation of *prakriti* description in Ayurveda, therefore, is supposed to give false quantitative values to different *dosha*. *Prakriti* examination by Patwardhan [9] succumbed to similar methodological pitfall where feature categories were identified and scaled to various *dosha* orders [9]. Prasher [10] adopted a similar process of *prakriti* analysis by opting multiple choice questionnaire, with each option referring to a property attributed to either of *vata*, *pitta*, or *kapha* [10]. Unfortunately, this pattern of *prakriti* evaluation remained prevalent in researches done so far in Ayurveda [13]. A recently developed software by CDAC is also not devoid of the similar pitfall of making a *prakriti* diagnosis [14].

A predetermination of feature class followed by search for their variable expressions and then the *dosha* preponderance is the prospective approach of making a *prakriti* diagnosis. A prospective approach, therefore, makes a *prakriti* diagnosis through compulsively selecting one among three variables from a feature class to determine either of the *dosha* prevalence. Incidentally, an unequal distribution of feature classes among dosha groups has given a way to craft artifact expressions to the places where they do not really exist. Meeting with a compulsive choice among a feature class to choose an expression to rate a *dosha* is supposed to give rise to false results due to mandatory reporting. Additionally, this is also noteworthy that in absence of a clear and convincing expression of features, common trends are to choose the modest options and to avoid the extremes. Therefore, a mandatory reporting does not necessarily infer positive features and instead may be an expression of the exclusion of others. This nonconviction when added with a compulsion to choose either of the available option is supposed to project false positive results in favor of some specific *dosha*. *Pitta*, for instance, being moderate in its physical features, has the highest possibility of being represented as false positive. This postulation is also supported through the *prakriti* distribution pattern observed among the studied population in few of the recent studies [9].

6.3 Diagnosing *Prakriti*: The Retrospective Approach

Against the currently utilized prospective model of *prakriti* diagnosis based upon feature identification followed by their *dosha* linking, a retrospective approach promises for more. The later model primarily proposes *dosha* recognition through identification of their cardinal features and checking for their availability through a binomial questionnaire (Yes/No). Eventually, this approach gives an equal opportunity for every feature either refused or accepted on account of their visibility. A retrospective approach of *prakriti* diagnosis is advantageous over prospective approach on two important grounds. Firstly, it offers a clear yes–no choice for the specific features making their selection unambiguous. Secondly, it also offers a liberty to refuse a feature by the observer if it is not clearly observable. Both of these factors significantly lower the possibility of misleading inferences arriving due to symptom overlap and compulsive reporting inherent to the prospective approach.

Why *dosha* represents an unequal distribution of observable features? Ayurveda proposes the theory of *dosha* property (*guna*) to answer this. Every *dosha* is proposed to have some inherent properties called as *guna*, and explicit phenotypical features of an individual are proposed to be the manifestation of these properties. A retrospective approach of *prakriti* diagnosis offers to identify the link of *dosha guna* to their physical manifestation. Eventually, through this way, *dosha* predominance can also be visualized differentially in reference to the *dosha* properties responsible for this predominance. *Charaka Samhita* gives the lead to identify *dosha* properties through physical expressions leading to manifestation of *prakriti* (Table 6.3).

6.4 Objective Identification of the Features for *Prakriti* Diagnosis

Prakriti identification features as described in *Charaka Samhita* (Table 6.3), when revisited for their objective verification, have given rise to an interesting observation. This was observed that the enlisted features are easy to be categorized on the basis of their objective verifiability. A prospective feature categorization may be sought as (1) Objectively verifiable features requiring a direct observation by the physician. Examples to this category are the features associated with physical built, height, complexion, etc. (2) Nonverifiable features requiring an interrogation from the patient. This class is primarily represented by the features pertaining to physiological and psychological attributes of a person. (3) There can also be a group of

Table 6.3 *Dosha guna* and their manifestations

No.	*Guna*	Features	Method of examination
(A) *Kapha*			
1	*Snigdha*	• Oily body	Inspection
2	*Shlakshna*	• Smooth body	Inspection
3	*Mridu*	• Soft texture	Inspection
		• Fair complexion	Inspection
		• Good-looking face features	Inspection
4	*Madhur*	• Good sexual induration	Interrogation
		• More offspring	Interrogation
5	*Sara*	• Compact body	Inspection
6	*Sandra*	• Well-formed body parts (proportionate)	Inspection
		• Well-nourished body parts	Inspection
7	*Manda*	• Slow physical movements	Inspection
		• Slow conversation	Inspection
		• Slow eating	Interrogation
8	*Staimitya*	• Delayed (well-thought) beginning of actions	Interrogation
		• Cool temperament	Interrogation
9	*Guru*	• Slow walking speed	Interrogation
10	*Sheeta*	• Less appetite	Interrogation
		• Less thirst	Interrogation
		• Less sweating	Interrogation
		• Less prone to heat-induced discomforts	Interrogation
11	*Picchila*	• Compact joints (not prominent)	Inspection
12	*Accha*	• Pleasing face	Inspection
		• Pleasing complexion	Inspection
		• Pleasing voice	Inspection
(B) *Pitta*			
1	*Ushna*	• Intolerant to heat	Interrogation
		• Soft textured	Inspection
		• Fair complexion	Inspection
		• Increased presence of moles	Inspection
		• Good appetite	Interrogation
		• Good thirst	Interrogation
		• Premature graying and fall of hair	Inspection
2	*Tikshna*	• Voracious eater and drinker (eat good quantity in a time)	Interrogation
		• Good digestive capability	Interrogation
		• Sharp reacting, argumentative	Interrogation
		• Intolerant to discomforts	Interrogation
3	*Drava*	• Lax and soft flesh and joints	Inspection
		• Profuse sweat, urine, and stool formation	Interrogation
4	*Visra*	• Increased and bad odor from armpit, head, and body	Interrogation
5	*Katu*	• Less sexual capacity	Interrogation
		• Less no. of children	Interrogation
6	*Amla*	• Less sexual capacity	Interrogation
		• Less no. of children	Interrogation

Table 6.3 (continued)

No.	*Guna*	Features	Method of examination
(C) *Vata*			
1	*Ruksha*	• Dry body	Inspection
		• Poorly formed and poorly nourished body	Inspection
		• Dry, poor, interrupted, and unpleasant voice	Inspection
		• Reduced sleep	Interrogation
2	*Laghu*	• Quick but incoherent movements	Interrogation
		• Quick but incoherent appetite	Interrogation
		• Quick but incoherent speech	Interrogation
3	*Chala*	• Unstable joints and body parts (moves them while sitting)	Inspection
4	*Bahu*	• Increased number of visible tendons and veins on extremities	Inspection
		• Overtalkative	Inspection
5	*Shighra*	• Quick indulgence in some activity	Interrogation
		• Increased amount of anxiety	Interrogation
		• Quick reactions in the form of attachment, detachment, or fearfulness	Interrogation
		• Quick understanding and grasping	Interrogation
		• Less memory	Interrogation
6	*Sheet*	• Intolerant to cold (does not like)	Interrogation
		• Prone to cold-induced ailments (common cold, URTI)	Interrogation
7	*Parush*	• Rough hair, nail, body, foot, and hand	Inspection
8	*Vishad*	• Prominent body parts (as joints)	Inspection
		• Crepitus in joints while moving	Interrogation

The guna and their features displayed here are selected as per the classical description of Charaka Samhita, Viman Sthan chapter 8/96–98

mix features which can either be physically verified and or be interrogated for. Question regarding the physical movements, increased presence of moles, premature graying and fall of hair, and understanding and grasping skills are examples to this category. If we measure the ratio of physically verifiable features against those who require an interrogation, we find that *vata* and *kapha* features come mainly from physically verifiable group whereas *pitta* comes from the interrogation group (Table 6.4).

This simple observation may have an important bearing in its relation to *prakriti* diagnosis. Firstly, it argues for the need of developing measures for a dependable identification of verifiable features (Table 6.5). Secondly, this observation also gives us an opportunity to revisit the conventional thought about *prakriti* considering their three major classes as independently identifiable set of constitutional components. Being represented by increased amount of physically verifiable features, *vata* and *kapha* presumably represent the morphological determinants of the body, whereas being represented by more nonverifiable features, *pitta* presumably represents the mental and metabolic determinants of the body. An implication of this observation, however, is yet to be ascertained.

Table 6.4 Objective classification of features in different *dosha* groups

Class of features	*Kapha* (%)	*Pitta* (%)	*Vata* (%)
Physically verifiable	65	20	64
Nonverifiable	37	86	54

Exceeds in percentage for some overlapping features

Table 6.5 Verifiable features for *prakriti* diagnosis and possible tests to verify them

Type of feature	Proposed test for verification
Body proportion	BMI
Complexion	Fitzpatrick scale, spectrophotometry, Von Luschan's chromatic scale
Skin moisture	Skinfold measurement
Skin fat	GSR

6.5 Developing a Standard Tool for *Prakriti* Diagnosis: What are the Primary Requisites?

To consider any diagnostic instrument as a help in clinical decision-making, most important is its validity and reliability. A content and construct validity, hence, requires a proper address in questionnaire-based models leading to *prakriti* diagnosis [15]. Furthermore, while constructing the questionnaire, ease of understanding, unambiguity, and application is also important. Once constructed, this can be cross-checked for its construct validity through observation of verifiable features by objective methods in parallel to the responses obtained through the questionnaire method. There are many postulated ways to an objective cross-check for verifiable features, and many more such ways can further be identified (Table 6.5).

Reliability of the *prakriti* diagnosis tool can be tested by subjecting the tool to reliability testing. A test–retest reliability is the one which is done by subjecting the same instrument to the same subject with a difference of few days. This test–retest reliability can further be strengthened by making an intrarater (when the repeat test is done by the same rater) and interrater (when the repeat test is done by some other rater) observations. The observations obtained can further be subjected to statistical methods like Pearson's correlation coefficient and Cohen's kappa coefficient of agreement to test them more critically.

6.6 Diagnosing *Prakriti*: What Could Be the Prototype Standard Model?

By visualizing the limitations of the existing methods of *prakriti* diagnosis, and also by identifying the basic requisites of making a standard tool to generate evidences, we can propose a prototype tool addressing the concerned issues. Considering the *prakriti* description based upon the properties of individual *dosha* type, a *prakriti* analysis questionnaire (PAQ) model can be prepared which essentially looks for the clear presence or absence of features. An arbitrary numerical value can be provided to each response obtained in order to get cumulative ratio of each *dosha* featured in an individual subset (Table 6.6). A liberty to accept or reject any feature in this proposed model eliminates the crux of compulsive reporting and consequent false-positive or false-negative inference in favoring or declining some particular *dosha*. The tool can further be verified through cross-testing the verifiable features and also through reliability testing, as discussed above.

6.7 Conclusions: Way Ahead for *Prakriti* Diagnosis in the Twenty-First Century?

Why do we need an evidence base to Ayurvedic practice? Do we still require an evidence base for a health-care practice which has proven its effects through historical evidence of its practice? These commonly raised arguments referring to the research needs in Ayurveda are required to be analyzed in relation to extended benefits of putting contemporary evidence base to the practice of Ayurveda, primarily for a prospective better health care and secondarily for enrichment and eventual growth of Ayurveda as a true science. Advantages of bringing evidence base to a medical practice are obvious, tangible, and numerous. This ultimately aims to deliver the advantages of rigorous researches in the field of medicine for the best possible patient care. A decision-making in medical practice shall therefore take the account of every possible and relevant information available which can make a change in the intervention aiming at ultimate betterment in proposed outcomes. An evidence base is therefore required to be adopted at every level of health-care practice from diagnostics to the therapeutic decision-making. Ayurveda too require a similar and thorough work to bring out an evidence base to its diagnostics primarily to support its fundamentals upon which a decision of therapeutic intervention can dependably be made.

Prakriti examination for its conceptual importance to Ayurvedic clinical practice requires effective and reliable tools of diagnosis, without which, it remains unable to offer any help in therapeutic decision-making in Ayurvedic practice. A prototype PAQ for *prakriti* diagnosis, hence, is proposed after a prudent analysis of limitation of existing models in use and methods required to fill the gap. This proposed prototype model, however, still requires to be tested on various parameters to test its validity and reliability. Once pilot tested, and suggested for possible limitations, it can go for further revisions till it is finally approved or rejected. If arrived at approval in course of its study, it can serve the purpose of being a handy tool for physician to retrieve dependable information regarding the patient's *prakriti* and its possible utilization in consequent Ayurvedic health care.

Moreover, and in concert with the properties of Ayurveda related to the genomic characteristic of the patient, we also submit that future research in complementary and alternative medicine will elucidate molecular genomic, proteomic, and

Table 6.6 Prototype *prakriti* analysis questionnaire (PAQ)

No.	*Guna*	Features	Yes/no (scores)
Kapha trait			
1	*Snigdha*	• Oily skin (scratch the mid-flexor aspect of rt. forearm with some blunt object. If mark is visible, it is dry, if not it is oily)	60
2	*Slakshna*	• Smooth skin	60
3	*Mridu*	• Less tolerant to difficulties	20
		• Fair complexion	20
		• Good-looking face features	20
4	*Madhur*[a]	• Good sexual capacity[b]	30
		• More offspring (0–2 = no, 3 or more = yes, including abortions or stillbirth)	30
5	*Sara*	• Compact muscular body[c]	30
		• Stable body (almost consistent body weight)	30
6	*Sandra*	• Well-formed, proportionate body parts	30
		• Well-nourished body parts	30
7	*Manda*	• Slow physical movements	20
		• Slow conversation	20
		• Slow eating	20
8	*Staimitya*	• Delayed (well-thought) beginning of actions	30
		• Cool temperament (less anxiety)	30
9	*Guru*	• Slow walking speed	60
10	*Sheeta*	• Less appetite	15
		• Less thirst	15
		• Less sweating	15
		• Tolerant to heat	15
11	*Picchila*	• Compact joints (not prominent)	60
12	*Accha*	• Pleasing face	20
		• Pleasing complexion	20
		• Pleasing voice	20
Total score[d]			
Pitta trait			
1	*Ushna*	• Intolerant to heat	15
		• Soft textured	15
		• Fair complexion	15
		• Increased presence of moles	15
		• Good appetite and thirst	15
		• Premature graying and fall of hair	15
2	*Tikshna*	• Voracious eater (eat good quantity in a time)	18
		• Voracious drinker (drink good quantity in a time)	18
		• Good digestive capability	18
		• Sharp reacting, argumentative	18
		• Intolerant to discomforts	18
3	*Drava*	• Lax and soft flesh and joints	45
		• Profuse sweat, urine, and stool formation	45
4	*Visra*	• Increased and bad odor from armpit, head, and body	90

Table 6.6 (continued)

No.	*Guna*	Features	Yes/no (scores)
5	*Katu*[a]	• Less sexual capacity[b]	45
		• Less no. of children (0–2 = yes, 3 or more = no, including abortions or stillbirth)	45
6	*Amla*[a]	• Less sexual induration[b]	45
		• Less no. of children (0–2 = yes, 3 or more = no, including abortions or stillbirth)	45
Total score[d]			
Vata trait			
1	*Ruksha*	• Dry skin	30
		• Poorly formed and poorly nourished body	30
		• Dry, poor, interrupted, and unpleasant voice	30
		• Reduced sleep	30
2	*Laghu*	• Quick but incoherent movements	40
		• Quick but incoherent appetite	40
		• Quick but incoherent speech	40
3	*Chala*	• Unstable joints and body parts (moves them while sitting)	120
4	*Bahu*	• Increased number of visible tendons and veins on extremities	60
		• Overtalkative	60
5	*Shighra*	• Quick indulgence in some activity	20
		• Increased amount of anxiety	20
		• Quick reactions in the form of attachment, detachment	20
		• Fearfulness or timidness	20
		• Quick understanding and grasping	20
		• Less memory	20
6	*Sheet*	• Intolerant to cold (does not like)	60
		• Prone to cold-induced ailments (common cold, URTI)	60
7	*Parush*	• Rough hair, nail, body, foot, and hand	120
8	*Vishad*	• Prominent body parts (as joints)	60
		• Crepitus in joints while moving	60
Total score[d]			

Note: Scores in PAQ are arbitrarily assigned in assumption that each *dosha* has an equal opportunity to be represented in the body. This is how we reached at proposing equal score to each *dosha*. Total score for each *dosha* was then distributed among the number of classical *guna* available to each *dosha*. Each *guna* in a specific *dosha* category thereby arrived at having an equal score. An individual *guna* score in a *dosha* category was then further subdivided as per the available features against each *guna*. This kind of scoring has given a proportionate weightage to each *guna* and their features in every *dosha* for the ease of understanding about their individual and cumulative role in determining a *prakriti*

[a]Quantity of semen is deleted as a feature of *Madhur (Kapha)*, *Katu*, and *Amla (Pitta)* properties because of its inability to be identified precisely in males and inapplicability to females

[b]These features are specific to married people. For unmarried people, alternative questions are to be framed

[c]Physical features like compact body and musculature are to be judged in accordance with the gender and geographical standards

[d]Total score is 960 for each *Dosha*. *Dosha* scores in every individual are to be calculated as per their availability, and then a predominance may be determined

epigenetic biomarkers of the Ayurvedic states and traits described above, in a manner similar to what is noted in the case of pathologies such as HIV/AIDS [16] and cancer [17]. A panel of biomarkers carefully articulated in the same manner could come together "to vote" [17] for *prakriti* parameters and come to form the fundamental of evidence-based Ayurveda-driven clinical intervention. Notably, few recent works on *prakriti* have already started building the evidences to test this hypothesis [18, 19].

Acknowledgments The author acknowledges Prof. Francesco Chiappelli, UCLA, for his intellectual help and support provided during the initial conceptualization of this chapter.

References

1. Ayurveda, Pubmed search for *Ayurveda* as a key word on http://www.ncbi.nlm.nih.gov/sites/entrez Accessed 28 Sept 2010
2. Valiathan MS (2006) Towards Ayurvedic biology: a decadal vision document. Indian academy of sciences, Bangalore
3. Valiathan MS (2006) Ayurveda: setting the house in order. Guest editorial. Curr Sci 90:5–6
4. Hankey A (2005) CAM modalities can stimulate advances in theoretical biology. Evid Based Complement Alternat Med 2:5–12
5. Mashelkar RA (2008) Second world Ayurveda congress (Theme: Ayurveda for the future)—inaugural address: part II. Evid Based Complement Alternat Med 5:243–245
6. Patwardhan B, Bodeker G (2008) Ayurvedic genomics: establishing a genetic basis for Mind Body Typologies. J Altern Complement Med 14:571–576
7. Rastogi S (2010) Building bridges between Ayurveda and modern science. Int J Ayurveda Res 1:41–46
8. Dahanukar SA, Thatte UM (1997) Current status of Ayurveda in phytomedicine. Phytomedicine 4:359–368
9. Patwardhan B, Joshi K, Chopra A (2005) Classification of human population based on HLA gene polymorphism and the concept of Prakriti in Ayurveda. J Altern Complement Med 11:349–353
10. Prasher B, Negi S, Aggarwal S, Mandal AK, Sethi TP, Deshmukh SR et al (2008) Whole genome expression and biochemical correlates of extreme constitutional types defined in Ayurveda. J Transl Med 6:48
11. Rastogi S (2009) Principles and practice of Ayurvedic rheumatology. Chaukhamba Sanskrit Pratishthan, Delhi
12. Joshi RR (2004) A biostatistical approach to Ayurveda: quantifying the tridosha. J Altern Complement Med 10:879–889
13. Rastogi S (1994) Development of an Ayurvedic therapeutic regimen for the management of rheumatoid disease. MD Thesis, IMS, BHU, Varanasi, India
14. C-DAC software for Ayurveda, Ayusoft (2010) Accessed at http://ayusoft.cdac.in/ Accessed on 28 Sept 2010
15. Rastogi S, Chiappelli F (2010) Bringing evidence basis to decision making in complementary and alternative medicine (CAM):Prakriti (Constitution) analysis in Ayurveda. In: Chiappelli F et al (eds) Evidence-based practice towards optimizing clinical outcomes. Springer, Heidelberg, pp 91–106
16. Chiappelli F, Shapshak P, Commins D, Singer E, Kangueane P, Minagar A, Oluwadara O, Prolo P, Pellionisz AJ (2008) Molecular epigenetics, chromatin, and NeuroAIDS/HIV: immunopathological implications. Bioinformation 3:47–52

17. Oluwadara O, Chiappelli F (2009) Biomarkers for early detection of high risk cancers: from gliomas to nasopharyngeal carcinoma. Bioinformation 3:332–339
18. Agarwal S, Negi S, Jha P, Singh PK, Stobdan T, Pasha MAQ, Ghosh S, Agarwal A, Consortium IGV, Prasher B, Mukerji M (2010) EGLN1 involvement in high altitude adaptation revealed through genetic analysis of extreme constitution types defined in Ayurveda. PNAS 107:18961–18966
19. Rizzo-Sierra CV (2011) Ayurvedic genomics, constitutional psychology and endocrinology: the missing connection. J Altern Complement Med 17:1–5

Chapter 7
Panchakarma: Ayurvedic Detoxification and Allied Therapies—Is There Any Evidence?

Sivarama Prasad Vinjamury, Manjusha Vinjamury, Sobhana Sucharitakul, and Ingebritt Ziegler

7.1 Introduction

Panchakarma is a collective term that indicates five independent procedures of detoxification to cleanse the body channels, along with many supportive therapies [1]. Literally, *Panchakarma* is made up of *Pancha* = "five" and *karma* = "procedure or action" (procedures of purification).

Ayurveda treats diseases using two different methods—*shodhana* and *shamana*. *Shodhana* means cleansing or detoxification of the body by expelling the deranged doshas. *Shamana* is pacification of symptoms without eliminating the morbid *doshas* [2, 3]. Typically, all treatment protocols ought to begin with *shodhana*, followed by *shamana* for optimal outcomes. When the body is saturated with toxins, the toxins interfere with the absorption of herbal medicines. Metaphorically, it is explained in terms of a delicious recipe being ruined when served in a filthy bowl. Furthermore, it is necessary to eliminate *ama*—accumulated

S.P. Vinjamury (✉)
Department of Fundamental Principles, Southern California University of Health Sciences, Whittier, CA, USA
e-mail: sivaramavinjamury@scuhs.edu

M. Vinjamury
Department of Ayurveda, Southern California University of Health Sciences and American University of Complementary Medicine, Cerritos, CA, USA
e-mail: acuveda@gmail.com

S. Sucharitakul
Department of Ayurveda, Acuveda Holistic Health Center, Los Angeles, CA, USA
e-mail: tippi_s@yahoo.com

I. Ziegler
Department of Fundamental Principles, Southern California University of Health Sciences, Grand Terrace, CA, USA
e-mail: ziegler.ingebritt@gmail.com

S. Rastogi (ed.), *Evidence-Based Practice in Complementary and Alternative Medicine*, DOI 10.1007/978-3-642-24565-7_7, © Springer-Verlag Berlin Heidelberg 2012

toxins in the channels—to re-establish the balance between basic causative factors: *dosha-dhatu-mala* [4].

Detailed descriptions of these unique detoxification and allied therapies are available in classical ayurvedic texts such as *Charaka Samhita*, *Susruta Samhita*, and *Ashtanga Hridaya* [5, 6]. Despite some minor differences, the authors agree upon the primary purpose of the five procedures [1, 2]. Subsequent authors and commentators have expanded on the process and scope for *panchakarma* [2]. Its broad application in various disorders is perhaps one of the reasons why *panchakarma* is becoming more popular and its utilization is increasing. However, there is a general lack of evidence to convince conventional medical practitioners to integrate these services in a regular hospital or clinic [7]. The evidence that is available on *panchakarma* does not match the large body of research done on various ayurvedic herbs over last 100 years [8].

The objective of this chapter is to describe the meaning and purpose of each of the five procedures of purification, as well as the allied therapies that are commonly used within *panchakarma* treatments by an ayurvedic practitioner. Furthermore, an attempt was made to review the evidence-based literature on each of these therapeutic interventions in order to provide the reader with information on how they are used in clinical practice and what the outcomes are.

7.2 Preparatory and Main Procedures

The five main procedures within panchakarma are: *vamana* (emesis), *virechana* (purgation), *nasya* (nasal instillation of herbal oils/powders), *basti* or *vasti* (herbal enema), and *raktamokshana* (bloodletting). Primarily, these practices are aimed at eliminating *ama* (toxins) from different parts of the body and cleansing the channels. For example, *vamana* and *virechana* facilitate elimination of morbid doshas from either end of the gastrointestinal tract; *nasya* helps to clear them via the nostrils.

Each procedure is performed in three phases [9]:

1. *Poorva karma*—preparatory methods
2. *Pradhana karma*—main procedure
3. *Paschat karma*—post-cleansing procedures that include dietary and behavioral regimen.

7.2.1 *Snehana and Swedana*

Preparatory methods include oleation: *snehapana* (intake of ghee/oil) and *abhyanga* (oil massage) followed by *swedana* (sudation). For internal oleation, one is made to drink ghee or oil for 3–7 days, essentially to lubricate the internal mucosa of the gastro-intestinal tract, as well as to loosen the toxins lodged within the tissues. During *swedana* (sudation), sweating is induced using herbal steam, herbal leaves, herbal powders tied in cloth bundles, and many other methods. This preliminary practice, which follows oleation, facilitates the movement of loosened toxins to the GI tract [10]. It is important to note that the above mentioned preparatory procedures may also sometimes be used as independent therapeutic procedures. Therefore, a very meticulous selection process is involved in developing a *panchakarma* protocol for each patient. The practitioner is required to consider multiple factors, such as *dosha* imbalance, condition of the patient, and/or ayurvedic constitution (*prakriti*). In general, it takes approximately 2–3 weeks to complete all three phases, depending upon the detoxification procedure selected.

7.2.2 *Vamana*

Vamana is "therapeutic emesis" performed to expel aggravated *kapha dosha* and *ama*. *Vamana* literally means "to expel out" or "to vomit." Prior to this cleansing procedure, the preparatory stage includes administration of *sneha* (oily substance) for 5–7 days using a graded dosage schedule. Additionally, external *snehana-swedana* procedures are performed on the fifth and sixth days. On the seventh day, *vamana* is induced by repeatedly administering certain herbal powders and concoctions followed by herbal teas or juices to facilitate the procedure. The patient is closely monitored throughout by observation and checking of vital signs. The end point is determined by the practitioner based on the patient's condition, ending *dosha* (*kapha*/*pitta*), and number of vomiting bouts.

In the post-procedure phase, cleaning and inhalation of herbal smoke are advised to clear the throat and nose. Light, warm diet such as watery rice porridge is indicated in this phase. It is recommended that transition to normal diet and lifestyle be gradual, as it takes over a week to replenish the body and re-establish *dosha* balance.

7.2.3 *Virechana*

Virechana is "purgation." It is aimed at expelling *ama* (undigested food/toxins) and excessive *pitta dosha* from the body. It is performed by giving purgative herbs to the patient after the preliminary practices of *snehana* and *swedana*. Similar to the *vamana* procedure above, the dosage of these herbs depends on the digestive power of the patient. Close monitoring of the vitals and patient's overall condition is very important. End point is decided based upon patient's condition and number of bowel movements. Excessive movements can be controlled by administering certain dietary and herbal preparations. The post-procedure regimen of diet and lifestyle is similar to *vamana*.

7.2.4 *Nasya*

Nasya karma is mainly intended to clean the channels in the head and neck region. The aggravated *kapha dosha*, which usually blocks the upper respiratory tract, is eliminated with the help of nasal instillation of herbal juices, oils, or powders. *Nasya karma* is classified into many types, but *shirovirechana* and *shodhana* types are the *nasyas* that are used for detoxification. Herbal smoke (*dhooma*) is also used for inhalation through the nose to remove sticky phlegm from the channels. The post-procedure regimens are not as stringent after *nasya*; however, it is necessary to follow certain restrictions in diet and lifestyle.

7.2.5 *Basti/Vasti*

Herbal enema, or *basti* (which is also pronounced and spelled as "*vasti*"), is very important among the five procedures. This procedure constitutes up to 50% of the whole Ayurvedic treatment for a patient with vata derangement. Of the three *doshas*, *vata* is the most powerful *dosha* as a disease causative factor. Like *nasya* therapy, *basti* is classified into many different types. *Shodhana* (detoxification) *karma* is performed mainly by *niruha* or *asthapana basti*. The protocol is determined according to the disease and the patient's condition. It may be administered for 3, 5, 8, 15, or 30 days continuously with alternate administration of the *anuvasana* type of *basti*. The post-procedure regimen of diet and lifestyle is somewhat less stringent than *vamana* and *virechana*, and is mostly dependent upon the type of *basti*.

7.2.6 *Raktamokshana*

Bloodletting treatment is performed to balance *rakta dosha* (blood). This therapy is carried out using several different devices. Based upon the type of device used, bloodletting is categorized into various types: *pracchana karma* (using tip of scalpel for pricking), *jalaukavacharana* (using leeches), and *siravyadha* (using needles). Of these, applying leeches is considered the safest and most comfortable, and is therefore the most popular type of *raktamokshana*. It is safe to use in all age groups and all types of people (Fig. 7.1, Tables 7.1 and 7.2).

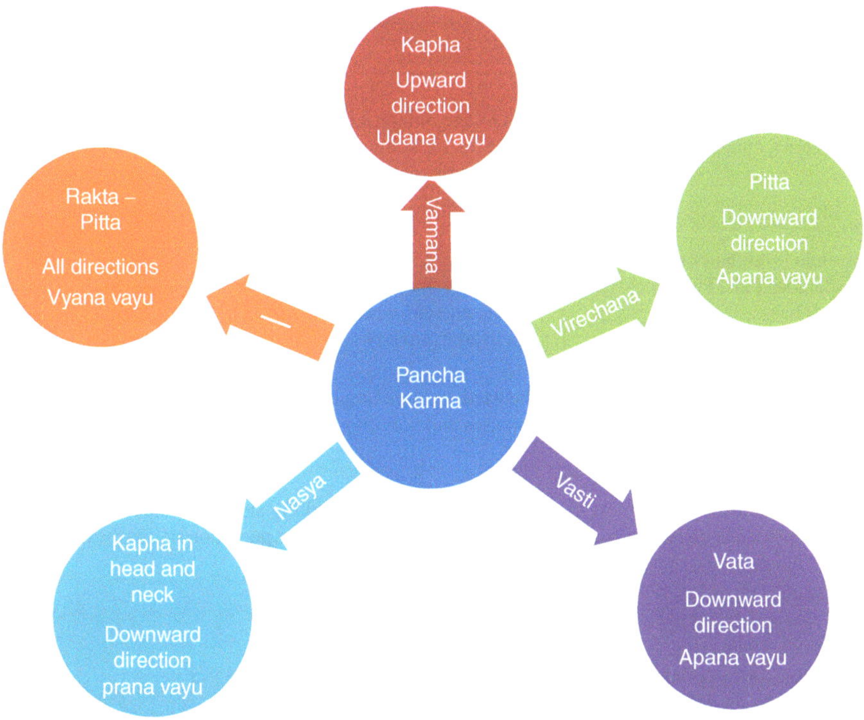

Fig. 7.1 *Panchakarma*

7.3 Allied Procedures

There are various *upakarmas*, or allied procedures/therapies, that fall under this category. Examples include *shirodhara* (ayurvedic oil dripping treatment), *shirobasti* (retention of warm herbal oil on the scalp with the help of a cap), *katibasti* (retention of warm herbal oil on the back with the help of a donut shaped bridge constructed with the help of dough), and *janubasti* (retention of warm herbal oil on the knee with the help of a donut shaped bridge constructed with the help of dough). These therapies are used as preparatory methods for the five main detoxification procedures or, most often, as independent therapeutic procedures to treat various local or systemic conditions. It is beyond the scope of this chapter to discuss the detailed procedures for each of these allied therapies.

Table 7.1 Indications and contraindications for *panchakarma*

Indications	Contraindications
Vamana	
Fever, cold, cough, skin diseases, asthma, epilepsy, anorexia	Very old age, infants/children, chronic fatigue, cardiac disease, chest injury, pregnancy, constipated, ascites, urinary retention, hemorrhage, splenomegaly, cataract, after fasting, parasite infestation, anxiety.
Virechana	
Chronic fever, herpes zoster, hemorrhoids, migraines, ear discharge	Hemorrhage, acute fever, alcoholism, indigestion, weak digestive fire, weak sense organs, after fasting, injured, weak and old, obese, emaciated, pregnant, recently delivered, anxiety
Basti	
Vatavyadhis—musculoskeletal system disorders, neurological deficits	Exhausted, chronic fatigue, indigestion, diarrhea, edema, nausea and vomiting, after *vamana*, *virechana*
Nasya	
Neurological disorders, psychological disorders, conditions of ear, nose, throat, eye, speech defect, delayed milestone, facial palsy	Indigestion, fasting, after taking alcohol, acute rhinitis, acute fever, poisoning, after purgation or diarrhea, asthma, hemorrhage, fainting
Raktamokshana	
Skin diseases, hypertension, menorrhagia, herpes zoster, boils, abscess, inflammatory disorders, gout	Edema, weak, emaciated, anemia, ascites
General contraindications for panchakarma	
Infants, old age, chronic disease, chronic fatigue pregnancy, cardiac and pulmonary diseases, cancer, HIV	
Time: on cloudy day, rainy, or during night panchakarma is not indicated	

Table 7.2 Indications for allied therapies (*upakarmas*)

Shirodhara	Insomnia, anxiety, stress, bipolar disorder, skin diseases
Shirobasti	Depression, bipolar disorder, epilepsy, MS, amnesia
Shali shastika pinda sweda	Chronic fatigue, fibromyalgia, emaciation, poliomyelitis, cerebral palsy, pseudomuscular dystrophy, hemiplegia, paraplegia
Choorna/patra pinda sweda	Fibromyalgia, arthritis, sciatica
Valuka pinda sweda	*Amavata* (rheumatoid arthritis), frozen shoulder
Udvartana	Heaviness, lethargy, cellulitis, obesity

7.4 Evidence Based *Panchakarma*

For our review, we conducted literature searches in PubMed, ABIM, Medknow, and eJIM using the following search terms: *Panchakarma, Shodhana chikitsa, vamana, virechana, nasya, basti, raktamokshana, ayurvedic detoxification, and others*. The complete list of search terms used is given above in Table 7.3. Our search was limited to articles published in English that are available in the National Library of Medicine or any other institutional library within the United States.

7.4.1 Studies on Vamana

A clinical study on *vamana* ($n=18$) for uncomplicated psoriasis reported highly significant outcomes in reduction of symptoms of scaling ($p<0.001$) in patients ranging in age from 12 to 70 years old [11]. The reduction in erythema, induration, itching, burning sensation, discoloration, and dryness of skin was also found to be highly significant ($p<0.001$ to $p<0.01$). In this study, vomiting was induced with *madanaphala*, *yastimadhu*, and *vaca*. Preparatory *snehana* and *swedana* was done 9 days prior to induction of vomiting.

The effectiveness of *vasantic vamana* and other *panchakarma* procedures including *virechana karma*, *vasti karma*, *nasya*, and *raktamokshana* on disorders of various systems was also reported. In one clinical trial ($n=30$), *vasantic vamana* followed by other *panchakarma* procedures and specific diet and lifestyle modification over a period of 1 month significantly improved the symptoms of skin, GI tract, respiratory tract, and *vata vikara* ($p<0.001$) [12].

Table 7.3 Databases, search terms and limits

Databases	Search terms		Limits
Pubmed	*Panchakarma*	*Upakarma*	Humans
ABIM	*Oleation therapy*	*Raktamokshana*	Clinical trial
eJIM	*Shodhana Chikitsa*	*Shirodhara*	Randomized controlled trial
Medknow	*Oil therapy*	*Jaluaka*	Review
	Ayurvedic detoxification	*Shirobasti*	English
	Abhyanga	*Leech therapy*	
	Vamana	*Shirolepa*	
	Swedana	*Poorva Karma*	
	Virechana	*Udwarthana*	
	Sudation	*Snehana*	
	Nasya	*Lepana*	
	Therapeutic sweating	*Snehapana*	
	Basti	*Keraliya Panchakarma*	
		Dhara	
		Pinda Sweda	

7.4.2 Studies on Virechana

Unlike studies on other types of *panchakarma*, studies on *virechana karma* included its use for longer periods, as opposed to the classical practice of a single administration of herbs after proper *snehana* and *swedana*.

A single blinded randomized controlled trial (RCT) ($n=42$) compared *virechana karma* integrated with oral administration of *Nyagrodhadi* pills (herbal formula for diabetes) with *Nyagrodhadi* pills alone in diabetic patients. The authors reported that the integrated treatment group improved significantly ($p<0.001$) more than the *Nyagrodhadi* pills only group, in both subjective and some objective measures used for assessing diabetes in this study [13]. However, there was no significant difference ($p<0.1$) in the fasting and postprandial blood sugar values between baseline and end of study within either group. In the combination group, *virechana karma* (*shodhana chikitsa*) preceded the administration of *Nyagrodhadi* pills (*shamana chikitsa*). The paper did not describe the herbs or the procedure used for *virechana karma*.

The benefits of *shodhana* treatment with *virechana karma* prior to symptomatic treatment (*shamana*) were noted in a patient with a history of 4 years recurrent eczema. The patient did not report any recurrence for 1 year after this *shodhana*/*shamana* approach, which included a combination of *panchakola phanta*, *panchatikta guggulu*, and *plain ghrita* for *sneha paana* followed by *trivrut leha* for *virechana* [14].

The effectiveness of *virechana karma* was also tested when given for longer periods as indicated in *amavata* (rheumatoid arthritis) [15]. *Gandharvahasthadi kwatha*, a decoction made with castor as one of the principal ingredients, was given to 60 patients diagnosed with *amavata*. The patients received 50 ml of the decoction for 21 days. The author reported clinical improvement in all of the patients (either cured or relieved, based on a scale developed by the investigators) in addition to reduction in erythrocytic sedimentation rate (ESR), C-reactive protein (CRP) levels, and seroconversion of RA factor. The improvement continued at the end of 1 year follow up in almost all of the patients.

Similar therapeutic benefits of daily *virechana karma* were reported [16] in a study on *nithyavirechana* and *nayopayam kashayam* for *tamaka shwasa* (bronchial asthma). In this single group pre-test post-test study ($n=20$), significant improvement ($p<0.001$) was noted in subjective symptoms such as the severity of disease based on self-report, shortness of breath, cough, effort of speech, and objective measures such as breath sounds and selected pulmonary function tests. *Eranda tailam* (castor oil) was administered as the agent for daily *virechana* (15–30 ml) in this study for 28 days. *Nayopayam kashayam* was given in 50 ml dosage twice per day during the same period. No information was available regarding follow-up and adverse events. The subjective improvements were determined with the help of a scale developed specifically by the investigators for this study. Information about its validity and reliability is missing.

7.4.3 Studies on Nasya

In a randomized clinical study on *nasya* ($n = 37$) for chronic cold, participants were given either *trayodashanga kwatha* with honey or *pradhamana nasya* with *trikatu* and *triphala churna*. The third group received a combination of *pradhamana nasya* followed by *trayodashanga kwatha* using the above described vehicles. The authors reported that the combination group had better symptom relief. Relief in other clinical features was also better in the combined group when compared to just *nasya* or herbal formula [17].

Similar findings were reported in another study on *nasya* for sinusitis [18]. In this study, an integrated approach was adopted. The treatment was comprised of external treatment of *anu tailam nasya* followed by inhalation of steam made up of *dasamoola kwatha*. Additionally, *tribhuvan kirti rasa*, an herbo-mineral formula, was given orally along with specific dietary advice for 90 days. The authors reported that the overall clinical success rate was 96.6%.

In addition to the studies on *nasya* for nose or sinus related symptoms, the therapeutic benefits of this procedure were also investigated in non-respiratory conditions. Bittar [19] investigated the efficacy of *virechana nasya* in subjects ($n = 25$) with history of intermittent chronic daily headache. Specifically the subjects had migrainous type of pain and had previous pharmacological treatment failures and were using over-the-counter (OTC) analgesics or other symptomatic/prophylactic drugs. In this study, *nasya* significantly improved ($p < 0.05$) the symptoms of chronic daily headache with an average drop in pain intensity of 63%. In this study, *nasya* was administered with either *ksheerabala* (101) or *anu tailam* according to the types of symptoms and patients, for either 7 or 14 days. Comparable dramatic outcomes were noted in another study on *nasya* and Bell's palsy. In this study ($n = 20$), both *anu taila* and *mashadi taila* were effective for this condition, with *anu taila* being slightly better. Both oils significantly relieved the symptoms of aphasia, closing of eyes and discomfort in eyes, tongue deviation, and drooling of saliva at the end of the study within each group. Preparatory *snehana* and *swedana* preceded *nasya karma* for the entire 15-day regimen. [20].

Positive outcomes and usefulness of *nasya karma* with *balavilwadi* ghee were demonstrated while treating dementia and Alzheimer's disease in a recent study conducted by Madhavikutty [21]. Similarly, the usefulness of *nasya karma* as a therapeutic method in treating hepatitis symptoms was also documented in a case report. A 23-year-old male presented with a total serum bilirubin of 34 mg/dl. *Avapidaka nasya* with the *svarasa* of *Luffa cylindrica* (*Koshataki*) was performed on the first and fourth day together with 14 days of *kshiradhara*. On the fourth day after the first administration, bilirubin level came down to 2.8 mg/dl, which was later stabilized with oral herbal therapy [22].

Although, the above studies are encouraging, their preliminary nature and limited sample sizes restrain us from making any generalizations based on the results (Tables 7.4 and 7.5).

Table 7.4 *Virechana* and *Basti*

Study	Design and sample size	Control, treatment, and duration	Outcome measures	(+/–)
Virechana				
Kumari et al. [13]	RCT $n=42$	Tx1: Oral administration of *Nyagrodhadi* pills Tx2: Virechana and *Nyagrodhadi* pills Duration: 30 days	Signs and symptoms F.B.S. P.P.B.S. Serum cholesterol Urine sugar	+
Hegde et al. [14]	Case study $n=1$	Tx: *Virechana* by *Trivrutta leha* along with the pre- and post-procedures Duration: 1 administration	Features of cellulites and eczematous changes	+
Srinivasulu [15]	Clinical study $n=60$	Tx: *Virechana* by *Gandharvahasthadi kwatha* Duration: 21 days	Scale developed by the investigators ESR and CRP levels	+
Prasad et al. [16]	Single group pre-test post-test study $n=20$	Tx: *Nithyavirechana* with *Eranda taila* along with oral administration of *Nayopayam kashayam* Duration: 28 days	Scale developed by the investigators	+
Basti/Vasti				
Krishnashastry et al. [23]	RCT $n=83$	Tx: *Vasti* with herbal mixture Placebo Gr: *Vasti* with sterile plain water Duration: 4 weeks	Customized assessment criteria developed by the investigators	+
Nair et al. [24]	Single group study $n=72$	Tx: *Vaitarana vasti* after 7 days of *patra pinda sweda* Duration: 7 days	Scale developed by the investigators	+
Gupta et al. [24]	RCT $n=30$	Tx1: *Vaitarana vasti* Tx2: Oral administration of *Sinhanada Guggulu* Tx:3 Combined Tx Duration: 30 days	Clinical, functional and hematological measurements	+

Shah et al. [26]	Clinical study $n=35$	Tx1: *Abhyanga* and *swedana* along with *Matra vasti* Tx2: *Abhyanga* and *swedana* along with *Matra vasti* with indigenous compound drug Duration: 3 weeks	Signs and symptoms scoring upon the severity	+
Karunagoda et al. [27]	Clinical study $n=40$	Tx1: *Matra basti* with *Dashamoola* oil Tx2: *Mastra basti* with plain sesame oil Duration: 7 days	Scoring of pain and associated symptoms	+
Khagram et al. [28]	RCT $n=118$	Tx1: *Matra basti* with *Brihat saindhavadi taila* along with oral administration of *Vatari Guggulu* Tx2: Oral administration of *Vatari Guggulu* Duration: 45 days	RA factors Biochemical and hematological factors Urine routine analysis Functional assessment	+
Tripathy et al. [29]	Clinical trial $n=15$	Tx1: *Dasamoola Ksheerapaka vasti* Tx2: Oral administration of *Amrataka* and *Parnabeeja* leaves paste with milk Tx3: Combined TX Duration: 30 days oral Tx. One *Vasti*	Subjective symptom scale developed by the investigators	+

Table 7.5 *Vamana*, *Nasya*, and *Raktamokshana*

Study	Design and sample size	Control, treatment, and duration	Outcome measures	(+/–)
Vamana				
Rai el al. [11]	Clinical study $n=18$	Tx: *Vamana* along with *snehana* and *swedana* Duration: one administration	PASI score	+
Rawal et al. [12]	Clinical research $n=30$	Tx1: *Vamana* Tx2: *Sampurana Panchakarma* Duration: 13–21 days for Tx1 29–39 days for Tx2	Cardinal signs and symptoms *Bahu dosh Lakshana* and fitness Graded symptoms Effect of the Tx	+
Nasya				
Chaudhari et al. [17]	RCT $n=37$	Tx1: Oral administration of *trayodashanga kwatha* with *madhu* Tx2: *Pradhamana nasya* with *trikatu*+*triphala churna* Tx3: Combined Tx Duration: 45 days for Tx1 Max of 7 *nasya* for Tx2 7 *nasya* followed by 45 days of *trayodashanga kwatha* for Tx3	Subjective improvement in clinical features Objective parameter (CRP level)	+
Panigrahi [18]	Randomized non-comparative trial $n=30$	Tx: Oral administration of *tribhvan kirti rasa* (Tablet) along with inhalation of steam of *dashamulakwath* (decoction) followed by *nasya* with *anu tailam* Duration: 45–90 days	Overall assessment of symptoms Overall assessment of efficacy recorded (after 3 months of Tx)	+
Bittar [19]	Preliminary study $n=25$	Tx: *Nasya* with *ksheerabala* (101) *tailam* for *vataja* and *pittaja* headache or *anutailam* for *kaphaja* and *sannipata* headache Duration: 7 days and 14 days for severe conditions	Laboratory results Total serum bilirubin	+

Thanki et al. [20]	Randomized clinical study $n=20$	Tx1: *Nasya* with *anu taila* Tx2: *Nasya* with *mashadi taila* Duration: 15 days	Scoring of cardinal signs Associated signs symptoms *Doshanubandhita Lakshanas* House classification system of facial paralysis	+
Anand [22]	Case study $n=1$	Tx: *Avapidaka nasya* with *savarasa* of *Luffa cylindrica* along with 14 days of *ksiradhara* Duration: two administrations on the first and fourth day	Laboratory results Total serum bilirubin	+
Madhavikutty [21]	Review Article	Tx: Purana ghrita / Balavilwadi ghrita for Nasya; Dhoopana (specific name not provided) for unmada, apasmara	N/A	N/A
Raktamokshana				
Michalsen et al. [30]	RCT $n=51$	C: Topical diclofenac regimen Tx: Leech therapy Duration: 28 days for C 1 administration for Tx Along with 91 days outcome comparison	Western Ontario and McMaster Universities Osteoarthritis Index Medical outcomes study	+
Rao et al. [31]	Open trial $n=7$	Tx: Leech therapy Duration: 6 administrations	Pre- and post-symptom observation	+
Pantakar et al. [32]	Case Reports	Tx: Leech Therapy		+

7.4.4 Studies on Basti (Vasti) Karma

Our search also resulted in a limited number of studies on *basti*. Krishnashastry et al. [23], in a randomized controlled trial, compared *vasti karma* with herbal mixture and sterile plain water in patients ($n=83$) with irritable bowel syndrome [23]. The herbal mixture was made up of a homogenized combination of the following herbs: *Vaca*, *Bilwa*, and Ashwagandha, with sesame oil and salt. Both groups received the interventions for 4 weeks and were followed for 12 weeks after the intervention period. Significant difference ($p<0.001$) in severity of abdominal pain, abdominal distension, and *vasti* retention time was reported in the treatment group when compared to the placebo group based on customized assessment criteria developed by the investigators. The article failed to report patient demographics, inclusion/exclusion criteria, randomization method adopted, and whether blinding was used. Similar beneficial results were also reported by Nair et al. [24] on the therapeutic effect of *vaitarana vasti* for sciatica due to inter-vertebral disc prolapse. In this single group study ($n=72$), the participants received sudation therapy with hot leaf bundles (*patra pinda sweda*) for 7 days prior to *vaitarana vasti karma*, which was also administered for 7 consecutive days. The *vasti* mixture included rock salt, molasses, tamarind, and sesame oil added to cow's milk. The authors reported improvement ($p<0.1$) in symptoms such as back pain, numbness, leg pain, and activities of daily living, as well as other items that were part of a scale developed by the study investigators. The study is limited by lack of a control group and follow-up data [24].

It was also noted that *vaitarana vasti* when combined with *simhanada guggulu* produced better improvement than either *vaitarana vasti* or *sinhanada guggulu* given alone in patients with rheumatoid arthritis for 30 days [25]. A three-armed RCT ($n=30$), which explored the efficacy of the above three interventions reported statistically significant ($p<0.001$ to $p<0.05$) improvement in clinical, functional, and hematological measurements between baseline and end of study within each group. In addition to the smaller sample size, the study is limited by lack of follow-up, between-group analysis, and failure to report patient demographics.

In addition to the studies on *kashaya vasti*, efficacy of *matra vasti* was also investigated in the management of *sandhivata* (osteoarthritis) and *kashtartava* (dysmenorrhea). In the osteoarthritis trial ($n=35$) by Shah et al. [26], the participants received either *matra vasti* alone or *matra vasti* and an indigenous herbal formula, depending upon the group assignment, for 3 weeks. In addition, all participants received *abhyanga* and *swedana* in this trial prior to giving *matra vasti* with *bala taila* (60 ml). It is interesting to note that the outcomes did not differ much between the groups, as both groups had significant within group improvements from baseline at the end of study [26]. The dysmenorrhea trial ($n=40$) by Karunagoda et al. [27] compared *matra vasti* between *dashamoola* oil and plain sesame oil (60 ml each). The results were similar to the osteoarthritis trial in that there was no significant difference between the groups, but within group significant differences ($p<0.001$) were reported. It is important to note here that such outcomes (lack of statistical significance between groups) are expected when two active treatments are compared [27]. The results of another RCT ($n=118$) that used *matra basti* with *brihat saindhavadi taila* in addition to *vatari guggulu* (an oral analgesic and anti-inflammatory herbal formula) for reducing the symptoms of rheumatoid arthritis indicate the benefits ($p<0.01$ to $p<0.001$) of *matra vasti* for another painful condition. However, the benefits were only marginally better than *vatari guggulu* given alone. Furthermore, the findings of this study were based on within group analysis, but not on between group analysis [28].

Effectiveness of *vasti* was also tested ón chronic amebic colitis in a small pilot study by Tripathy et al. [29]. In this three armed clinical trial ($n=15$) *dasamoola ksheerapaka vasti* was compared with *amrataka* and *parnabeeja* leaves paste (30 g) given orally with milk. The third group received both *vasti* and the oral herbal formula. Although some improvements were reported in certain symptoms, the authors did not notice significant differences between the groups. Besides the sample size, this study is beset with weaknesses such as poor diagnostic criteria, treatment protocol, and nonstandardized outcome measures [29].

7.4.5 Studies on Raktamokshana

The most common type of bloodletting that has been investigated systematically is leech therapy. Our search did not retrieve studies on other types of bloodletting.

Michelsen et al. [30] reported in a randomized controlled trial ($n=51$) that leech therapy provided more significant improvements in the symptoms of osteoarthritis of the knee than the topical diclofenac therapy [30]. The primary end point, pain at day 7, was reduced from a mean of 53.5 ± 13.7 to 19.3 ± 12.2 after leech therapy compared with 51.5 ± 16.8 to 42.4 ± 19.7 with topical diclofenac. Furthermore, there was a remarkable improvement in function, stiffness, and total arthritis symptoms throughout the 91 day follow-up period in the leech therapy group when compared to the diclofenac group. In this trial, leech therapy was administered only once (4–6 leeches applied locally), whereas the diclofenac gel was applied twice a day for 28 days in the control group.

The benefits of leech therapy in non-pain related conditions such as leukoderma and Buerger's disease were also investigated. Bloodletting in these conditions is indicated because these are considered as diseases related to blood or *raktavaha srotas*. The usefulness of leech therapy for *svritra* or *leukoderma* was investigated in a case series [31]. In this small trial, positive changes in skin pigmentation were noted in four out of seven patients (age group 13–48 years). In one case, the white patch was fully covered with new pigmentation. New 5–8 pigmentation spots of 0.2–0.4 mm size appeared on each affected patch in 3 cases and only changed in color from white to light pink without producing any pigmentation in the rest of the cases. Hemoglobin levels pre and post leech applications with a mean of reduction of 0.43% was also observed. In this study, 2–3 leeches were applied six times once a week for 6 weeks over the affected area for a period of 30–45 min.

A discussion on the application of leeches in Buerger's disease by Patankar et al. [32] reported that *raktamokshanam* provided excellent results in several patients who underwent leech therapy [32]. Specific details of the studies were not available in this review article. However, the authors recommended more rigorous clinical trials in this area.

7.4.6 Studies on Panchakarma (All Procedures Included)

During our literature search, we also identified a few studies that included more than one procedure as an intervention for the treatment groups. We reviewed them independently below. These studies were either single group studies or randomized controlled trials. The control group interventions were often active other forms of treatment for the same condition. Unless the sample sizes are properly calculated and statistically powered, it is difficult to find between group differences.

A clinical study investigating the efficacy of *Shodhana* therapy in rheumatoid arthritis ($n=15$) provided *snehapana*, *swedana*, *virechana*, and *basti karma* within a period of 32 days. Significant improvement in pain, morning stiffness, joint swelling, and joint tenderness was observed at the end of the trial period. Furthermore, functional improvement was also noted by way of improved grip strength and walking time. The improvement continued during the 6-month follow-up period in 8 of the 15 patients with no signs of relapse. However, three patients had acute exacerbation within 3 months [33]. Another study ($n=80$) that also adopted *snehapana*, *swedana*, *virechana*, *and basti karma* for paraplegia reported marginal improvement in the panchakarma group when compared to shamana group that received Ashwagandha kwatha with *Gorochanadi gulika* internally and *Balashwagandhadi taila* for Abhyanga. Patients were assessed for disability to walk and raise the legs, sensory impairment, and control over bowels and bladder. At the end of the intervention period of 60 days both groups showed significant improvement, but the panchakarma group demonstrated more improvement in muscle power and bowel/bladder control [34].

Results of another RCT ($n=150$) reiterate similar benefits of panchakarma in hemiplegia patients. Namboodiri et al. [35] compared panchakarma and shamana therapy in this three-armed study. The panchakarma group received *snehapana*, *swedana*, *virechana*, *basti*, *and nasya* therapies while the shamana groups received either the combination of *bhadradarvyadi kwatha*, *dhanwantharam gulika*, and *mahamasha thaila abhyanga* or the combination of *ekangaveera rasa* internally along with *pinda sweda* for 14 days. The total study duration was 60 days, by which the panchakarma group improved better than the two control groups [35]. Another study ($n=112$) that adopted the combined therapy that included s*nehana*, *swedana*, *virechana*, and *basti* treatment with *mashadi kashaya* and *taila* for hemiplegia also demonstrated similar improvement when compared to the comparison group that received colored water and oil for *vasti* [36]. A retrospective data analysis based upon the observation of patients of *Pakshaghata* (hemiplegia) for a decade validates that a multi-therapy *panchakarma* treatment that includes cleansing prior to tonification produced better results than plain *shamana* therapy alone [37]. The combination of *snehana*, *swedana*, and *basti karma* also provided better relief in sciatica patients than those who received *shamana* treatment alone. This study ($n = 61$) had a 50% drop out rate, but all those who continued improved [38].

Effectiveness of multi-therapy *panchakarma* was also investigated in psychological disorders such as major depressive disorder [39]. In a randomized controlled trial ($n = 80$), participants were divided into four groups: (1) *vamana* therapy group; (2) *shamana* therapy group, which received herbo-mineral pill, *Unmada gajankusha rasa* 250 mg bid for 3 months; (3) *vamana* and the herbo-mineral pill group; and (4) Western medicine group, which received fluoxetine 20 mg once a day for 3 months. Hamilton Depression rating scale as well as clinical assessment were utilized to determine the improvement in symptoms. A between group analysis revealed that the *vamana* group patients demonstrated significant improvement ($p < 0.01$) than the fluoxetine group. Similarly, the group that received both *vamana* followed by the herbo-mineral pill improved significantly ($p < 0.01$) than the pill only group. It is interesting to note that there was no significant difference ($p > 0.05$) between the combination group and the fluoxetine group. Both groups improved similarly. In this study, the participants were not equally divided into the four groups. The herbo-mineral group and the fluoxetine group had 30 each and the two *vamana* based groups had 10 each.

A prospective longitudinal evaluation (pre test-post test) of ayurvedic detoxification procedure on 15 healthy individuals was conducted by Herron and Fagan [40]. In this study, a comprehensive 2-week program of detoxification was adopted. It included: internal and external oleation, herbal steam bath, purgation, and herbal oil enema. Each session lasted 2.5–3 h. All participants continued with oil massage at home for 6–8 weeks. The investigators observed for lipophil-mediated reduction of toxicants such as dichlorodiphenyldichloroethylene (DDE) and polychlorinated biphenyls (PCBs) in the study participants when compared to 40 control subjects. After treatment, mean levels of PCBs (46%) and beta-HCH (58%) declined significantly in the study subjects to suggest that lipophil-mediated detoxification may be an effective method to reduce fat soluble toxicants inside our bodies [40].

7.4.7 Studies on Upakarmas (Allied Procedures)

7.4.7.1 *Shirodhara*

Shirodhara is an ayurvedic oil dripping therapy. It is one of the most popular ayurvedic treatment methods in the West due to its noninvasive nature. In addition to medicated oils, medicated buttermilk, milk, and some herbal concoctions are also used for 30–60 min.

Pokharel et al. [41] reported that *shirodhara* with lukewarm milk when combined with a proprietary herbal blend Insomrid® is more effective in reducing insomnia than *shirodhara* or Insomrid® given alone. In this study ($n = 30$), Insomrid® tablets were given with warm milk for 30 days, *shirodhara* was done for 15 days, and the combination group received both Tab. Insomrid® and *shirodhara* simultaneously in the same dose and schedule as mentioned above [41].

In a three-armed randomized controlled trial on menopause ($n = 43$), *shirodhara* was compared with internal use of either estrogen or *saraswatarishta*. The authors reported that *shirodhara* showed better effect in improving the emotional state of menopausal women as compared to the other two groups. The dosage schedule of interventions adopted in this study was: estrogen 0.025 mg once a day, *saraswatarishta* 20 ml twice a day before meals for 45 days. In this study, *shirodhara* was performed for 30 min a day for 45 days with a gap of 3 days after every 7 days of treatment [42]. Similar encouraging outcomes were also obtained in a case series ($n = 10$) when *shirodhara* was added to conventional ayurvedic treatments such as *shirovasti*, *abhyanga*, *swedana*, and oral herbal treatments in the treatment of degenerative cerebellar ataxia [43].

Shirodhara with *mucukanda kashaya* when combined with *anu taila nasya* and *jatamansi* powder orally significantly reduced chronic headache symptoms as opposed to each of the above interventions given separately. In this RCT ($n = 72$), the investigators performed *shirodhara* for 30 min daily and applied two drops of *anu taila* for *nasya karma* daily for 21 days. However, *jatamansi* powder (6 g orally) was given for 3 months to the subjects in the *jatamansi* group alone. The combined group also received all the above treatments for 21 days only [44].

In the recent past, a group of Japanese researchers lead by Kazuo Uebaba studied the physiological and psychoneuroimmunologic effects of *shirodhara* in different subjects. This group developed a healing robot to perform *shirodhara* in a computerized reproducible manner. Five experiments on physiological changes of both subjects and technicians during manual *shirodhara*, standardization of oil weight between the manual and robotic *shirodhara*, physio-psychological changes during *shirodhara* by the healing robot in relation to anxiety and altered state of consciousness (ASC), anxiolytic effect of the robotic therapy, and impact of different dripping media on the experiences of *shirodhara* were investigated. The results showed that *shirodhara* induced bradycardia and lower tidal volume and CO_2 output ($p < 0.05$), and the state of anxiety decreased abruptly ($p < 0.005$). ASC scores were highest in the domain of trance, passiveness, timeless sensation, wordless sensation, and concentration. ASC scores and anxiolytic effects showed a significant correlation ($p < 0.01$). The authors report that successive *shirodhara* treatments reduced tension and anxiety of anxious subjects in 1 month. However, similar positive changes were not noted in the EEGs of the technicians, who performed *shirodhara* manually. Their EEGs indicated a stressful state which may also justify the utility of the healing robot as an assistant to the technicians [45].

Another randomized controlled ($n = 16$) by Uebaba et al. [45] compared *shirodhara* treatment and control supine position with monitoring of physiologic, biochemical, immunologic, and psychometric parameters including anxiety and altered states of consciousness (ASC). The results showed that *shirodhara* treatment showed lowered level of state anxiety and higher levels of ASC. The correlation between anxiolysis and the depth of ASC was significant in *shirodhara* treatment group ($p<0.05$). NK cell activity after *shirodhara* treatment also showed significant correlation with anxiolysis and the depth of Trance of ASC ($p<0.05$ and $p<0.01$, respectively). However there was no significant difference by two-way ANOVA. The treatments were administered for 30 min and used plain sesame oil and the robotics to regulate oil dripping during *shirodhara* [46]. A subsequent study by Xu et al. from the same group also demonstrated that *shirodhara* performed with medicated sesame oil produced larger correlation between anxiolysis and improved ASC than plain sesame oil *shirodhara* or just lying in supine position. Simple increased correlation was observed between psycho-physiologic effects and the elevated foot skin temperature in the medicated oil *shirodhara* than plain sesame oil *shirodhara* and supine position. In this study lavender essential oil was mixed with sesame oil to make it medicated oil. This study ($n=16$) adopted a randomized cross-over design and used all standardized outcome measures [47]. Nevertheless, the results of all the above experiments on *shirodhara* by this group need to be interpreted with caution due to the small sample sizes and the study on healthy subjects.

7.4.7.2 *Shirovasti*

Shirovasti is a form of independent *snehana*, wherein warm medicated oil is made to stay on the scalp for 30–45 min. In this technique, a leather cloth 20″ × 18″ is wrapped around the head of the patient with the top open to allow pouring oil. This therapy is predominantly used for conditions that originate from brain or head.

We identified only one study on *shirovasti*. In this study 30 patients with Parkinson's disease received either *shirovasti* with *mandukaparni ghrita* or the herbo-mineral formula, *kampavatari rasa*. Both groups received 5 g of *Mucuna pruriens* powder internally. Although symptoms in both groups improved significantly over time, the *shirovasti* group showed better improvement than the oral pills only group. Positive outcomes were noted in speech, posture, emotional stability, and bradykinesia [48]. *Mandukaparni ghrita* was made up of Mandukaparni herb and cow's ghee only. The dosage of *kampavatari rasa* was 250 mg twice a day.

7.4.7.3 *Agnikarma*

Agnikarma is cauterization. Application of severe heat that would burn the skin or local tissue is occasionally practiced by ayurvedic practitioners specially trained in certain surgical techniques to reduce pain and cure non-healing ulcers. The efficacy of *agnikarma* was tested in a comparative study ($n=40$) for sciatica. *Agnikarma* significantly reduced pain ($p<0.01$) and improved straight-leg raising (SLR) test ($p<0.01$) compared to the control group that was treated with *katibasti* using *ksheerabala* oil. In this study, *agnikarma* was administered on the 1st, 8th and 15th day while *katibasti* was administered once daily for 7 days continuously. The author also cited the limitations of the study as small sample size and lack of follow-up for longer periods [49].

7.4.7.4 *Uttara Vasti*

Uttara vasti is per urethral administration of medicated oil to treat urinary disorders. In women, per vaginal administration of oils, primarily done to treat gynecological disorders, is also known as *uttaravasti*. A randomized controlled clinical trial ($n=36$) compared *uttara vasti* ($n=28$) with a commonly used nonsteroidal anti-inflammatory drug ($n=8$) in primary dysmenorrhea. Significant relief in the intensity of pain and less painful successive cycles was observed in the *uttara vasti* group than the NSAID group. This improvement within *uttara vasti* group continued during follow-up period too. Significant improvement ($p<0.001$) was noted between baseline and second follow up in all the symptoms, except diarrhea, backache, and vaginal pain. Pain relief was also noted in the NSAID group, but only with frequent dosage and bad side effects such as burning sensation in stomach, nausea, and vomiting. The trial utilized *Operculina turpethum* (Trivrit) and *Allium sativum* (Lasuna) oil for *uttara vasti*, which was administered for 3 days from the ninth day of menses for three menstrual cycles. Tablet Meftal-Spas was administered twice a day during the menstrual cycle for 3 days to the control group [50].

Similar positive outcomes were also noted in another clinical study ($n=30$) on leukorrhea (*svetapradara*). This trial compared *uttara vasti* with *lodhra kwatha* and *dhatakyadi yoga* given orally ($n=15$) with oral herbal medicine alone ($n=15$). The combination group demonstrated significant improvement in all the cardinal symptoms ($p<0.001$) and that it is more beneficial with 62.86 percentage of relief compared to 45.90 of the oral therapy only [51].

7.4.7.5 *Snehana* and *Swedana*

Although *snehana* and *swedana* (oleation and sudation) are essentially used during preparatory phase of *panchakarma*, their use as independent allied treatment methods is widespread in ayurvedic practice. In such an instance, the drastic elimination procedures are not included in the treatment protocol.

In a three-armed clinical trial, *snehana* and *swedana* together were compared to an ayurvedic herbal formula, *ashwagandha guggulu* or to an integrated group. The third group received both the pills and underwent *snehana* and *swedana* for osteoarthritis ($n=30$). For *snehana*, *panchaguna taila* was used as an external application. *Swedana* was provided with steam generated by boiling *dashamoola kwatha* for 90 days. Significant improvements ($p<0.0001$) in pain, swelling, and stiffness were noted within each group over time, but the authors reported marginally better improvements in the groups, which underwent *snehana* and *swedana* [52].

Similar results were obtained with 21 days of *snehana* with *nirgundi taila* and *swedana* with *patra pinda* (leaves bundle) were combined with *trayodashang guggulu* and *vishatinduka vati* orally for sciatica. Some of the limitations of this trial include lack of comparison group and the short duration of the trial [53].

Another clinical trial on the efficacy of *snehana* and *swedana* on osteoarthritis of the knee reemphasizes the value of these allied treatments when provided along with oral herbal analgesics and physical therapy. This three-armed study ($n=30$) demonstrated that an integrated approach that included three interventions—*snehana, swedana* externally, *lakshadi guggulu* orally, and physical therapy (traction)—is relatively better than the latter two interventions given independently for 28 days. The improvement in this study was assessed by the score based upon the severity of the following signs and symptoms: joint pain, edema, tenderness, restriction of movement, stiffness, local crepitation, and walking time [54]. The small sample size and non-reliable outcome measures limit a broader application of the results of this study. The usefulness of *snehana* and *swedana* as a primary treatment method in the management of *vata vyadhi*, specifically low back pain, has also been established [55]. All these studies demonstrate the significance and specific function of *snehana* and *swedana* in the management of pain related conditions.

Pinda sweda, a specialized type of *swedana* that includes applying heat with cooked rice bundles dipped in warm milk and *dashamoola kashaya*, has been shown to decrease creatine kinase (CK) levels in a patient with Duchenne's muscular dystrophy. In this progressive condition, the authors also noted improvement in muscle power at the end of 6 weeks of treatment with *pinda sweda*. This single case report does indicate the promise of this treatment for such chronic progressive condition and calls for more attention and larger clinical trials [56].

In an interesting pilot study on *snehana* alone ($n=20$), two methods of internal oleation, *achasneha* (ingestion of oil or ghee in a graded dose for 7 days) and *vicarana sneha* (ingestion of small amounts of oil/ghee twice a day for 30 days) were compared. *Bhadradarvadi tailam*, given as *vicarana sneha*, was more effective ($p<0.0001$) than *achasneha* in relieving the symptoms of sciatica, although both methods reduced the symptoms [57]. The effects of *snehapana* on the lipid profile of patients were demonstrated by another pilot study ($n=10$). In this study, the patients consumed between 104 and 163 ml of *sneha* within 5–7 days and the type of *sneha* was individualized. One of the following was used as the *sneha* for this study: *ksheerabala taila*, *dashamoolabala taila*, *indukanta ghrita*, and *murchana taila*. All the patients received *swedana* with steam and *virechana* at the end of *snehapana*. There was a significant reduction ($p<0.0001$) in total serum cholesterol and increase in HDL cholesterol [58].

Results of a small case series ($n=6$) on ichthyosis vulgaris (dry scaly skin) also suggest the extended effects of *snehana* and *swedana* in conditions other than pain. This pilot trial utilized *avagaha sweda* induced by cow's urine as the medium for steam generation and *yashtimadhu taila* for *snehana* for 30 days of treatment. A significant improvement (60–82%) was noticed in the clinical features such as roughness, scaling, mal odor, pruritus, and hair change [59].

7.5 Summary and Conclusions

The purpose of this chapter is to provide a brief overview of ayurvedic detoxification therapies and allied therapies as well as to review the research literature available on these therapies. This review is intended to inform the reader of the current evidence on these therapies to help them understand their strengths and weaknesses based on the limited information available.

Panchakarma is one of the most important treatment methods in Ayurveda that is used to restore balance to the body through five different cleansing methods. Its proper administration ensures that the body will be more receptive to other remedies, making them more effective with minimal doses [9]. The collective five-fold therapeutic approach can be used for preventive and rejuvenative purposes as well [60]. Furthermore, it has been shown to be helpful as a program for behavior change by assisting one's expected and reported adherence to new and healthier behavior patterns [10]. These benefits support the use of *panchakarma* for everyone, including healthy persons. The meticulous three phase process is comprised of careful preparation of a person before undergoing drastic cleansing methods, followed by the main procedures and the final phase of restoration and systematic rebuilding of *agni* and energy [60]. These processes are tweaked and adjusted per individual needs to match the person's disease and/or body constitution.

The literature review does indicate that almost all the procedures under the umbrella of *panchakarma* have been investigated—some of them very thoroughly. However, previous literature reviews done on this topic indicate an overall poor quality and paucity of clinical studies [7]. Our review supports this viewpoint. While there are several studies on *vasti karma* and *nasya karma*, the studies on *vamana* and many allied therapies are very limited in number. Regardless, a majority of the studies we reviewed showed that the main procedures, *vamana*, *virechana*, *nasya*, *vasti*, and *raktamokshana* and the allied therapies, such as *shirodhara*, are useful and have been shown to be significantly better or equal to the controls they were compared against. The significant levels ranged from $p<0.05$ to $p<0.0001$. Nonetheless, several of these studies are beset with limitations and are of poor quality. A common limitation that was seen across all the studies was the small sample sizes that were as low as just five in each group. Secondly, the randomization method adopted in assigning participants to either group was not explained in the randomized controlled trials. Thirdly, the outcome measures were often developed for the study by the authors and did not validate them. Fourthly, neither the diagnostic criteria nor the trial duration were supported with literature in these trials. Fifthly, there was no description of blinding protocol or its evaluation at the end of the studies to determine absence of bias. It was also noted that some studies had no control group, no clear inclusion/exclusion criteria, and no details about patient demographics or baseline characteristics.

Last but not least, the majority of the trials did not describe the compliance and dropout rates and presence or absence of adverse events. In view of these limitations, we have to be careful in interpreting the findings of these studies and generalizing the results.

Despite the limitations, however, *panchakarma* and the allied therapies have a definitive role in the management of diseases from an ayurvedic perspective. The findings from the preliminary and pilot studies are encouraging and pave the way for future large clinical trials. It is recommended that well-designed rigorous clinical trials with sufficient sample sizes be conducted using a whole system approach to study this complex treatment method.

References

1. Joshi SV (2005) Ayurveda & panchakarma. Motilal Banarasidas, New Delhi
2. Singh RH (2002) Panchakarma therapy. Chowkhanba Sanskrit Series Office, Varanasi
3. Sharma H, Chandola HM, Singh G, Basisht G (2007) Utilization of ayurveda in health care: an approach for prevention, health promotion, and treatment of disease. Part 1—ayurveda, the science of life. J Altern Complement Med 13:1011–1019
4. Warrier PS (1991) Chikitsa Sangraham. Arya vaidy sala Kottakkal, Kerala
5. Sharma PV (1983) Charaka Samhita. Chaukhambha Orientalia, Varanasi
6. Bhishagratna KK, Mitra D (1998) Sushruta Samhita. Chowkhambha Sanskrit Series Office, Varanasi
7. Rastogi S (2011) Panchakarma: exploring through evidences. Light Ayurveda J 9:30–36
8. Sharma H, Chandola HM, Singh G, Basisht G (2007) Utilization of ayurveda in health care: an approach for prevention, health promotion, and treatment of disease. Part 2— ayurveda in primary health care. J Altern Complement Med 13:1135–1150
9. Chaube A, Prajapati P, Dixit SK (1996) Pharmaceutical processing in Panchakarma vis-a-vis Poliomyelitis. Anc Sci Life 17:50–59
10. Conboy LA, Edshteyn I, Garivaltis H (2009) Ayurveda and panchakarma: measuring the effects of a holistic health intervention. Scientific World Journal 9:272–280
11. Rai PK, Singh OP, Rai NP, Singh SK (2008) Efficacy of vamana in the management of kitibha (psoriasis). Aryavaidyan 22:9–42
12. Rawal M, Chudasma KM, Vyas RV, Parmar BP (2010) Effect of vasantic vaman and other panchakarma procedures on disorders of various systems. AYU 31:319–323
13. Kumari J, Mehta CS, Shukla VD, Dave AR, Shingala TM (2010) A comparative clinical study of Nyagrodhadi Ghanavati and virechana karma in the management of Madhumeha. AYU 31:300–304
14. Hegde P, Hemanth DT, Emmi SV, Shipla MP, Pradeep SS, Santosh YM (2010) A case discussion on eczema. Int J Ayurveda Res 1:268–270
15. Srinivasulu M (1998) Role of virechana karma in amavata by Gandharahastadi kwatha. J Res Ayurveda Siddha 19:132
16. Prasad MS, Ramachandran AP, Acharya GS, Kamath TS (2010) Evaluation of the role of Nithyavirechana and Nayopayam kashaya in Tamaka Shwasa. AYU 31:294–299
17. Chaudhari V, Rajagopala M, Mistry S, Vaghela DB (2010) Role of Pradhamana Nasya and Trayodashanga Kwatha in the management of Dushta Pratishyaya with special reference to chronic sinusitis. AYU 31:325–331
18. Panigrahi HK (2006) Efficacy of Ayurvedic medicine in the treatment of uncomplicated chronic sinusitis. Anc Sci Life 16:6–11
19. Bittar G (1997) A preliminary study on the efficacy of Nasya (errhine) in the management of chronic daily headache. Aryavaidyan 10:208–213
20. Thanki KH, Joshi NP, Shah NB (2009) A comparative study of Anu Taila and Mashadi taila Nasya on Ardita (Facial Paralysis). AYU 30:201–204
21. Madhavikutty P (2000) The role of nasya and dhoopa in Dementia and Alzheimer's disease. Aryavaidyan 13:228–233

22. Anand PKV (2006) Role of virecana nasya in the management of jaundice— a case study. Aryavaidyan 19:176–179
23. Krishnasastry M, Yadava RK, Singh RH (1996) Effect of Vasti therapy in the management of irritable syndrome (Pakwasayagata Vata Vyadhi). J Res Ayurveda Siddha 17:16–25
24. Nair PKS, Madhavkutty P, Namboodiri PKS, Tewari NS (2001) Therapeutic effect of vaitarana vasti (Vangesena) in inter vertebral disc prolapse with sciatica and related problems. J Res Ayurveda Siddha 22:120–130
25. Gupta A, Sharma RS, Sharma AK (2000) Clinical evaluation of vasti chikitsa in the management of amavata (rheumatoid arthritis). J Res Ayurveda Siddha 21:165–175
26. Shah MR, Mehta CS, Shukla VD, Dave AR, Bhatt NN (2010) A clinical study of Matra Vasti and an Ayurvedic indigenous compound drug in the management of Sandhigatavata (Osteoarthritis). AYU 31:210–217
27. Karunagoda K, Shukla K, Donga S, Tanna C, Dei LP (2010) A comparative study of Dashamoola Taila Matra Basti and Tila Taila Matra Basti in Kashtartava (dysmenorrhea). AYU 31:305–310
28. Khagram R, Mehta CS, Shukla VD, Dave AR (2010) Clinical effect of Matra Basti and Vatari Guggulu in the management of Amavata (rheumatoid arthritis). AYU 31:343–350
29. Tripathy KA, Kar AC, Tewari SK (1997) Effects of Ayurvedic treatment on amoebic colitis. Anc Sci Life 17:28–31
30. Michelsen A, Klotz S, Lüdtke R, Moebius S, Spahn G, Dobos GJ (2003) Effectiveness of leech therapy in osteoarthritis of the knee: a randomized, controlled trial. Ann Intern Med 139:724–730
31. Rao MM, Deep VC, Padhi MM, Das B, Nanda GC, Sahu DP (2006) Application of leech therapy in the management of Svitra (Leukoderma). Aryavaidyan 19:144–147
32. Patankar U, Shakya AK, Sharma SS (2006) Application of leech in Buerger's disease—a critical study. Aryavaidyan 19:81–85
33. Nair PKS, Sankarankutty P (1993) Evaluation of the efficacy of classical Sodhana therapy in the management of rheumatoid arthritis. J Res Ayurveda Siddha 24:115–124
34. Madhavikutty P, Namboodiri PKN, Tewari NS (2000) Shamana therapy versus panchakarma therapy in the management of pangu (paraplegia). J Res Ayurveda Siddha 21:112–125
35. Namboodiri PKN, Pillai NGK, Nair PKS, Sethu KS, Prabhakaran VA, Vijayan NP (1999) Classical panchakarma therapy vis-à-vis samana therapy in the management of pakshaghata (hemiplegia)—a comparative study. J Res Ayurveda Siddha 20:54–71
36. Pillai SM, Vijayan NP, Bhagavathy KC, Santhakumari K, Bhattathiri PPN, Bhaskaran KP (1980) Effect of Panchakarma treatment with Masadiyoga on Pakshavadha. J Res Ayurveda Siddha 1:301–328
37. Nair PKS, Namboodiri PKN (1998) Role of Panchakarma in the management of Pakshaghata (Hemiplegia). J Res Ayurveda Siddha 19:22–23
38. Prasad RD, Tyagi MK (1999) Clinical evaluation of drug therapy associated with Panchakarma in the management of Gridhrasi (Sciatica). J Res Ayurveda Siddha 20:78–82
39. Dubey S, Tripathi JS, Gupta S, Reddy KRC (2010) A comparative clinical trial on the role of Panchakarma therapy and Unmada Gajankusha Rasa in the case of major depressive disorder vis-à-vis kaphaja Unmada. AYU 31:205–209
40. Herron RE, Fagan JB (2002) Altern Ther Health Med 8:40–51
41. Pokharel S, Sharma AK (2010) Evaluation of Insomrid Tablet and Shirodhara in the management of Anidra (Insomnia). AYU 31:40–47
42. Santwani K, Shukla VD, Santwani MA, Thaker G (2010) An assessment of Manasika Bhavas in menopausal syndrome and its management. AYU 31:311–318
43. Sriranjini SJ, Pal PK, Devidas KV, Ganpathy S (2009) Improvement of balance in progressive degenerative cerebellar ataxias after Ayurvedic therapy: a preliminary report. Neurol India 57:166–171
44. Gupta R, Singh RH (2001) A clinical study on Ayurvedic management of chronic daily headache with special reference to sirodhara and sirovirecana. J Res Ayurveda Siddha 12:81–94

45. Uebaba K, Xu FH, Tagawa M et al (2005) Using a healing robot for scientific study of shirodhara. IEEE Eng Med Biol Mag 24:69–78
46. Uebaba K, Xu FH, Ogawa H, Tatsuse T, Wang BH, Hisajima T, Venkatraman S (2008) Psychoneuroimmunologic effects of Ayurvedic oil-dripping treatment. J Altern Complement Med 14:1189–1198
47. Xu F, Uebaba K, Ogawa H, Tatsuse T, Wang BH, Hisajima T, Venkatraman S (2008) Pharmaco-physio-psychologic effect of Ayurvedic oil-dripping treatment using an essential oil from Lavendula angustifolia. J Altern Complement Med 14:947–956
48. Chandre R, Tripathi JS (2007) Role of sirovasti in the management of Kampavata vis-à-vis Parkinsonism. Aryavaidyan 21:25–29
49. Bali Y, Vijayasarathi EJ, Venkatesh BA (2010) Efficacy of Agnikarma over the padakanistakam (little toe) and Katibasti in Gridhrasi: a comparative study. Int J Ayurveda Res 1:223–230
50. Jahan S, Sujatha N, Neelam (2010) Role of Uttara Vasti with Trivrit and Lasuna oil in the management of primary dysmenorrheal. AYU 31(2):228–231
51. Shukla M, Tiwari A, Sharma S (2010) Principle verification of svetapradara vis-à-vis leucorrhoea with Dhatakyadi yoga and Lodhrakvatha uttara basti. Aryavaidyan 23:85–91
52. Pathak B, Dwivedi KK, Shukla KP (1992) Clinical evaluation of Snehana, Swedana and an Ayurvedic compound drug in Sandhivata vis-a-vis Osteroarthiritis. J Res Edu Ind Med April–June:27–34
53. Nanda GC, Padhi MM, Chopra KK (1998) Effect of Trayodashang Guggulu and Vishatinduka vati along with abhyanga and swedana in the management of Gridhrasi (sciatica). J Res in Ayurveda and Siddha 14:116–121
54. Rajoria K, Singh SK, Sharma RS, Sharma SN (2010) Clinical study on Laksha Guggulu, Snehana, Swedana & traction in osteoarthritis (knee joint). AYU 31:80–87
55. Rehlan RK (2005) Role of Snehana and Swedana in the management of Vatavyadhi with special reference to back-ache. Aryavaidyan 18:235–239
56. Rastogi S, Singh RH (1996) Duchennes muscular dystrophy—management through Pinda Sweda therapy. J Res Ayurveda Siddha 17:105–111
57. Nair R, Vijayan NP, Indirakumari S et al (1985) Snehapana effect of Bhadradarvadi Taila in Gridhrasi. J Res Ayurveda Siddha 5:149–162
58. Nair RB, Nair PKS, Madhavikutty P et al (2002) Effect of Snehapana on the lipid profile of patients with rheumatic and neurological disorders. J Res Ayurveda Siddha 23:1–9
59. Dash D (2007) The management of Ichthyosis with Gomutra avagaha and Yashtimadhutaila abhyanga. Aryavaidyan 20–4:228–231
60. Gupta M, Shaw BP (2009) Uses of medicinal plants in Panchakarma Ayurvedic therapy. Indian J Tradit Knowledge 8:372–378

Chapter 8
Gut and Joint Interconnections: A Reappraisal to Ayurvedic Understanding of Joint Diseases

Sanjeev Rastogi and Ranjana Rastogi

8.1 Introduction

Ayurveda, in true representation to disease prevalence pattern among human population, is marked by vivid elaboration to various common clinical entities. Infective conditions predominantly marked by fever and noninfective degenerative and metabolic conditions like diabetes, anemia, jaundice, and joint diseases are among few conditions described in Ayurveda in great details. Among them all, joint diseases make a proportionate sum to the net patient input to any Ayurvedic clinic seen in India [1, 2]. Among joint conditions commonly seen in Ayurvedic clinics, predominant ones are the diseases marked by joint pain, inflammation, and limitation to movements. Patients having joint pathologies visiting Ayurvedic outdoors are invariably found to have few common features. They are chronically disabled, are prediagnosed, and are marked with deformities, depression, and dependence [3, 4]. It is less common to find a newly diagnosed patient with joint disease in an Ayurvedic clinic. Ayurveda works admirably in joint afflictions; this layman's belief becomes an observable fact when we see a large number of these patients waiting for their turn of consultation or panch-karma therapy in an Ayurvedic setting [5]. Although an unavailability of dependable and safe remedy to many of these conditions through conventional medicine and a countrywide deficit of trained rheumatologists for their early admiration substantiates to escalating number of joint patients in Ayurvedic outdoors, it does not reduce the prima facie impression of effectiveness of Ayurvedic therapy in such conditions.

S. Rastogi (✉)
PG Department of Kaya Chikitsa, State Ayurvedic College, Lucknow University, Lucknow, Uttar Pradesh, India
e-mail: rastogisanjeev@rediffmail.com

R. Rastogi
Department of Obstetrics and Gynaecology, Vatsala Hospital, Lucknow, Uttar Pradesh, India
e-mail: rastogiranjana2010@rediffmail.com

S. Rastogi (ed.), *Evidence-Based Practice in Complementary and Alternative Medicine*,
DOI 10.1007/978-3-642-24565-7_8,

What should we expect from Ayurveda in a joint condition where the contemporary system of medicine is away from reaching to a dependable and reasonable management plan and where a patient is marked with lost hopes and fortunes of being recovered [3]. For obvious reasons of complexities associated with joint diseases, the expectations from Ayurveda for intervention in such conditions should be made balanced plausibly and pragmatically. Any plausibility of Ayurvedic interventions to act upon joint diseases lies onto its unique propatient understanding of a disease and its original gut–joint pathology theory, based on which Ayurveda holds promises of further exploration of its principles especially in the segment of joint pathologies to complement the existing management protocols within various joint diseases.

Food, its type, digestion process, and postdigestion physiology have remained the key aspects to an Ayurvedic understanding of health and subsequent pathogenesis. Besides their role to many other diseases, they are found to have a special bearing in joint diseases. Ayurveda groups inflammatory diseases of joint under the umbrella term of Amavata and proposes diet, digestion, and postdigestive mechanisms for being major incriminators to its pathogenesis. An association of diet with arthritis has remained a subject of debate since long. We have come across various studies where exacerbation of arthritis symptoms was observed by certain inclusion diets and similarly a remission was observed through exclusion diets [6–9]. Due to a huge variability in food consumption pattern across the globe, we however could not yet reach to a consensus for what are the foods that may lead to arthritis. This is, however, more or less agreed that a small component of all arthritis may get worsened and relieved by some diets [10]. There have also been the studies identifying an increased intestinal permeability in reference to excessive use of NSAIDs or otherwise as a cause to increased immunological gut responses in reference to various dietary antigens [11].

Ayurvedic understanding of diet in relation to joint pathology goes deeper than identifying type of food for arthritis symptom exacerbations. It actually points out to certain mechanism through which a normal food can also be converted as a precursor to various pathologies. Incidentally, a good account of lifestyle diseases including those afflicting the joints are found to have evidence-based links to trivial dietary faults existing for a considerable period of time.

Unfortunately, mere proposal of a hypothesis to understand a disease process may not really help to the actual disease management. In light of theoretical proposals and observations referring to clinical practice of Ayurvedic rheumatology, Ayurveda is required to realize more honestly what is still undone on their part of joint disease understanding and management. To be more honest, it requires paving ways to translate its founding principles of joint disease in galore to treat them more effectively. Ayurveda requires realizing the expectations of the patients who are making most of its clientele and requires finding ways to come true to those expectations. Needless to say, a thorough research with a clear vision of translating its conceptual excellence into utilizable repertory is the only way forward.

Contemporary researches to explore the rheumatologic conditions in Ayurveda have so far been diversified. By and large these researches are found limited to the exploration of possible clinical utility of herbal or herbomineral compounds alone or in addition to panch-karma procedures in various joint conditions [12]. Failing to find any admirable result through these clinical researches, of late, Ayurvedic rheumatology research has shifted from individual treatments to the development of a complete management plan, often a cocktail regimen, desirous to give some impact upon patients by adopting variable combination of a drug in oral or local forms, a diet, and a physico-biological procedure aptly called as panch-karma. Whatever idea of research is adopted so far to explore the subject of Ayurvedic rheumatology, it failed to contribute, and therefore despite of a huge patient input, it could not pave ways to the development of a dependable understanding and subsequent treatment protocols in Ayurvedic rheumatology. Forthcoming sections of this chapter are in realization to this important missing aspect of Ayurvedic rheumatology.

Considering the fundamentals of Ayurvedic pathogenesis, a disease may find its origin through multilevel imbalances to human physiology. These imbalances could be diversified, affecting various physiological functions like metabolism, digestion, absorption, circulation, synthesis, and elimination. *Agni* (fire of transformation) irregularity coupled with irregular functions of three founding physiological principles, namely, *vata*, *pitta*, and *kapha*, mark the basis of any pathogenesis in Ayurveda. Further to it, Ayurveda also identifies a few exclusive *hetu* or *nidana* (etiological factors) for most diseases. Diet forms an exclusive component to these etiological elaborations in Ayurveda.

Planning a dependable management in a disease condition thereby largely depends upon the understanding of its etiopathogenesis. It is therefore mandatory to reappraise Ayurvedic pathophysiological understanding to various rheumatologic conditions to design a definitive treatment protocol malleable as per the specific causes. *Amavata*, a syndromic entity in Ayurveda, is found to have reasonable resemblances with various inflammatory arthritic conditions [13]. Being one important representative to the subject of rheumatology, in terms of its prognosis and also in terms of its prevalence [5], *Amavata* is largely taken up as a clinical prototype in Ayurvedic rheumatology. A thorough reappraisal to its etiopathological understanding, therefore, is presumed essential to tailor an effective plan of its management and also to various other joint conditions where a similar etiopathogenesis is presumably involved.

8.2 *Amavata*: An Interplay of *Ama* and *Vata*

Amavata, an Ayurvedic parallel to rheumatologic syndromes, does not have a mention in the triad of ancient Ayurvedic classics (*Charaka Samhita*, *Sushruta Samhita*, *and Ashtanga Samgraha*). It finds its first ever mention as a syndrome in *Madhava Nidana* (sixth century AD), a text dedicated to Ayurvedic clinical diagnostics [14]. Thereafter, however, *Amavata* could find a regular mention to Ayurvedic texts and has become an indispensible part of Ayurvedic clinical medicine study and practice. This is interesting to note here about the apparent absence of this disease in particular from classical triads and its relative late entry into the Ayurvedic curriculum. Does it point out to some specific emergence–prevalence–incidence pattern to the disease which may have a relation to changes in local dietary, social, or environmental customs? Defining *Amavata*, *Madhava* explained it as a disease characterized by simultaneous vitiation of *ama* and *vata*, a duo of pathological entities, vitiating independently but in unison leading to a pathology complex enough to be explained through either of them alone.

8.2.1 Ayurvedic Understanding of a Disease Pathogenesis

Ayurveda proposes a novel mechanism to the beginning of a disease process in any individual. It identifies the same factors responsible for a disease process whom otherwise are responsible for the preservation of health during their normal occurrence and functioning. This proposal has a beautiful resemblance to the concept of eco-balancing where a definitive sum of one entity is found responsible for a sustainable eco-health and failing to which a population is presumed to suffer from a cascade of anomalies related directly or indirectly to the primary imbalance [15].

8.2.2 Etiology of Amavata

Etiological description of *Amavata* in Ayurveda renders a divergent spectrum of factors presumably leading to its origin. Dietary factors, metabolic status, physical activities done prior or immediately after the food intake, and average physical activities in general are principal components of this spectrum. An etiology to Amavata as depicted by *Madhava* clearly identifies two distinct roots to it. These are:

1. *Amavata* in metabolically and physically less active people who are also engaged in incompatible dietary practices. *Madhava* describes this as "*Viruddhaaharacheshtasya mandagnernischalasya cha*," a condition marked by a preexisting *mandagni* and hypoactive physical state clubbed with an eagerness to go for *viruddh-ahara*. This description of *Madhava* tries to differentiate one set of etiology from the other where a different set of etiology is found responsible to *Amavata*.
2. *Amavata* in physically and metabolically active people who are also having a practice of indulging into physical activities just after having heavy fatty meals. *Madhava* defines this state as "*Snigdhama bhuktavato hyannam vyayamam kurvatastatha*."

This set of etiology proposes the involvement of people with a good metabolic status and appetite and also with much agility. An exercise session following a heavy fatty meal which is presumed to be the reason of *Amavata* in these cases, incidentally, reminds us to the stressful urban working environments where one is constantly under substantial work stress and, as a consequence, is bound to rush to work even immediately after meals.

We can find that Ayurveda, through its etiopathogenesis, explores the possibilities of heterogeneous pathologies to the syndrome of *Amavata*. Any such possibility further gives us a clue as to why the presentation, responses to the treatment, and ultimate prognosis in *Amavata* are not identical in any two apparently similar cases. This divergent etiology of *Amavata* also explains about the heterogeneous spectrum of rheumatologic disease profile and their afflicting population in general.

8.2.3 *Ama*: The Primary Root to Rheumatologic Diseases

Ama is a novel concept of Ayurveda which adequately elaborates various rheumatologic pathogenesis marked by features of stiffness, heaviness, fever, swelling, and pain. *Ama* literally stands for something which is unripe. From physiological perspectives, production of *ama* refers to the under-operative state of *agni* leading to liberation of inadequately processed end products. These end products, being inadequately processed, have a macromolecular structure, which is bigger and grosser than those end products which might have produced if a complete processing would have taken place. *Ama*, thereby, owing to its macromolecular structure, in general, is told to have a clogging property with a predilection to block the *srotas* (fine conduits of the body), an important step through which most *ama*-related symptoms begin manifesting.

As *ama* is the produce of hypometabolic state, adequately referred as *mandagni* in Ayurveda, it can have multiple forms, depending upon the level of its origin. It can be produced in gastrointestinal tract where an inadequate digestion may give rise to production of macromolecular substances largely antigenic in nature for their under-processing into simpler forms. It can also be generated at tissue level where substrates are exposed to enzymatic actions for their conversion into ultimately utilizable forms in tissues. An under-processing of substrates at tissue level is proposed to give rise to *ama* at tissue level which is also referred to as *dhatu gata ama*.

8.2.3.1 Causes of *Ama* Production

Ayurveda identifies various dietary irregularities as the primary reason to *ama* production and subsequently to many *ama*-related diseases. Among all, an excessive intake of food is found to be the principal cause to such pathology (*Atimatram punah sarvadoshaprakopanama – Charaka Vimana* 2/7). An occasional excessive intake, however, produces transient symptoms only which are local to gastrointestinal tract and may not have a sustainable systemic effect required for the production of joint diseases.

Table 8.1 Food and its intake-related factors which may cause *Ama* production

Food quality–related factors	*Guru* (difficult to digest)
	Ruksha (dry mainly due to lack of fat)
	Sheet (cold)
	Shushka (dry mainly due to lack of hydration)
Food appearance–related factors	*Dwishta* (which is not liked in appearance)
Food effect–related factors	*Vishtambhi* (causing gastric discomfort)
	Vidahi (causing burning in abdomen)
Food preparation–related factors	*Ashuchi* (unclean)
Food composition–related factors	*Viruddha ahara* (incompatible food)
Food intake–related factors	*Akal* (food intake at improper time)
Psychological status at the time of food intake	*Kama* (extremely desirous)
	Krodha (angry), *Lobha* (lust), *Moha* (attachment), *Irshya* (jealous)
	Lajja (shameful), *Shoka* (grief)
	Abhimana (proud)
	Udvega (anxious)
	Bhaya (fearful)
	Up-*tapta* (sad)

Explaining further about the causes of *ama* production, *Charaka* identifies various other diet and its intake-related factors ultimate to *ama* production. Principal ones among them are shown in Table 8.1.

By observing the causes of *ama* production, it is apparent that besides quality of the food, an intake method and mood status at the time of food intake can also play a great role in determination of ultimate outcome to the consumed food. Effects of various psychological factors, especially the stress upon intestinal functioning, have increasingly been recognized [16]. A sustained stress is found to give rise to observable microscopic changes into gut epithelium and to its subsequent physiology. In many experimental studies, various types of physical and psychological stress are found to induce dysfunction of intestinal barrier, resulting in enhanced intake of potentially noxious material (e.g., antigens, toxins, and other proinflammatory molecule) from the gut lumen into the bloodstream [17]. This gives a very interesting proposition to see if these noxious materials play the role of ama as a progenitor to joint diseases as perceived in Ayurveda.

8.2.3.2 *Mandagni*: The Hypodigestive State

Mandagni is another Ayurvedic conceptualization for the possible reasoning to *ama* production. *Agni* is proposed to be the principal factor responsible for transformations in the body. As per its site of action, it is variously named as *Jatharagni* (transforming factor in gut), *Bhutagni* (transforming factor in substrates while they are in transition), and *Dhatvagni* (transforming factor in tissues responsible for active utilization of substrates to build up tissue). This is interesting to elaborate upon what *mandagni* is and how this may lead to production of *ama*. As we are aware, to

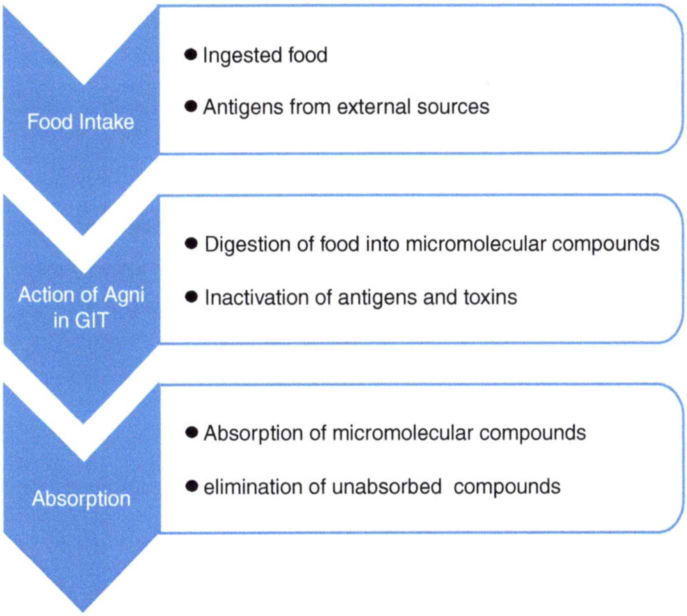

Fig. 8.1 Normal digestive physiology

complete the process of any transformation, an adequacy of *agni* is required; it is clear that if *agni* is inadequate, the produce of it would not be of the desired consistency. These macromolecular substances which are produced by incomplete processing of substrates are nothing but *ama* (unripe) for their potential to be broken further into smaller components (Figs. 8.1 and 8.2).

Mandagni or a hypodigestive state thereby is found to be operational at two levels which are mutually interdependent. At one end, it acts through a deficient enzyme state, leading to inadequate processing of the substrates and thereby producing inadequately treated end products of enzymatic reactions (Fig. 8.3). On the other hand, it also points out to an integral pathology to gut mucosa which is supposedly responsible for the poor enzymatic secretions. An inadequate secretion may also be consequential to food intake, food quality, or food composition–related factors, as is discussed earlier (Table 8.1). Through both of its operational mechanisms, mandagni gives rise to the following pathology:

1. Inadequate handling with the ingested substances
2. Enhanced uptake of improperly treated macromolecular substances into the systemic circulation

In whatever way the *ama* is produced, due to its increased influx in the gut mucosa in reference to *mandagni*-related epithelial changes, it makes the surrounding immune system exposed to various new antigens, a pathology which marks the beginning to various autoimmune disorders.

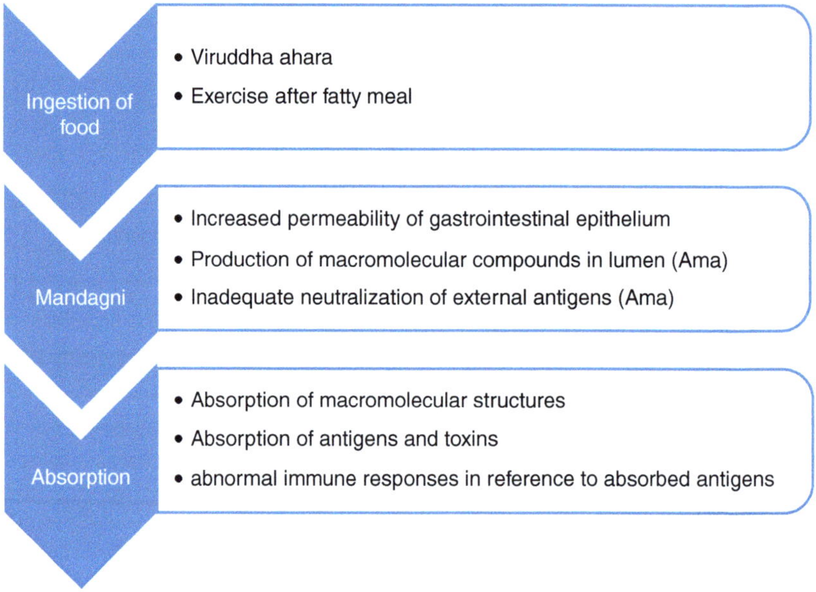

Fig. 8.2 Digestive physiology referring to production of *Ama* and subsequent pathology

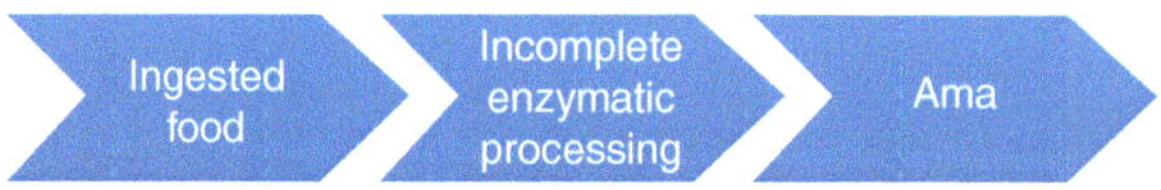

Fig. 8.3 Production of *Ama* through incomplete enzymatic processing of ingested food

An inadequate processing of food leading to production of *ama* can also be a result of reduced contact between food and enzymes, a factor which is aptly described in subsequent etiology to *Amavata*. An exercise following a fatty meal may lead to a rapid transit of food from the gut, making it less exposed to enzymatic activity. The result would again be the production of substrates none other than *ama*.

8.3 Etiopathogenesis of *Amavata*

Describing further to etiology of *Amavata*, *Madhava* stressed upon two principal etiologies predominant either to sedentary people marked with *mandagni* and habitual to *viruddh-ahara* or to active but stressed people who are compelled to make physical activities immediately after meals, especially the ones which contain fat. Interestingly, we can clearly say that these two etiologies are nothing but the two distinct mechanisms of producing *ama*, which once produced, chooses a common pathway to develop *Amavata*-related manifestations. This would also be interesting to elaborate these two distinct etiopathogenesis of *Amavata* in light of recent advances made in the field of digestive physiology. But before elaborating it further, it is important to have a look at the common pathway through which *Amavata* finally manifests.

8.3.1 Pathogenesis in Amavata

Once the *ama* acquires a sustainable formation and subsequent accumulation in the gastrointestinal tract due to either of its two principal etiologies, it goes further to subsequent morbid changes. *Ama* produced and accumulated in such ways is subsequently subjected to internalization and migration towards the places which are rich in substances having a property similar to that of *ama*. For general considerations, *kapha* has a reasonable resemblance to that of *ama*, and therefore, this movement of *ama* is largely directed towards *kapha* predominant places in the body. *Vata* plays an important role in *ama* internalization and also in its further movements within the body.

Accumulating further and reaching to a critical level, *ama* then flows through arteries where it gets an opportunity to react with various preexisting substrates of *vata–pitta–kapha* distinctions. This interaction gives rise to diverse products having profound adherence as a common feature. An *ama* produce of this variety quickly develops weakness and heaviness in the body as a forerunner to *Amavata*. A *vata* and *ama* accumulation following to this in joints mainly to the lumbo-saccral region gradually cause a stiffness to the whole body. This is how *Amavata* begins.

A few points conceptualized to *Amavata* pathogenesis in *Ayurveda* are truly phenomenal. *Ama*, the principal causative factor to *Amavata*, is said to be produced through variable ways. Once *ama* acquires a sustainable production owing to regularity of its etiology, it does not remain in gastrointestinal tract alone but, under the influence of *vata*, starts getting internalized to body tissues. *Vata* here depicts the factors which promote internalization of *ama* through the intestinal mucosa. A small amount of *ama* internalized in such a way remains limited to gut surrounding tissue and causes immune changes at local level. Under normal circumstances, the gut epithelium allows only minute quantity of intact antigens to cross into the mucosa, where they interact with the mucosal immune system to downregulate inflammation [17]. It is, however, important to observe that if *ama* is produced in higher quantities, it may absorb to reach to intestinal portal system. Once internalized, *ama* is subjected to interactions with various preexisting substrates having *vata–pitta–kapha* properties. As a consequence, *ama* is further converted into its highly adherent form. Interestingly, by considering *ama* as macromolecular antigenic substances, we can also presume exposure of these antigens to preexisting T lymphocytes in the peripheral circulation [18]. An antigen–T lymphocyte complex is then further exposed to immune reactions, leading to the ultimate production of antibodies against such antigens which are having a gross cross-reactivity, especially to *ama*-resembling substances of which *kapha* is the most important to be considered [19].

Table 8.2 General features of *Amavata*

Feature	Interpretation
Angamarda	Body ache
Aruchi	Loss of appetite
Trishna	Thirst
Aalasya	Malaise
Gaurava	Heaviness
Jvara	Fever
Apaka	Indigestion
Shunata-anganaam	Swelling in various body parts

8.3.2 Symptomatology in Amavata

Amavata in general is manifested through a variety of symptoms which are produced through a clogging of microconduits of body through *ama*. Besides this, *ama*, the principal morbid product in *Amavata* itself, has properties which promote inflammation in connection to its adherence with various preexisting tissues in the body. General features of *Amavata* as given in Ayurvedic texts are shown in Table 8.2.

It is important to understand that in *Amavata*, because of intangible nature of inherent pathogenesis and also because of need of accumulation of etiological factors to a critical level before *Amavata* is actually manifested, a time gap between etiological exposure and a symptom manifestation is obvious and can never be clearly predicted.

The symptom profile and intensity in *Amavata* and their time concordance in reference to etiological exposures are therefore variable in reference to various confounding factors like individual capacity to handle various noxious substances and individual response in reference to that exposure.

Once the pathogenesis of *Amavata* gets matured, it is manifested through various musculoskeletal symptoms which become the hallmark to this disease (Table 8.3). An association to *vata*, *pitta*, or *kapha* to disease-causing factors in *Amavata* further gives rise to a few identical features typical to these factors. Thereby an association of pitta is marked with burning and tenderness, *vata* with pain, and *kapha* with heaviness and itching (Table 8.4).

8.4 Reappraising *Amavata* Etiology to Contemporary Understanding

As we have understood so far, *Amavata* is found to have two distinct etiologies. It either initiates among people who are less active, have poor digestive capacities, and are habituated to *viruddha ahara* or among people who are active but stressed. The typical etiology narrated for latter subgroup is an exercise schedule just after heavy meals containing fat.

Table 8.3 Specific symptoms of *Amavata*

Features	Contemporary meaning
Saruja sandhi shotha	Painful swelling at joints
Hasta, Pada, Shiro Gulpha, Trika Jaanu, Uru Sandhi	Hand, foot, cervical, ankle, sacral, knee, and hip joints
Rujyatetyarthah vyaviddha iva vrishchike	Intense pain like a scorpion bite
Agni-daurbalya	Indigestion
Praseka	Excessive salivation
Aruchi	Loss of appetite
Gaurava	Heaviness
Utsaha hani	Loss of interest
Vairasya	Loss of taste
Daah	Burning
Bahu-mutrata	Polyurea
Kukshi kathinata	Hardness in abdomen
Shula	Pain in abdomen
Nidra viparyaya	Sleep diversion
Trit	Thirst
Chardi	Vomiting
Bhrama	Giddiness
Murcha	Syncope
Hrid griha	Heaviness in heart
Vida Vibaddhata	Constipation
Jadya	Stiffness
Aantra kujana	Increased sound in abdomen
Aanaha	Abdominal distention

Table 8.4 *Dosha* specific features in *Amavata*

Dosha	Features
Pitta	*Daha, Raga*
Vata	*Shula*
Kapha	*Stimit, Guru, Kandu*

This is interesting to elaborate these two distinct etiologies of *Amavata* in reference to their contemporary significance as per recent understanding of human physiology.

8.4.1 *Amavata Among People with Mandagni–Nischalata–Viruddha ahara*

A distinct subgroup of people characterized by less active routines, poor digestive capacities, added with habitual *viruddha ahara* intake is identified in Ayurveda as susceptible to *Amavata*. As the group is characterized by three independent pathological factors which are able to cause independent pathologies at their own, this is interesting to see as to how they interact together to give rise to a more complicated pathology like *Amavata*.

Mandagni can arise independently as a feature in response to various dietary or routine responses. It can also arise as a response to *Nishchalata*, an independent factor identified as a cause to *Amavata*. As we have understood so far, *mandagni* or the hypoactive metabolic state can manifest at gastrointestinal tract level through a reduction in independent or cumulative enzyme quantity secreted in response to the dietary intakes. Any such deficiency will lead to an inadequate transformation of dietary intake into the subsequent end products; the result will be the production of *ama*. A further quest into *mandagni* gives us a clue that *mandagni* itself is not limited to transiently reduced enzymatic secretions but simultaneously also involves the factors which cause a permanent deficit into the enzyme secretion mechanism. An important mechanism which may be involved in mandagni-related features could be a gradual destruction of intestinal mucosal cells responsible for enzyme secretion and also a poor intramural plexus response to dietary stimuli, leading to a neurohormonal mechanism for enzymatic secretions. Interestingly, dietary lectins from common dietary staples like cereal grains and legumes are found to have influence upon structure and function of enterocytes and lymphocytes [20, 21]. Wheat germ agglutinin and lectin in general are found bound to gut brush border epithelial cells, causing damage to the base of villi through disarrangement of cytoskeleton, increased endocytosis, and shortening of the microvilli [20–22]. The structural changes induced by this agglutinin on intestinal epithelial cells elicit functional changes including increased permeability [23] which may facilitate the passage of undegraded dietary antigens into systemic circulation [21]. This is important to reappraise if this could be the possible mechanism of working of *mandagni* and *ama* in reference to *Amavata* pathogenesis.

Nischalata or poor physical activity can reciprocally be associated to *mandagni*. A sedentary lifestyle eventually reduces the energy expenditure and subsequent energy requirements of human body. If it is sustained longer, it may lead to a sustained low energy transaction or *mandagni*. A mandagni of independent origin, in turn, can also cause *nischalata* as a consequence to poor digestion and subsequent production of *ama*.

Viruddha ahara is another important factor which contributes to the pathogenesis of *Amavata*. *Viruddha ahara* classically represents the combination of food which is incompatible if taken together. This dietary incompatibility as per Ayurveda is operational not only at level of food composition but also at levels like *Matra* (quantity), *Guna* (property), *Karma* (action), *Kala* (time duration), or *Sanskara* (qualitative transformations) of food. An incompatibility, therefore, may substantiate through any such factor making a food unsuitable to human consumption.

Viruddha ahara is proposed to give rise to many transient and stable clinical features. *Charaka* defines *viruddha ahara* for three of its distinct properties [24]:

1. Characters opposite to *dhatu*
2. *Dosha* vitiating property
3. Remains in the body even after the *dosha* vitiation

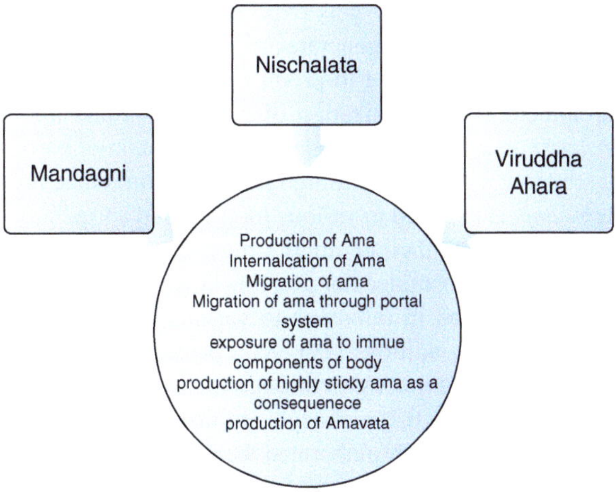

Fig. 8.4 An interplay of *Mandagni–Nischalata–Viruddha ahara* leading to *Amavata*

This clearly marks out the property of *viruddha ahara* for their stable antigenic properties leading to chronic and lasting illnesses.

In reference to *viruddha ahara*, it is also important to understand that a method of intake also can turn a wholesome food into the incompatible ones. Mental state of the person who is consuming the food plays a very important role in determining the net outcome to a dietary intake. Although acting primarily through *agni*, it can make the consumed food incompatible due to the poor enzymatic action and subsequent production of end products which are not compatible with body tissue. A net interplay of *mandagni–nischalata–viruddha ahara* can be speculated, as shown in Fig. 8.4. Once the *ama* is produced subsequent to etiological exposures, it acquires a common pathway to cause the disease. *Ama* produced gradually gets internalized under the influence of *vata*. This internalization of *ama* is variously facilitated by many factors coacting at the gut mucosa–lumen interface. Under normal circumstances, gut epithelium controls internalization of large antigenic molecules through an intestinal barrier function. This barrier includes physical diffusion barrier, regulated physiological and enzymatic barrier, and immunological barrier which are under neurohormonal control and can be affected by various mechanisms like stress and dietary intakes. A continuous epithelial cell layer interconnected with tight junctions restricts both transcellular and paracellular permeation of molecules, thus constituting the principal component of intestinal barrier. In addition, the epithelium exerts an important physiological defense by secretion of fluid and mucus, together with secretory IgA, into the lumen to dilute, wash away, and bind noxious substances [17]. A mechanism which operates to cause intestinal barrier dysfunction may be complex and may involve either of the barriers we discussed. A loosening at the mucosal tight junctions, besides direct cellular damages in response to stress or incompatible intakes, becomes one plausible mechanism through which ama can find a way to get internalized to the gut peripheral tissue. This tissue is invariably rich in lymphatics and gives a reason to Ayurvedic perception of *ama* migration to the places which are similar to *kapha*. Any *ama* which gets internalized in such a way to gut periphery gets exposed to various immune factors operating locally. As a consequence, it generates local immune reactions causing local inflammation, a phenomena required to produce gut immunity physiologically but can facilitate architectural disorganization of gut mucosa and thereby can augment *mandagni*. A large quantity of *ama* added with a substantial barrier dysfunction may give *ama* a way to get absorbed through portal system. Once internalized through portal system, *ama* is exposed to various food-related antigens and also to various indigenous proteins. Due to their complex structure, *ama* is presumed to have a cross-reactivity to various macromolecular proteins intrinsically available in the body, a phenomena recently studied in reference to various dietary proteins and their antigenicity in autoimmune conditions [19]. As a primary immune reaction, *ama* is exposed and trapped by T lymphocytes through their target receptors. Once trapped, *ama* is presented further to B lymphocytes to produce antibodies against such *ama* antigens. Ayurveda beautifully elaborated the whole phenomena as an *ama–vata–pitta–kapha* interaction leading to huge production of highly adherent and disease-causing type of *ama*.

8.4.2 Amavata Among Snigdha–Bhuktavato–Vyayama People

Another etiology speculated for *Amavata* is for people where *mandagni* is not a primary pathology and where *ama* is produced through a mechanism of escaping enzymatic action upon dietary components because of their rapid transit. *Snigdha ahara* itself has an affinity for being rapidly transmitted. An exercise following a fatty meal elaborates about the mental and social state of the person who is consuming food. A compulsion to go for work immediately after meals is a good example which elaborates the Ayurvedic *snigdha–bhuktavato–vyayama* proposition of *Amavata*. Interestingly, a rapid transit not only gives a poor exposure of enzymes upon their respective substrates, it also reduces the neutralization of various dietary toxins through respective action of many neutralizing factors in the gut lumen. The result is the production of *ama* which could be a net sum of inadequately digested end products and also inadequately neutralized toxins.

A habit or a compulsion of intruding into exercise after meals more adequately is expressed through the stress which might be related to one's profession. A continuous stress gives rise to certain phenomenal changes to gut mucosa in reference to its permeability and absorptive capacity. Under stress, macromolecular molecules from the gut are found easily internalized into the gut mucosa, a phenomena which is less commonly observed in a normal unstressed mucosa.

It is therefore easy to speculate that under stress, a person is more liable to have increased production of *ama* as a combination to inadequately processed end products of digestion and also to inadequately neutralized dietary toxins. At the same time, it is also noteworthy that under stress, this *ama* gets a better opportunity to get internalized into the gut mucosa, a phenomena which is crucial for the genesis of *Amavata* subsequently (Fig. 8.5).

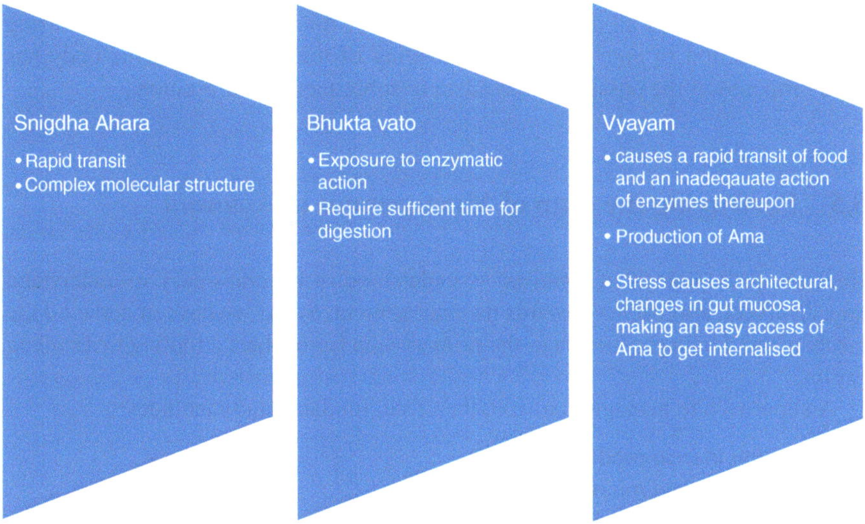

Fig. 8.5 Pathogenesis of *Amavata* among *Snigdha–Bhuktavato–Vyayama* people

8.4.3 Final Pathway to Amavata Production

We can find that production of *ama* may have different pathways, but once it is produced and internalized, it adopts a common pathway of reacting with body tissue, ultimately leading to production of *Amavata*.

Ama, once internalized, is usually migrated to the gut periphery, a tissue which is usually rich in lymphatics. Ayurveda perceives it as the primary migration of *ama* to *kapha* predominant tissue. This migration is supposed to give rise to local reactions which can also augment the architectural changes in gut mucosa. In case of sustained and copious production of *ama*, it can get absorbed through the portal system of intestine, a mechanism which makes *ama* exposed to more diversified and systemic actions. During its migration through portal system, *ama* gets opportunities to react with various body tissues, of which more important are the T lymphocytes. *Ama* trapped through T lymphocytes is further presented to B lymphocytes for a subsequent production of antibodies against trapped *ama*. Interestingly, *ama* or the macromolecular antigens internalized in such a way are found to have a cross-reactivity with various tissue proteins due to molecular mimicry [25]. Antibodies, therefore, produced against such *ama* particles are presumed to act against many self-proteins too, a mechanism through which a cascade of autoimmune disease begins.

Ama, after its reaction to *vata–pitta–kapha*, is proposed to become highly adherent (*picchila*) and noxious, an elaboration which truly fits to the subsequent antibody production in reference to *ama* presentation to B lymphocytes. This *ama* has a high affinity to body tissue which is adequately elaborated through its clogging *picchila* property.

Ayurveda portrays all the subsequent events of *Amavata* pathogenesis referring to the production of *picchila ama*. A clogging of microconduits of the body has been proposed as the possible mechanism to subsequent manifestations.

8.5 Portraying the Plan of Management in *Amavata*

Once the pathogenesis of *Amavata* is understood, it becomes easy to understand how Ayurveda approaches towards its management. So far we have understood the mechanism of *ama* production as the primary step from where a footing to *Amavata* begins.

An approach to manage *Amavata*, therefore, fundamentally includes:

1. Reduction in *ama* production
2. Reduction in *ama* internalization
3. Dissociation of internalized *ama*

8.5.1 Reduction in Ama Production

A reduction in *ama* production could be the primary step to handle *Amavata*. As *ama* is the outcome of *mandagni*, a recorrection of *agni* could be considered as the primary step to deal with *Amavata*. This is important to understand that a recorrection of *agni* here essentially involves an architectural correction of intestinal mucosa which is ultimately responsible for the enzyme secretions. We are aware that intestinal mucosa observes a regular shedding off phenomena with its renewal at regular intervals. By avoiding the mechanisms which may be involved in gut mucosal destruction and by adopting a supportive mechanism to protect gut mucosal lining, a restoration of gut mucosa and subsequently *agni* may be approached.

At the same time, we also need to understand that a supplementation in the form of additional enzymes from external sources or the drugs which may stimulate the enzymatic secretions may not be an efficient remedy to *mandagni* as it would either transiently patch up the problem instead of making a correction, or it would stimulate the compromised mucosa for more enzyme production, a measure which will augment the cell destruction in long run.

A *mandagni* correction, therefore, in *Amavata* should only be approached, initially by avoidance of etiological factors which are causing a *mandagni* and subsequently by exposing the intestinal mucosa to dietary substrates which may promote tissue restoration. The best approach is to begin with food which requires simple digestion. This food is called *laghu* (the food which requires less time to get digested) in Ayurveda.

For restoration of *agni*, it is also important that *agni* be given a chance to recover on its own by providing it a period of rest. This can be approached through a reduction in daily calorie intake in comparison to the presumptive expenditure. A relative negative energy balance for few days is proposed to help elimination of stored junks within the tissue, thereby making the system more clean. Ayurveda approaches to relative negative energy balance through *laghvasana* (less food intake) and *langhana* (fasting). Interestingly, both of these approaches are considered as cornerstones of *Amavata* management in Ayurveda. Interestingly, beneficial effects of fasting and vegetarian diet upon markers of rheumatoid arthritis are now been identified through many researches including the systematic reviews [26–30].

A reduction in *ama* production should also be approached through reduction of intakes which are *ama* promotive. *Viruddha ahara* and *snigdha ahara* are such intakes which themselves are *ama* promotive. They thereby are required to be reduced. An observation of reduced symptom intensity among rheumatoid arthritis patients consuming a vegetarian diet substantiates this management approach [26–29]. Activities which are *ama* promotive should also be reduced at the same time when we are trying to reduce *ama* through dietary corrections. A sedentary lifestyle with minimum of physical activities or a stressful lifestyle where one is compelled to be involved in extraneous physical activities just after food intake should, therefore, also be avoided.

8.5.2 Reduction in Ama Internalization

Through the discussions of preceding parts of this chapter, we are aware that internalization of *ama* is primarily dependent upon architectural changes to the gut mucosa in reference to *mandagni* or stress. A reduction of *ama* internalization, thereby, can only be achieved if an architectural correction to gut mucosa is approached. To initiate with, this is important to avoid the factors like stress and *viruddha ahara* which may promote the mucosal destruction.

Besides this, the gut mucosa is also required to be provided with enough rest to get an opportunity to restore its deficits, if there are any. Conventionally, this is being done with the observance of *langhana* (fasting) or *lagvasana* (relative fasting).

8.5.3 Dissociation of Internalized Ama

Simultaneous to reduction in *ama* production and its internalization, among established cases of *Amavata*, we also required to deal with *ama* which is already internalized and has interacted with body tissue to generate noxious and adherent form of *ama*.

A dissociation of the macromolecular structures of *ama* into smaller fractions which independently may not have the adherence property of *ama* is commonly employed approach of Ayurveda to dismantle internalized macromolecular *ama*.

The herbs rich in *katu* (bitter), *tikta* (pungent taste), and *lavana* (salt) *rasa* (taste) are found good to offer dissociative effects to *ama*. Ayurvedic formulations offering *dipana* (ignition) and *pachana* (dissociation) effects are mainly composed of components which are predominant in these *rasa*.

A comprehensive management plan of *Amavata*, therefore, can be tailored around the idea of *ama* formation, its internalization, and its reaction to body tissue. Essentially, a reversal to *Amavata* pathology should also be sought to the same order.

An important thing which needs to be stressed at this juncture is the presumption of time which may be required to give an observable effect among *Amavata* patients through an Ayurvedic *Amavata* management protocol. We need to reiterate here about prospective etiopathogenesis and level of ama which might be present in individual cases. If there are no good reasons to produce explicit amount of *ama* and if the *agni* is not compromised, possibly the recovery may be faster in comparison to a person where there are ample opportunities for *ama* to surface because of preexisting *mandagni* added with dietary inputs promotive to *ama* production.

If *ama* is available in ample amount and has interacted well to the body tissue, it is obvious to think that this would take longer to be recovered in comparison to other conditions where *ama* remained less offensive. Furthermore, due to huge variability to the *ama*–tissue interaction, an *ama* produce may also be variable in terms of its dissociability. This gives us a reason to understand huge individual variation to Ayurvedic treatment response among *Amavata* patients.

To sum up, we need to reiterate that a management plan to *Amavata* should be confronted at various fronts simultaneously. Obviously and for this reason too, a management to *Amavata* is time-consuming and cumbersome, a phenomena which is routinely observed in the clinical practice of Ayurvedic rheumatology.

8.6 Conclusion

Rheumatoid arthritis in particular and various autoimmune arthritic conditions in general are still the big challenges to the human health-care system. *Amavata* in Ayurveda is conceptualized as a group of conditions marked predominantly by joint afflictions besides many other systemic manifestations. It is for this reason that *Amavata* is often placed parallel to what is understood about rheumatoid arthritis in modern medicine. Interestingly, it is not only their symptom resemblance but rather a pathogenesis too which gives us a clue to think for a common wisdom behind the understanding of autoimmune joint conditions within these two streams of health care. Ayurveda, since antiquity, argued for a gut initiative to *Amavata*, a phenomena explored only lately through the contemporary science. These explorations have dissected into the gut–joint interactions to find a feasibility of generating a joint disease in the future. It is found that architectural changes at gut epithelium are primarily responsible to many immunological changes in the body which may further initiate the process of more complex autoimmune reactions due to their properties of molecular mimicry and cross-reactivity. *Mandagni*, a beautiful elaboration of hypodigestive state from Ayurveda, further explains about possible architectural changes in gut lumen which subsequently may lead to a hypoenzymatic condition, a prerequisite to *ama* production. Ayurvedic management approach to *Amavata* comprehensively handles the issues individually involved in its pathogenesis. At this juncture, we can conclude that an evidence base to Ayurvedic management of *Amavata* is almost ripe on the conceptual grounds. It only requires to be tested clinically and experimentally to give it a more sharpened effect so as to offer a more pragmatic, dependable, reproducible, and biological approach to deal with various autoimmune joint conditions.

Deciphering the Ayurvedic attributes of a pathogenesis in tune to the contemporary knowledge is the foremost prerequisite of articulating a trustworthy Ayurvedic intervention protocol in any condition [31]. Making a hypothesis based upon classical thoughts and associating it judicially with contemporary knowledge serves as a foundation to an evidence-based synthesis. If sustained and subjected to rigorous methods of scientific enquiry, it may ultimately help in modulating evidence-based Ayurveda [32, 33]. *Amavata* exposition in this purview may prove to be a milestone in unearthing the ways of synthesizing evidence base to Ayurveda.

References

1. Rastogi S, Singh RH (1999) Identifying the stress area for future research in Ayurveda—a demographic study. New Approaches Med Health 6:20–28
2. Rastogi S, Hemchandra RR, Singh RH (2006) Institutional practice of Ayurvedic system of medicine: survey analysis to discuss the strategies for its optimal utilization. Ayush Tomorrow 1:1–19
3. Rastogi S (2009) Principles and practice of Ayurvedic rheumatology. Chaukhambha Sanskrit Pratishthan, Delhi
4. Rastogi S (2009) Special features of rheumatoid arthritis in patients visiting an Ayurvedic hospital. New Approaches Med Health 17:23–29
5. Malviya AN (1994) Prevalence of rheumatic diseases in India: results of a population survey. J Indian Rheum Assoc 2:13–17
6. Hicklin JA et al (1980) The effect of diet in rheumatoid arthritis. Clin Allergy 10:463
7. Panush RS et al (1986) Food induced arthritis. Arthritis Rheum 29:220–226
8. Kroker GP, Stroud RM, Marshall RT et al (1984) Fasting and rheumatoid arthritis, a multicentric study. Clin Ecol 2:137–144
9. Kremer J (1985) Effects of manipulation of dietary fatty acids on clinical manifestation of rheumatoid arthritis. Lancet 1:184–187
10. Darlington LG (1986) Placebo controlled, blind study of dietary manipulation therapy in rheumatoid arthritis. Lancet 1:236–238
11. Jenkins RT (1987) Increased intestinal permeability in patients with rheumatoid arthritis: as side effect of oral NSAID therapy? Br J Rheumatol 26:103–107
12. Baghel MS (2005) Researches in Ayurveda. Mridu Ayurvedic publication and sales, Jamnagar
13. Rastogi S (2009) Development of diagnostic criteria for Amavata: inferences from a clinical study. J Res Ayur Siddha 30:1–10
14. Upadhyaya YN (ed) (1993) Madhava Nidana. Chaukhambha Sanskrit Sansthan, Varanasi
15. Rastogi S, Singh RH, Ramchandani MH, Chiappelli F (2011) Global warming in 21st century: propositions from Ayurveda, a traditional health care system. In: Cossia JM (ed) Global warming in 21st century. Nova science publishing Inc, New York, pp 143–163

16. Bennett EJ, Tennant CG, Piesse C, Badcock CA, Kellow JE (1998) Level of chronic life stress predicts clinical outcome in irritable bowel syndrome. Gut 43:256–261
17. Soderholm JD, Perdue MH (2001) Stress and the gastrointestinal tract II. Stress and intestinal barrier function. Am J Physiol Gastrointest Liver Physiol 280:G7–G13
18. Cordain L, Toohey L, Smith MJ, Hickey MS (2000) Modulation of immune function by dietary lectins in rheumatoid arthritis. Br J Nutr 83:207–217
19. Hvatum M, Kanerud L, Hallgren R, Brandtzaeg P (2006) The gut joint axis: cross reactive food antibodies in rheumatoid arthritis. Gut 55:1240–1247
20. Liener IE (1986) Nutritional significance of lectins: properties, functions and applications in biology and medicine. Academic, Orlando
21. Pusztai A (1993) Dietary lectins are metabolic signals for the gut and modulate immune and hormone functions. Eur J Clin Nutr 47:691–699
22. Sjolander A, Magnusson KE, Latkovik S (1986) Morphological changes of rat small intestine after short time exposure to concanavalin A or wheat germ agglutinin. Cell Struct Funct 11:285–293
23. Sjolander A, Magnusson KE, Latkovik S (1984) The effect of concanavalin A or wheat germ agglutinin on the ultrastructure and permeability of rat intestine. Int Arch Allergy Appl Immunol 75:230–236
24. Tripathi BN (ed) (1991) Charaka Samhita, Sutra Sthana 26/81. Chaukhambha orientalia, Varanasi
25. Albani S, Carson DA (1996) A multistep molecular mimicry hypothesis for the pathogenesis of rheumatoid arthritis. Immunol Today 17:466–470
26. Kjeldsen-Kragh J, Haugen M, Borchgrevink CF, Laerum E, Eek M, Mowinkel P, Hovi K, Forre O (1991) Controlled trial of fasting and one-year vegetarian diet in rheumatoid arthritis. Lancet 338:899–902
27. Kjeldsen-Kragh J, Mellbye OJ, Haugen M, Mollnes TE, Hammer HB, Sioud M, Forre O (1995) Changes in laboratory variables in rheumatoid arthritis patients during a trial of fasting and one-year vegetarian diet. Scand J Rheumatol 24:85–93
28. Fujita A, Hashimoto Y, Nakahara K, Tanaka T, Okuda T, Koda M (1999) Effects of a low calorie vegan diet on disease activity and general conditions in patients with rheumatoid arthritis [article in Japanese]. Rinsho Byori 47:554–560
29. Muller H, de Toledo FW, Resch KL (2001) Fasting followed by vegetarian diet in patients with rheumatoid arthritis: a systematic review. Scand J Rheumatol 30:1–10
30. Michalsen A, Weidenhammer W, Melchart D, Langhorst J, Saha J, Dobos G (2002) Short-term therapeutic fasting in the treatment of chronic pain and fatigue syndromes—well-being and side effects with and without mineral supplements [article in German]. Forsch Komplementarmed Klass Naturheilkd 9:221–227
31. Mashelkar RA (2008) Second World AAyurveda Congress (Theme: Ayurveda for the Future)—Inaugural Address: Part I. Evid Based Complement Altern Med 5:243–245. doi:10.1093/ecam/nen014
32. Valiathan MS, Thatte U (2010) Ayurveda: the time to experiment. Int J Ayur Res 1:3
33. Vaidya AB, Raut AA (2006) Evidences based Ayurveda sorting fact from fantasy. In: Ayurveda and its scientific aspects—opportunities for globalisation. Department of AYUSH and C. S. I. R, New Delhi, pp 1–39

Chapter 9
Ayurvedic Approach to Cardiovascular Diseases: Delineating the Literary and Clinical Evidences

Sanjeev Rastogi, Rajiv Rastogi, and P.S. Srivastav

9.1 Introduction

Ayurveda is a comprehensive, traditional health care wisdom rooting from Indian subcontinent and witnessing a global reach in the contemporary world. This global reach of traditional health care wisdom in general is consequential to the submission of inefficiency observed by and large of conventional health care models in finding efficient cures to various age and lifestyle-related disorders and also to various idiopathic illnesses where the causes and subsequently the cures are not truly straightforward. Conventional health care model, as a result, is compelled to go for a restructuring to its own dictums of disease interventions for inclusion of more naive, comprehensive, docile, dependable, ecofriendly, sustainable, human, and real-life solutions within its own ambit of disease understanding and management. Standing close to its literal meaning (*ayu* = life, *veda* = discipline of study or knowledge, a more appropriate English translation of Ayurveda could be vivo-logy), Ayurveda, through a conglomeration of various nature-driven preventive and curative approaches referring to human health comes as a natural ally to join conventional medical science for providing a more comprehensive care to humanity. Eventually, this comprehensive approach not only cares for physical health but also equally cares to mental, social, and spiritual components of health which are integral to total quality of life (TQL) determination in toto [1].

A quest of being healthy and subsequently to look for the causes and cures of diseases is as old as the origin of human. Initiated subsequent to this natural quest,

S. Rastogi (✉) • P.S. Srivastav
PG Department of Kaya Chikitsa, State Ayurvedic College, Lucknow University, Lucknow, Uttar Pradesh, India
e-mail: rastogisanjeev@rediffmail.com

R. Rastogi
Department of Ayush, Central Council for Research in Yoga and Naturopathy, MOH&FW, New Delhi, India

S. Rastogi (ed.), *Evidence-Based Practice in Complementary and Alternative Medicine*, 159
DOI 10.1007/978-3-642-24565-7_9, © Springer-Verlag Berlin Heidelberg 2012

a process of information accumulation through continuous experimentation and observation of natural processes was observed throughout the ages. In early Vedic periods (*Atharvaveda* circa 1500 BC), this knowledge accumulation took the shape of a more defined discipline of study which was further refined and enriched in early historic period marked by the exponential growth of various philosophical schools throughout the globe [2, 3]. Passing through a history of over 3,500 years, Ayurveda, besides few other indigenously derived medicines, still caters to the need of over 80% of domestic population in India [4] and also comprises a major traditional health care approach among many Asian countries [5].

9.2 Fundamentals of Health and Disease: The Ayurvedic Perspectives

Contrary to many other medical systems, talking exclusively about diseases and their management as a mean to restore health, Ayurveda has its own approach of considering preservation of health as its primary motive. Subsequently, it has paid a considerable attention to understand what the health is and how this can be preserved by observing some simple protocols. While talking about human health, Ayurveda simultaneously has a purely individualistic approach by linking the subtle details of human prakriti (constitution) to disease propensity and prognosis besides having a composite approach of linking microcosm with macrocosm through its unity of individual and cosmos principle (*loka-purusha samya* theory) [6]. Ayurvedic health care fundamentals can principally be grouped as (1) those defining the dynamic interaction between macrocosm and microcosm and (2) those defining the vital activities of an individual body.

9.2.1 Conceptualizing a Reciprocal Relation Between Macrocosm with Microcosm: Theory of Loka-Purusha Samya

A conceptualization of *lok* (universe), *purush* (individual), and *samya* (resemblance) is an Ayurvedic dictum which seeks multiple applications to living systems besides its application to health and disease. Man is considered as a miniature replica of cosmos with all its essential constituents and functions. The constituent elements of the universe and those of the smaller universe within the human body are identical, and their responses to varied stimuli are also identical. Ayurvedic theory of origin of life, which largely is a derivative of *Sankhya* school of thought, considers the life as a culmination of *A-vyakta* (invisible) building material into more *vyakta* (visible) forms through a directed process of condensation and combination of various primary elements called as *mahabhuta*. Owing to the limitation of human perception, these *mahabhuta* are counted to be five and are perceived through their special attributes by special senses. This idea of origin of life has become the basis of theory of *panchamahabhuta* which established every living or nonliving constituted of the same primary elements where a proportional difference among these elements in different objects defining differentiating physical or physiological features. It is this identity of composition which underlies the central dogma of Ayurvedic therapeutics that mandates a selective choice of food and drugs for a desired effect of health maintenance to diseases cure [7]. It was believed that this principle could hardly operate in the absence of perceived similarity between the substances in the external and internal to man. The man and the cosmos here look to be in an energy-based dynamic relation where the flow is directed from higher to lower levels [2].

9.2.2 *Prakriti*: The Basis for Being in Health or Disease

Expanding its dictum of origin of life, Ayurveda proposes every individual to be composed of a specific set and subset of *panch bhautic* components. Every set specific to an individual is thought to be determined genetically (as per the *panch bhautic* predominance in sperm and ova) with partial influences of maternal nutrition, age of mother, and environmental factors. Individual vital attributes and subsequently its socioeconomic gains are proposed largely to be determined by the primary set of *panch mahabhut* of an individual called as *prakriti*. This is further proposed that to be in health, this is important to maintain the primary set of five elements balanced, and therefore, a regimen of diet and routine is important to be observed. Any imbalance incriminated deliberately or casually leads to imbalance and subsequently to disease. A principle of treatment in this respect is as simple as the eruption of the disease is. This is to observe the means which can help reestablish the lost balance. Ayurveda has laid huge importance upon diet and routine for the proposed pathogenesis of a disease or as a requisite for being in health. Fundamentally, it is owing to their five elemental propositions, but can we make some further scientific inferences through these abstract principles? A differential expression of genes is known to influence human health and behavior. How a differential five elemental composition may find a place through expression of differential vital characteristics of an individual is interesting to be explored in light of theory of differential gene expression. We also know about epigenetic principles explaining for environmental and dietary influences upon differential gene expression. This would be interesting to see further if the Ayurvedic idea of preserving ones *prakriti* to remain in health has any relation with differential expression or suppression of genes through various dietary and environmental means. Evidences are accumulating to find *prakriti* association to some specific genetically determined metabolic regulators which finally determine the fate of ingested food and, subsequently, their effects upon body [6, 8].

Table 9.1 Correlating functional attributes to *mahabhuta* and *tridosha*

Functional attributes	*Mahabhuta*	*Dosha*
Transport	*Akash, vayu*	*Vata*
Disintegration	*Agni*	*Pitta*
Synthesis	*Jala, prithvi*	*Kapha*

9.2.3 Intervening in a Disease: Identifying the Pathology and Determining the Tools of Intervention

As vital manifestations are said to be the mandates of *prakriti* and, in turn, to be of *panchamahabhuta,* a *prakriti* or eventually a compositional imbalance could possibly be identified by observing the anomalies of vital functions and by contrasting them to the functions of the same individual in health. Principal functions of a living unit, i.e., transport, disintegration, and synthesis, are proposed to be the attributes of different *mahabhuta* (Table 9.1). As per their functional specificity, these are further called as *tridosha (vata, pitta,* and *kapha*), determining a specific set of function ruled by a specific set of *mahabhuta.* By identifying the subtle changes in functional attributes, an abnormal status of *mahabhuta* could be known. This is how a diagnosis is proposed to be made in Ayurveda. An anomaly of *mahabhuta* can either be in the form of excess or deficit; therefore, the restoration is inclined toward making a rebalance through countering or supplementing the incriminated one. As an offshoot to the *panchabhautic* theory, establishing an identical composition to every substance, every substance was further identified as a potential medicine. This is subsequent to the identification of an elemental imbalance as cause of disease and elemental predominance among various substances of cosmos including herbs, minerals, metals, and animal derivatives.

Within the huge repertory of nature, which substance for which disease? This was yet to be determined before an intervention could truly be made. An elemental predominance of herbs or nonliving substances is not possible to be identified through their vital functions. Therefore, it required an attribute which may truly be representative to the elemental composition of the object at one hand with a clear perceptibility through conventional senses on the other. Intercepting beautifully at this stage, Ayurveda proposes a novel idea of identifying elemental composition and thereby the pharmacological properties of a substance by its taste (Table 9.2). *Rasa* (taste) as the principal attribute from a substance, further supplemented with *guna* (quality), *virya* (potency), *vipaka* (aftertaste), and *prabhava,* determines the pharmacological properties of a substance. Eventually, a drug choice in Ayurveda is made as per the elemental imbalances leading to symptoms and choosing the substance supposed to make the elemental rebalance to restore health. An elemental basis to taste and subsequently to its pharmacology has remained a subject of debate in modern pharmacology. Brunton (1985) proposed an atomic weight basis to the taste by observing that similar tastes are produced by combinations which contain elements such as lithium, sodium, and potassium, showing a periodic recurrence of

Table 9.2 *Rasa* and its elemental composition

Rasa	Elemental composition
Madhura	*Jala, prithvi*
Amla	*Prithvi, agni*
Lavana	*Jala, agni*
Katu	*Vayu, agni*
Tikta	*Vayu, akasha*
Kashaya	*Vayu, prithvi*

ordinary physical properties. Among the carbon compounds, those which produce similar tastes are found to contain a common "group" of elements. Thus, organic acids contain the group COOH, the sweet substances $CH_2{\cdot}OH$ [9]. A proposal of Ayurveda for an identical composition behind an identical taste therefore cannot easily be overruled. Further convincing evidences regarding the relation of taste and its pharmacology were proposed by observation of similar pharmacological properties to similar tasting substances [10, 11].

9.3 Cardiovascular Diseases: Ayurvedic Viewpoint

Ayurvedic classics present an elaborate description of cardiovascular system and the diseases originating through it. Interestingly, while talking about possible etiologies to cardiovascular diseases, a substantial stress has been laid upon stress-inducing factors, and therefore its avoidance through observation of a righteous conduct is promoted as an important intervention to cardiac diseases.

9.3.1 Cardiovascular System: Anatomic-Physiological Correlates in Ayurveda

Hridaya, the Ayurvedic synonym for heart (derived from the Sanskrit word *hrit,* having an epistemological resemblance to heart), is defined as an organ which has a capacity to receive and to disburse [12]. Enumerated as an organ, it is further said to be a place of vitality and consciousness by its consideration among ten vital places of body (*das pranaytananani*). Describing its gross anatomy, *Sushruta* resembles it with inverted lotus having a property of expansion and shrinkage during work and rest similar to the changing diurnal dimension of lotus flower and also projecting arch of aorta from apex similar to the peduncle of lotus flower [13] (Fig. 9.1).

Extending further within the description of system, a heart is said to be an organ where ten composite openings either in the form of arteries (*mahamula*) or veins (*mahaphala*) exist. A circulation in human body is said to exist at three stages

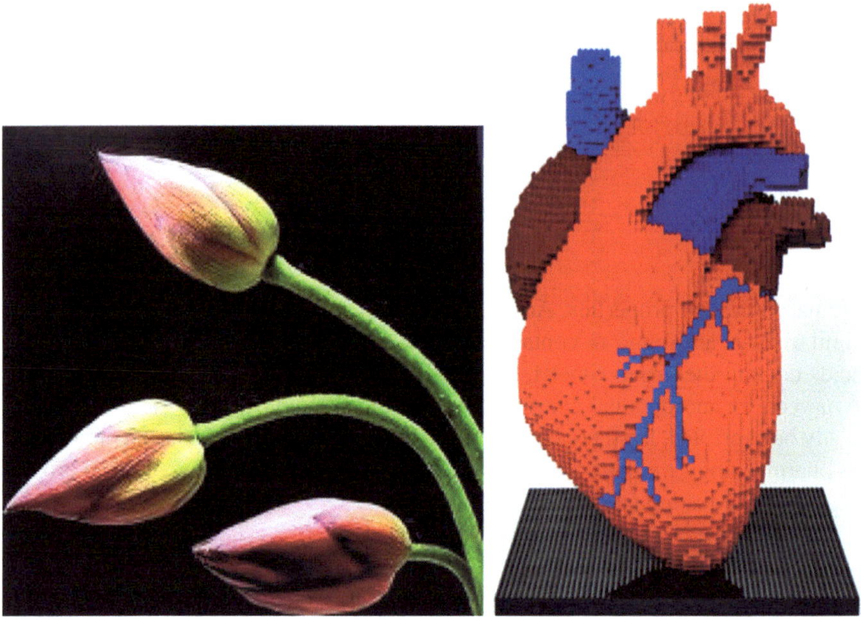

Fig. 9.1 Inverted lotus and its resemblance to anatomical features of heart as described in Ayurveda (With permission from Nathan Sawaya, The art of the brick, downloaded from http://www.brick-artist.com/contact.html downloaded on 18 Aug 2010)

Table 9.3 Three primary vessels, their functions and resemblance to conventional vascular structures

Primary vessel	Function	Resembling conventional vascular structure
Dhamani	Circulation through active pumping	Artery
Srotas	Percolation of blood through secretion	Capillary
Sira	Passive circulation of blood	Vein

through three distinct vessels, namely, *dhamani* (the one which pumps to make the flow of blood), *srotas* (the one which percolates blood), and *sira* (the one which slips the blood). This directional flow of blood as described in Ayurveda has a good resemblance to that of modern artery-capillary-vein circulation (Table 9.3).

Heart is said to be the place of *oja* (vital essence) which is perceived as nutrients flowing in blood. As heart pumps the blood throughout the body, it is also pumping *oja,* and hence, the vessels coming out from this are also called as *ojovaha* (*vaha* = permitting to flow). Heart is further said to be the seat of activities of whole body, brain, sense organs, and their perceptions for essentiality of a good circulation to ensure these all (*Charaka Samhita Sutra Sthana* 30/5).[1]

[1]Shadangama angamvigyanam indriyadyartha panchakam/Atma cha sagunashchetashchintyaam cha hridi sanshritam//charaka samhita sutra sthana 30/5.

Considering this importance, heart in Ayurveda is considered as a *marma* (vital seat) where a trauma, either blunt or invading, can result in syncope or even death (Ch.Su.30/6).[2]

The pumping action of heart is performed by *vyan vayu* which results in blood circulation to nourish the tissues (*dhatus*). The heart and the arteries along with the *buddhi, indriya,* and *mana* are under the control of *prana vayu* (A.S.Su20).

9.3.2 Diseases of Heart

This is important to appreciate in the beginning only that a disease classification in Ayurveda carries a syndromic approach where in case of obscurity of the pathogenesis, the symptoms and signs form the basis of a disease nomenclature. In Ayurveda, it is the generalization and not the obscurity of the pathogenesis which forms the basis of this approach. A disease name in Ayurveda therefore, in no way, stands parallel to what is understood in modern medicine in terms of pathogenesis to a similar name. This distinct style of Ayurvedic disease description warrants for two important inferences. The first is that a disease as described in Ayurveda may not be taken granted for a disease in conventional understanding merely on the basis of their nomenclature resemblance. The other and clinically more important inference is that a disease entity description in Ayurveda, if it is seen from conventional perspectives, is not limited to the specified disease chapter of ancient Ayurvedic text books but is available in a scattered form to many other places.

As Ayurvedic disease nomenclature is primarily focused on presenting symptom or the site of symptoms, a disease from modern perspective because of multiplicity of symptoms may find its description in multiple chapters in Ayurveda focusing upon specific symptoms. Referring this to heart disease, we find that a description of heart disease from modern perspective is not limited to the chapter of *Hrida Roga* in Ayurveda, but instead, it is widely scattered through the description of *shvasa, hicca, shotha*, and *pandu* also besides its primary description available within the cognizance of *hrida roga*.

9.3.2.1 General Causes of *Hrida Roga*

Among various causes identified to precipitate a heart disease, most appreciable ones as per Ayurveda are *vyayama* (excessive exercise), *tikshna ahara* (pungent diet), excessive use of *virechana* (purging), *vasti* (medicated enema), or *vamana* (emesis). Some primary diseases leading to emaciation, excessive worry, stress, fear, and a direct trauma to heart may also lead to a heart disease. By observing the

---

[2]Tasyopaghatanmurchayam bhedan marana mricchati/yadwi tata sparshavigyanam dhari tattatra samshritam//charaka samhita, Sutra sthana 30/6.

enumerated causes of heart diseases as are appreciated in Ayurveda, this is easy to infer that Ayurveda considers the etiological factors in reference to practical manifestation of a disease. A pathological understanding follows only to this primary observation. For causes described here as a reason to heart disease, most are concerned with water and nutrition depletion from the body either though an excessive loss (*vaman, virechana, vasti,* excessive exercise, trauma) or a reduced intake (emaciation, stress, fear, worry). All these causes ultimately lead to a depletive state where the functions of the heart (Sect. 8.3.1) are not adequately met, hence mimicking a heart disease. This is difficult to find that if among these many causes, anyone can essentially and finally qualify to terminate into a real cardiac pathology. This is also important to observe that contrary to contemporary understanding of risk factors to cardiac diseases, besides psychological factors, Ayurveda does not mention any other factor in its vivid list of etiology to heart diseases. Of most important among all is the nonobservance of obesity and dietary excess from the list of risk factor to heart disease among descriptions of Ayurveda. This important observation raises a question against the linking of fundamental understanding of heart disease in both the streams of medicine. This puts further emphasis to our previous connotation of Ayurvedic descriptions for being more functional compared to the modern understanding which is primarily pathological. This fundamental difference to the understanding of etiopathogenesis of heart disease in both the streams of medicine forms the basis to their differential approach which is often contrasting to each other. Contrary to the modern approach of treating heart disease which is marked by a salt, oil, and fat reduction, Ayurvedic medicaments used in this condition are predominantly marked by an excess of salt, oil, and fat.

9.3.2.2 Type of *Hrida Roga* in Ayurveda

Ayurveda identifies five distinct kinds of heart diseases as per their clinical description. This disease classification is essentially the etiological classification where the symptoms originating as result of some specific cause are grouped under the head of disease. As per the *doshic* distinction of causes, the heart diseases of Ayurveda can either be grouped as that caused by independent causations (*vata, pitta,* and *kapha*) or a combination (*tridoshaja*) or else as a complication (*krimija*). Heart disease description as is given in Ayurveda has a thorough resemblance to many typical presentations available to conventional cardiac diseases. Therefore, this would be of worth to explore the Ayurvedic presentation of cardiac diseases with their possible correlates in modern science. Among all, *vataja* and *krimija hrida roga* have special resemblance to modern understanding of angina and infarction, respectively.

Vataja Hrida Roga

A *vataja hrida roga* is proposed to be precipitated by grief, fasting, exercise, and dry, less, and zero-oil foods. Presenting symptoms are trembling or tightening around heart, loss of consciousness, lack of responsiveness, or rigidity. The pain perceived is of greater intensity (*Charaka Samhita Sutra Sthana* 17/30–31).[3] A *vataja hrida roga* presentation as is given in Ayurveda has a typical resemblance to the unstable or stable angina presentations which may be precipitated through a variety of mechanisms including factors promoting catecholamine secretions and consequently increasing myocardial oxygen demand [14]. Various etiological factors described in *vataja hrida roga* satisfy to this proposition of mechanism for precipitation of angina pain.

Krimija Hrida Roga

Charaka has given a very elaborate description of pathogenesis in *krimija hrida roga,* its possible clinical presentation and prognosis. A heart disease when composed of all three possible *doshas* (*tridoshaja*) and a person having such a disease (the one who has angina), if indulges ignorantly in repeated consumption of *til* (sesame), milk and its products (*kshira*), and *guda* (raw sugar) or like substances, develops some outgrowths (*granthi*) within arteries of the heart. These outgrowths gradually, while being in touch with nutritional part of blood (rasa), liquify. This liquified portion of outgrowth gives rise to the growth of various worms which eat up the heart (*Charaka Samhita, Sutra Sthana.* 17/37–40). This description of Ayurveda regarding pathogenesis of *krimij hrida roga* has a striking resemblance to the pathogenesis of evolution of atheroma, development of a lipid-rich necrotic center of atheromatous lesion, and plaque rupture to develop microthrombi or large occlusive or nonocclusive mural thrombi [15]. In case of occlusion of thrombi to an arterial lumen, it leads to the development of infarction. Symptoms caused by *krimija hrida roga* are said to be of acute onset, difficult to manage, and characterized by severe pain often of piercing or cutting nature and requiring urgent management. These features are further having a resemblance to acute myocardial infarction presentations as it is understood to modern science.

9.3.2.3 Preventing Heart Diseases: Ayurvedic Wisdom

Considering its importance as a vital organ which governs the systemic circulation, Ayurveda pays a special attention to save the heart from trauma directly or indirectly and also from various factors which may in turn become a precipitation factor for various heart diseases. Surprisingly, while advising for care to heart, *Charaka* further says to save cardiac arteries too through observation of certain do's and don'ts. It is said to avoid various stress-causing factors and to effortfully promote

[3]Shokopavasavyayamarukshashushkaalpa bhojanai/vayuravishya hridayam janayatuttama rujam// Vepathu veshtanam stambha pramoha shunyata dara/hradi vatature rupam jeerne cha atyarthavedana//Charaka samhita Sutra Sthana 17/30–31.

the consumption of substances which are cardiopromotive and thereby helping in the maintenance of normal integration of cardiac vessels. An *amla* (sour) taste in general is considered as cardioprotective. Endorsing it further, *Charaka* has identified a group of ten natural substances which are predominantly sour in taste under *hridya* (cardioprotective) division. Without making a convincing remark, this is interesting to find ASA (acetyl salicylic acid) as a cardioprotective primarily because of its antiplatelet aggregation substance. Incidentally, ASA happens to be a week acid having a clear sour taste. While talking about pathogenesis in *krimija hrida roga, Charaka* has stressed the people who, despite of having a *hrida roga,* still indulge in consuming substances like sesame, milk, and sugar-rich substances as more prone for *krimija hrida roga*. This description is much similar to the current-day dietary instructions which are required to prevent a heart disease.

At this point, Charak's wisdom for prevention of cardiovascular diseases is worth mentioning, "One who wishes to protect his heart (*mahat*), arteries (*mahamoolas*) and vitality (*ojas*) should avoid the causes which produce grieved mood and perform intentionally with the diets and doings which are *hriddya* (cardio protective), *ojasya* (vitality raising) and *srotas prasadanam* (pleasing to channels). They should follow a calm (*prasham*) and self investigating (*gyanam*) life style" (C.Su.30/13–14).

9.3.2.4 Treating Heart Diseases: Ayurvedic Principles

Besides advocating for various measures to prevent heart diseases through careful observance of certain cardio supportive acts, Ayurveda further describes a few pharmacological interventions to deal with *vataja* and *krimija hrida roga*. This is evident through a literary review that rock salt (*saindhava lavana*), sour substances, *shunthi* (zingiber), and *pushkara mula* (inula root) are fairly taken up as a dependable component of heart disease management in Ayurveda. Besides this, a use of sesame oil or *ghrit* (purified butter) processed with herbs is also often recommended as a respite. A carefully designed and customized *shodhana* (biopurification) is also recommended for heart disease. Fasting and use of digestives following a *shodhana* are advocated in *krimija hrida roga.*

9.4 Contemporary Evidences for Ayurvedic Therapy to Various Cardiological Conditions

9.4.1 Evidences Through Classical Researches

Despite of its contemporary importance, an Ayurvedic description of cardiac disease has rarely been subjected to a critical analysis. In the absence of a clear correlation with heart diseases from conventional point of view and with that of

Ayurveda, it is difficult to apply convincingly the medicine described in one text to the notion it is perceived by another. In a broader sense, Ayurvedic description of heart diseases seems not limited to the diseases of heart but, instead, encompasses a broad range of conditions in and around heart and also the pathologies directly or indirectly affecting the function of heart. It is for this reason, many conditions where primary pathology is a circulatory deficit are also considered as *hrida roga* in Ayurveda.

Many attempts have been made to correlate various Ayurvedic *hrida roga* conditions to their modern parallels. Because of inadequacy to their research models, none however could reach to a conclusive submission.

Researches in cardiac diseases in reference to the exploration of efficacy of individual compounds and comparative effectiveness research to multidrug therapy had been attempted primarily at various postgraduate research institutes of Ayurveda in India. These researches are by and large exploratory throughout the country and are limited to find clinical effect of certain compounds in certain cardiac conditions. In spite of their genuine focus upon exploratory analysis of various Ayurvedic compounds for their possible clinical utility, in lack of good research protocols, it could not contribute to growth of *hrida roga* understanding in Ayurveda. The other part of the research at the same time was done by biomedical scientists who worked with one or few isolated herbal isolates for their possible effects upon established cardiac pathologies.

Conditions commonly approached by Ayurvedic research institute in India for their research in cardiology were hypertension, congestive heart failure, hyperlipidemia, and ischemic heart disease. These conditions were tried to be treated with various classical Ayurvedic compounds either as a pilot, a control, and a combination treatment protocol.

Unavailability of these researches conducted at various research institutes of Ayurveda in India is another problem which interferes with making of a systematic review based upon researches conducted at various places in India. Most of these works are in the form of doctoral or postdoctoral research works and are available only through a physical search. Following are the glimpses of works done at State Ayurvedic College, Lucknow, India, where the postgraduate researches in Ayurveda are conducted for over 35 years.

In initial studies, congestive heart failure was tried with *hridaya chintamani rasa, satavarjunadi yoga,* and *arjunadi kashaya.* In few controlled studies, the results were found comparable to and not better than control, which was the standard regimen of digoxin in most studies [16–18].

In a study on hyperlipidemia with *arogyavardhini*, an Ayurvedic herbometallic compound, a comparison was made to *arogyavardhini* where metallic components were removed. The study reported a substantial reduction to serum cholesterol level among patients treated, however no significant difference among both variety of *arogyavardhini* either with or without metal [19].

Studies upon hypertension were largely conducted in the pilot form. Trials conducted with *sarpagandhadi yoga* are marked with inconsistent reports of inconclusive findings [20] to a significant fall in blood pressure [21]. Further reports upon hypertension with *jatamansi yoga* and alcoholic extract of *Coleus forskohlii* Briq root observed significant blood pressure reduction in trial [22–24]; however, in some studies, a contrary results have also been observed [25]. A further work upon ischemic heart disease in 1988 through *pushkar brahmi guggul* as the trial drug could not find any noticeable results [26].

9.4.2 Evidences Through Biomedical Researches

There are no clinical trials listed at NIH in reference to Ayurvedic treatment proposal to any cardiological condition [27]. Similarly, till date, there are no Cochrane reviews enlisted in the Cochrane Library in reference to Ayurvedic therapy in cardiac disease [28]. A Pubmed search for "Ayurveda and cardiovascular disease" as search words identified ten entries. Among them, however, none qualified to be identified as evidence to Ayurvedic interventions in cardiovascular disease [29]. This observation found cardiology as a naive subject of research in Ayurveda from contemporary point of view.

An advent of reserpine in India as an active component from *sarpagandha* (*Rauwolfia serpentina*), and its successful use in reducing the blood pressure, initially tried to bring Ayurveda from folklore to biomedical laboratories. As early as in 1931, Bose and Sen reported antihypertensive effects of *sarpagandha*, a herb known to Ayurveda since centuries for its traditional use in mania and psychosis [30]. Its therapeutic effect to mania was later presumed to be an attribution to its blood pressure–reducing capacity. A further interest to reserpine however lost to the observations of intractable depression following its regular use until it is renewed recently, when observation of more clear mechanism of its action is made.

Terminalia arjuna has been another herb from Ayurveda which attracted sufficient attention of biomedical scientist for its possible favorable actions upon various cardiac pathologies. Bharani (1995) in a double-blind, placebo-controlled crossover study upon effect of Terminalia bark extract upon patients of refractory congestive heart failure shown the stable improvement in symptoms and signs of heart failure along with improvement in left ventricular ejection-phase indices with definite improvement in quality of life [31]. *Terminalia arjuna* has also been favorably investigated for its antioxidant and hypocholesterolemic effects in a randomized placebo-controlled trial. This study found antioxidant effects of *arjuna* equivalent to vit. E [32]. Arjuna bark has also been investigated for its possible role in chronic stable angina in another double-blind, placebo-controlled crossover study [33]. An antiplatelet action to arjuna bark has also been reported recently [34].

Commiphora wightii (*guggulu*) is another commonly used Ayurvedic herb resin which has been extensively researched for its antihyperlipidemic actions. A monograph of all the major citations of its use has been published [35]. Satyavati, Dwarakanath, Sukhdev, and Nityanand have extensively studied the hypolipidemic effect of *C. wightii*. The product has also been marketed and widely used [36, 37]. The side effects of the plant have also been documented. The mechanism of its toxicity, however, is yet to be ascertained.

9.5 Future of Research in Ayurvedic Cardiology

What is the evidence basis to use of Ayurvedic drugs in various cardiac and related conditions? When we ask this question to ourselves, we are sure to find a million of questions unanswered, a thousand of them unattempted, and only a handful approaches moving in the direction of real evidence-based practice. Ayurvedic practice of medicine is largely based upon certain key principles of identifying a pathogenesis and corresponding offers toward its management. Ayurveda elaborates beautifully to the concepts of health and disease by their exposition through theory of *panchamahabhuta* and *tridosha*. It further identifies an intricate interrelationship between microcosm and macrocosm and explores their possible interaction toward health and disease. Ayurveda further elaborates admirably the clinical sign and symptoms to most clinical entities as are known today. On the contrary, a pathogenesis (*samprapti*), in reference to specific clinical entities, is rather poorly understood to a critical mind and so is its treatment approach.

A therapy in Ayurveda is proposed to occur in two principal ways:

1. *Dosha pratyaneek*: A treatment based upon logics of pathogenesis and its management through identification of the drugs which logically act against the actual pathogenesis
2. *Vyadhi pratyaneek*: A treatment based upon direct action of a drug upon certain clinical entity without taking a note for the pathogenesis of the disease and pharmacological properties of the drug from Ayurvedic perspective

A rationality of the former application can be drawn in clinical practice if the pathogenesis and the pharmacological action of a drug are previously known. This forms the evidence base to the selection of a drug in a particular condition as per Ayurvedic principles. It is in this context, must also be noted, that any approach which utilizes the former principle of choosing a drug in a particular condition should also require to take an account of any variability of drug actions in reference to their contemporary availability. Needless to say, any deviation to pathology status from the one that is classically drawn should also be taken into account.

The other approach of a disease management in Ayurveda requires more rigorous evidences to prove its worth. Various medicines in Ayurveda are described to work through their *prabhava* (special action). In these drugs, an Ayurvedic pharmacological rationale to their usage cannot be established. This is easy to find that in the absence of pharmacological rationales, establishment of their clinical efficacy is the single largest prerequisite justifying their uses. We can easily find that this can be done only through rigorous clinical trial of the drugs commonly used in Ayurveda on the basis of their *prabhava*.

Talking specific to cardiovascular diseases, Ayurveda needs to work at many fronts simultaneously. It requires to find what is the actual relationship between *hrida roga* and contemporary understanding of cardiac diseases. It also has to identify what is the rationale of identifying various etiological factors crucial to the birth of a *hrida roga*. Similarly, it has to find the rationale of advocating various oil-, fat-, and salt-rich preparations in context to heart diseases especially when the same are considered as the risk factors to the same clinical conditions by contemporary medical science.

Through the clinical experiences, various other herbs, like *karaveer* and *punarnava*, and minerals or metals, like *mandura*, have also been observed for their good effects upon cardiovascular system. These experiences are required to be enriched by proper documentations arriving through rigorous clinical trials to bring forth the undaunted evidences.

Besides active drug intervention, lifestyle modifications, stress reduction, and avoidance of precipitating factors have also been recognized globally for their potential to impede and even revert a cardiac pathogenesis. Interestingly, Ayurveda identifies lifestyle codes as one among its founding principles to assure a healthy life. *Charaka* has beautiful elaborations of the idea in the form of *achara rasayana* and through elaborations of qualifying conditions if someone wishes to remain healthy. These principles though in general are the rules of good living, at the same time they also have a potential for a disease reversal. It is particularly true in reference to cardiac diseases.

It at the same time should also be understood that a few Ayurvedic herbs have also been noted for their toxicological potential upon heart. Most notable herb among them is aconite (*vatsanabha*), a frequently used herb in Ayurvedic preparations having digestive and antipyretic properties. We have come across many case reports where a morbid cardiac arrhythmia is reported after consumption of aconite-containing Ayurvedic preparations [38, 39]. Without getting further into these reports to see who is guilty, the manufacturer, the prescriber, or the patient, we simply need to understand that there are potentially toxic drugs in Ayurveda in reference to their effect upon cardiovascular system, and thereby, a caution is required to be observed while prescribing them. This observation becomes more relevant when we see an ever-increasing use of CAM in conjunction with conventional medicine without getting them searched for potential herb-drug interactions. Cardiovascular diseases, for their increasing prevalence and also for their stable nature, offer more caution to be exercised in this regard [40, 41].

Cardiovascular morbidities are going to become the largest cause of morbidities to human population in near future [42]. This is supposed to amount second only to cancer. In light of currently observed epidemiological shift of diseases in a global perspective, where lifestyle, degenerative, and mutagenic pathologies are outreaching infective pathologies, conventional practices of medicine are largely found inadequate, and need of a pragmatic, human, natural, and close to real-life situation approach of medicine is directly felt [43]. Ayurveda having a potential to comply for this emerging void in practice of medicine, needs to be tested rigorously for its thoughtful, rationale, potential, and evidence-based use to serve what is most deserved at the time. Accumulating evidences about optimal medical therapy (OMT) including lifestyle modifications in cases of stable coronary diseases for their comparable effectiveness to invasive procedures like percutaneous coronary intervention (PCI) [44] are strong enough to persuade for thinking more seriously toward the lifestyle and natural alternatives to cardiovascular disease management. In one landmark trial, Manchanda et al. [45] found that Yoga lifestyle is a feasible and cost-effective intervention in patients with advanced coronary artery disease. Yogendra et al. [46] revealed that Yoga-based lifestyle modifications helped in regression of coronary lesions and in improving myocardial perfusion. Srivastava [47] noted a reduction of SBP, DBP, heart rate, and body fat%, total cholesterol, triglycerides, and LDL after regular yogic practices.

In light of accumulating evidences, both primary and secondary, Ayurveda, inclusive of yoga and naturopathy for its comprehensive and inclusive approach, seems to be a promising complement to the existing knowledge about cardiovascular diseases [48].

References

1. Rastogi S (2009) Ayurveda for comprehensive health care. Indian J Med Ethics 6:101–102
2. Valiathan MS (2009) An Ayurvedic view of life. Curr Sci 96:1186–1192
3. Singh RH (2010) Exploring larger evidence-base for contemporary Ayurveda. Int J Ayurveda Res 1:65–66
4. Kales SN, Saper RB (2009) Ayurvedic lead poisoning: an under-recognized, international problem. Indian J Med Sci 63:379–381
5. Traditional medicine. Downloaded from http://www.who.int/mediacentre/factsheets/fs134/en/. Accessed on 16 July 2011
6. Rastogi S, Chiappelli F (2010) Bringing evidence basis to decision making in Complementary and Alternative Medicine (CAM): Prakriti (constitution) analysis in Ayurveda. In: Chiappelli F, Caldeira Brant XM, Neagos N, Oluwadara OO, Ramchandani MH (eds) Evidence-based practice toward optimizing clinical outcomes. Springer, Berlin Heidelberg, pp 91–106
7. Rastogi S (2010) Building bridges between Ayurveda and modern science. Int J Ayurveda Res 1:41–46
8. Ghodke Y, Joshi K, Patwardhan B (2011) Traditional medicine to modern pharmacogenomics: Ayurveda Prakriti type and CYP2C19 gene poly morphism associated with the metabolic variability. Evid Based Complement Altern Med. Article ID 249528, DOI:10.1093/ecam/nep 206
9. Brunton TL (1885) A text-book of pharmacology, therapeutics and materia medica. Macmillan and Co., London
10. Beauchamp GK, Keast RS, Morel D, Lin J, Pika J, Han Q et al (2005) Breslin phytochemistry: ibuprofen-like activity in extra-virgin olive oil. Nature 437:45–46
11. Joshi K, Hankey A, Patwardhan B (2007) Traditional phytochemistry: identification of drug by 'taste'. Evid Based ComplementAltern Med 4:145–148
12. Tripathi BN (ed) (1983) Charaka Samhita Sutra Sthana 30/3. Chaukhambha Surbharti Prakashana, Varanasi

13. Shastri AD (ed) (2007) Sushruta Samhita, Sharira Sthana 4/31. Chaukhambha Sanskrit Sanssthana, Varanasi
14. Alaeddini J, Shirani J (2009) Anginapectoris. Downloaded from http://emedicine.medscape.com/article/150215-overviewAnginaPectoris/. Accessed on 17 July 2011
15. Davies MJ (1997) The composition of coronary artery plaques. N Engl J Med 336: 1312–1314
16. Yadav RK (1978) A clinical study of an indigenous compound on sannipataja hrida roga with special reference to congestive heart failure. M.D. thesis, SAC, Lucknow University, India
17. Birthray MK (1981) Clinical ayurvedic studies on congestive heart failure. M.D. thesis, SAC, Lucknow, India
18. Chandel PS (1983) Clinical classical studies and effect of herbal compounds (Arjunadi kashaya) on Hridaroga—Congestive cardiac failure., M.D. thesis, SAC, Lucknow University, India
19. Nigam RP (1981) A clinical trial of arogyavardhini (Herbal) in cases of raised rakta gata sneha (Hyperlipidaemia). M.D. thesis, SAC, Lucknow University, India
20. Dwivedi P (1983) Effect of sarpagandhadi yoga and savasana on hypertension with a comparative study to vyana prakop. M.D. thesis, SAC, Lucknow University, India
21. Raguvanshi K (1987) Clinical evaluation of sarpagandhadi compound on hypertension. M.D. thesis, SAC, Lucknow University, India
22. Srivastava VS (1985), Effect of jatamansyadi yoga on essential hypertension a clinical study. M.D. thesis, SAC, Lucknow University, India
23. Kumar R (1991) Further observation on the effect of alcoholic extract of coleus Forskohlii Briq root in cases of hypertension. M.D. thesis, SAC, Lucknow University, India
24. Jain JK (1988) Observation on the effect of alcoholic extract of Coleus forskohlii briq root in cases of hypertension. M.D. thesis, SAC, Lucknow University, India
25. Srivastav PS (1978) Therapeutic trial of Coleus forskohlii Briq (Changla jari) on the patients of systemic arterial hypertension. M.D. thesis, SAC, Lucknow University, India
26. Sharma H, Chandola HM, Singh G, Basisht G (2007) Utilisation of Ayurveda in Health care: An approach for prevention, health promotion and treatment of disease. Part 2-Ayurveda in primary health care. J Alt Comp Med 13:1135–1150
27. Clinical trials on Ayurveda. Available at http://clinicaltrials.gov/ct2/results?term=cardiovascu lar+diseases+and+Ayurveda+. Last accessed on 20 May 2011
28. Cochrane review on Ayurveda. Available at http://www.cochrane.org/search/site/cardiovascular%20disease%20and%20Ayurveda. Last accessed on 23 May 2011
29. Ayurveda and cardiovascular disease. Available at http://www.ncbi.nlm.nih.gov/pubmed. Last accessed on 17 Sept 2011
30. Sen G, Bose KC (1931) Rauwolfia serpentina, a new Indian drug for insanity and high blood pressure. Indian Med World 2:194
31. Bharani A, Ganguli A, Bhargava KD (1995) Salutary effect of *Terminalia Arjuna* in patients with severe refractory heart failure. Int J Cardiol l49:191–199
32. Gupta R, Singhal S, Goyle A, Sharma VN (2001) Antioxidant and hypocholesterolaemic effects of Terminalia arjuna tree-bark powder: a randomised placebo-controlled trial. J Assoc Physicians India 49:231–235
33. Bharani A, Ganguli A, Mathur LK, Jamra Y, Raman PG (2002) Efficacy of Terminalia arjuna in chronic stable angina: a double-blind, placebo-controlled, crossover study comparing Terminalia arjuna with isosorbide mononitrate. Indian Heart J 54:170–175
34. Malik N, Dhawan V, Bahl A, Kaul D (2009) Inhibitory effect of Terminalia arjuna on platelet activation in vitro in healthy subjects and in patients of coronary heart disease. Platelets 20:183–190
35. Apte V (1998) Monograph on *Guggul* and *Guggul kalpa* (monograph in Marathi). Mumbai
36. Satyavati GV, Dwarakanath C, Tripathi SN (1969) Experimental studies on the hypocholesterolemic effect of *Commiphora mukul* Engl (*Guggul*). Indian J Med Res 57:1950–1952
37. Nityanand S, Kapoor NK (1971) Hypocholesterolemic effect of *Commiphora mukul* resin (Guggal). Indian J Exp Biol 9:376–379

38. Rastogi S, Ranjana, Singh RH (2007) Adverse effects of Ayurvedic drugs: an overview of causes and possibilities in reference to a case of Vatsanabha (Aconite) overdosing. Int J Risk Saf Med 19:117–125
39. Dhesi P, Ng R, Shehata MM, Shah PK (2010) Ventricular tachycardia after ingestion of Ayurveda herbal antidiarrhoeal preparation containing aconitum. Arch Intern Med 170:303–305
40. Yeh GY, Davis RB, Phillips RS (2006) Use of complementary therapies in patients with cardiovascular disease. Am J Cardiol 98:673–680
41. Miller KL, Liebowitz RS, Newby LK (2004) Complementary and alternative medicine in cardiovascular disease: a review of biologically based approaches. Am Heart J 147:401–411
42. Available at http://www.cdc.gov/heartdisease/statistics.htm. Last accessed on 20 Nov 2010
43. Mamtani R, Mamtani R (2005) Ayurveda and yoga in cardiovascular diseases. Cardiol Rev 13:155–162
44. Boden WE, O'Rourke RA, Teo KK, Hartigan PM et al (2007) Optimal medical therapy with or without PCI for stable coronary disease. N Engl J Med 356:1503–1516
45. Manchanda SC, Narang R, Reddy KS, Sachdeva U, Prabhakaran D, Dharmanand S, Rajani M, Bijlani R (2000) Retardation of coronary atherosclerosis with yoga lifestyle intervention. J Assoc Physicians India 48:687–694
46. Yogendra J, Yogendra HJ, Ambardekar S, Lele RD, Shetty S, Dave M, Husein N (2004) Beneficial effects of yoga lifestyle on reversibility of ischemic heart disease: caring heart project of international board of yoga. J Assoc Physicians India 52:283–289
47. Pal A, Srivastava N, Tiwari S, Verma NS, Narain VS, Agrawal GG, Natu SM, Kumar K (2011) Effect of yogic practices on lipid profile and body fat composition in patients of coronary artery disease. Complement Ther Med 19:122–127
48. Rastogi R (2011) Naturopathic and yogic intervention in the management of coronary artery disease. Light Ayur J 10:49–54

Chapter 10
Rasayana Therapy and Rejuvenation

Ram Harsh Singh and Sanjeev Rastogi

10.1 Introduction: What Is Ayurveda?

Ayurveda is the oldest system of life science, health care, and cure originating from India. It is based on its own fundamental principles, diagnostics, and therapeutics. It makes a unique holistic approach to the understanding of the structure and function of the body including the pathology and its manifestations which is distinctly different than that conceived in conventional modern medical sciences. The ancient classical knowledge of Ayurveda has been passed on to the present times through two sets of authentic classic texts with three books each, popularly known as (1) *Brihattrayi*, i.e., three big books and (2) *Laghuttrayi*, i.e., three small books. Three big books are (1) *Caraka Samhita* (700 BC), (2) *Susruta Samhita* (600 BC), and (3) *Vagbhatta Samhitas*, namely, *Astanga Samgraha* and *Astanga Hridaya* (AD 300). The three small books are (1) *Madhav Nidan* (AD 900), (2) *Sharangdhara Samhita* (AD 1300), and (3) *Bhav Prakash* (AD 1600). All these texts have been written in Samskrit, now translated in many modern languages including Hindi and English along with many commentaries. As such, these texts are now easily accessible for the scientists and scholars of present time for their scientific inquiries and research leads. Even in the classical period, Ayurveda was practiced professionally as a very developed science of life and medicine in eight specialized branches, namely, (1) *kayachikitsa* or internal medicine; (2) *salya tantra* or surgery; (3) *shalakya tantra* or ENT and ophthalmology; (4) *kaumarabhritya* or obstetrics, gynecology, and pediatrics; (5) *agada*

R.H. Singh (✉)
Department of Kaya Chikitsa, Institute of Medical Sciences,
Banaras Hindu University, Varanasi, India
e-mail: rh_singh2001@yahoo.com

S. Rastogi
PG Department of Kaya Chikitsa, State Ayurvedic College, Lucknow University, Lucknow,
Uttar Pradesh, India
e-mail: rastogisanjeev@rediffmail.com

S. Rastogi (ed.), *Evidence-Based Practice in Complementary and Alternative Medicine*,
DOI 10.1007/978-3-642-24565-7_10, © Springer-Verlag Berlin Heidelberg 2012

tantra or toxicology; (6) *bhutavidya* or psychiatry and demonology; (7) *rasayana* or rejuvenation and geriatrics; and (8) *vajikarana or* sexology and reproduction.

A critical study of these texts reveals that Ayurveda was already a very developed science of life, health care, and cure. The concepts, theories, and practices as recorded in Ayurveda seem to have been established through observational studies with the help of scientific parameters, i.e., *pramanas*, namely, (1) *pratyaksa* or direct physical observation; (2) *anuman* or inferential evidence; (3) *aptopadesa*, i.e., scriptural evidence; and (4) *yukti pramana* or planned experimental evidence. Besides this structured scriptural evidence base, Ayurveda also enjoys a rich experience-based evidence through long-standing popular use in the hands of Ayurvedic practitioners. However, this primary evidence needs to be supported by new scientific evidence [1–6].

10.2 What Is *Rasayana*?

As stated earlier, Ayurveda, the science of life and longevity, has been practiced in India since inception in an *astangic* form through its eight specialty branches. One of the eight branches is specially devoted to the uplift of nutrition, immunoenhancement, and longevity. It is called *rasayana tantra*. This chapter will discuss in detail the definition and scope of *rasayana*, mode of action of *rasayana* measures, their classification and range of application, methodology of its use and its indications, contraindications, and complementary uses besides certain observations on future potential development of *rasayana* therapy in newer areas in modern times. The following are the classical textual references on *rasayana* therapy [7–14]:

- *Caraka Samhita Cikitsa Sthana Chapter 1, Pada 1–4*
  1. *Abhayamalakiya Rasayana*
  2. *Prana Kamiya Rasayana*
  3. *Karapracitiya Rasayana*
  4. *Ayurveda Samutthaniya Rasayana*
- *Susruta Samhita Cikitsa Sthana Chapter 27–30*
  27. *Sarvopaghata Shamaniya Rasayana*
  28. *Medhayuskamiya Rasayana*
  29. *Swabhawa Vyadhi Pratisedhaniya Rasayana*
  30. *Nivritta Santapiya RasÁyana*
- *Astanga Hridaya Uttar Tantra Chapter 39*

10.2.1 Definition and Scope of Rasayana

The word *rasayana* (*rasa* + *ayana*) refers to procurement of nourishment for formation of best qualities of *dhatus*, i.e., cells and tissues of the body, which leads in turn to an improved physiological state, better immunity, biostrength, mental competence, and longevity. Thus, *rasayana therapy* has a comprehensive scope for positive

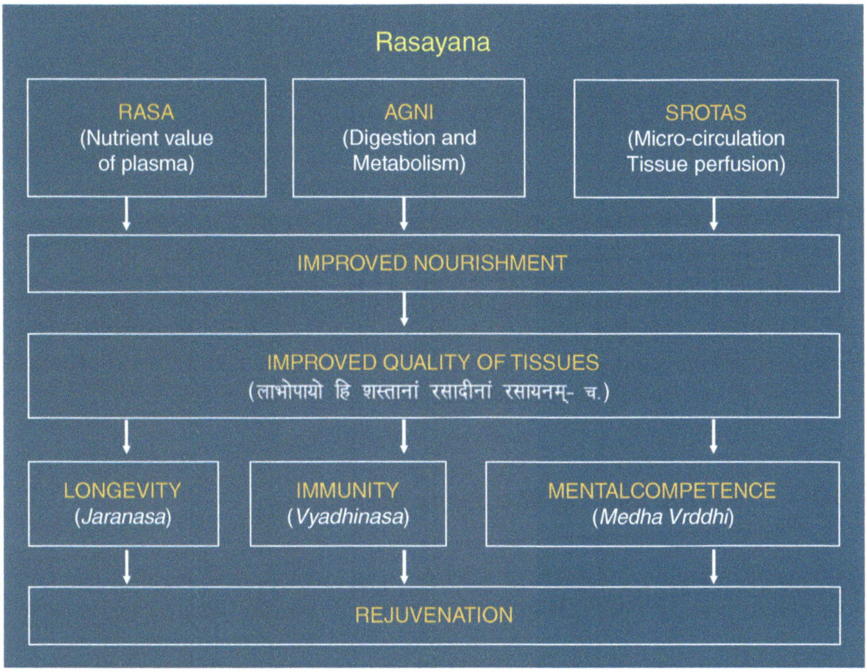

Fig. 10.1 Proposed mechanisms of action of *rasayana*

nutrition, immunoenhancement, longevity, and sustenance of mental and sensorial competence. Besides promotion of mental and physical health and rejuvenation potential, *rasayana therapy* affords a preventive role against all range of diseases through improved immunity and biostrength. Thus, *rasayana therapy* is the essential component of Ayurvedic geriatrics and geriatric health care.

10.2.2 Mechanism of Action

The *rasayana* procedures and *rasayana* drugs produce their therapeutic effect in the mind-body system through either or all of the following three mechanisms (Fig. 10.1):

1. At the level of *rasa* by directly acting as a nutrient in itself, enriching the nutrient value of *posaka rasa* in the plasma. The examples are a range of nutrient *rasayanas* like *shatavari*, *sharkara*, *ghrita*, *mukta*, etc.
2. At the level of *agni* by enhancing the biofire system of the body with improvement of the digestive and metabolic functions, further promoting the nutritional status as may be seen in case of *rasayanas* like *pippali and shunthi.*
3. At the level of *srotas*, i.e., microcirculation, by inducing *srotoprasadana* effect, improving the competence of the inner transport system, microcirculation, and tissue perfusion, such as *guggulu rasayana*.

Rasayana drugs are also proposed to promote tissue longevity through some more novel mechanisms like:

- Reduction of toxin/metabolic waste load within the cell through their reduced production or increased scavenging
- Ensuring the efficient use of energy within the cell requiring less substrate consumption leading to reduced requirement and reduced waste production
- Initiation of self-repairs by providing essential nutrients participating in regeneration directly or through promotion of latent enzyme systems

While acting through the abovementioned three probable routes, the *rasayana remedies* create a positive nutritional status in the body, assist in healthier tissue formation, immunocompetence, optimum mental stamina, and longevity. Such an improved biological state is considered as *kayakalpa or rejuvenation.*

10.2.3 Classification of Rasayana Measures

Rasayana is not a mere remedy or a recipe. It is a rejuvenative regimen and is an approach to positive health. It includes elements of positive lifestyle and conduct, healthy dietetics, and rejuvenative herbs and minerals. *Rasayana* is practiced as a routine open lifestyle form or as an intensive indoor regimen, depending upon the need of and the feasibility for a client. The *rasayana* therapy can be classified as below:

A. As per method of use:
   1. *Vatatapika rasayana* or a casual outdoor practice
   2. *Kutipraveshika rasayana* or intensive indoor regimen (inclusive of *panchakarma*) using a specially designed *trigarbha rasayana kuti* or therapy chamber

B. As per scope of application:
   1. *Kamya rasayana*—for promotion of health of the healthy, further subclassified as:
      (a) *Sri kamya*—to promote luster and beauty
      (b) *Prana kamya*—to promote longevity
      (c) *Medha kamya*— to promote mental competence
   2. *Naimittika rasayana*— to induce biostrength in a diseased person to fight better with his existing disease

C. *Adjunct rasayana*— nonrecipe rejuvenative regimen to be practiced alone or as an adjunct for all forms of *rasayana* therapy, remedies, and recipes
   1. *Achara rasayana*— healthy rejuvenative positive lifestyle
   2. *Ajasrika rasayana*— daily dietary *rasayana* approach consuming *sattvika*, nourishing elements of diet

10.2.3.1 Age-Specific *Rasayana*

Ayurveda considers aging as the *swabhawa* or the nature of a living being. The mind-body system has been conceived to last for a time-bound span of 100–120 years.

Table 10.1 Age-related biolosses and some suggested *rasayana drugs*

S. no.	Decades of life span (years)	Natural biolosses	Suggested *rasayana*
1	0–10	Balya—corpulence	*Gambhari, ksira, ghrita*
2	11–20	Vriddhi—growth	*Bala, amalaki*
3	21–30	Chhabi—luster	*Àmalaki, haridra*
4	31–40	Medha—intellect	*Brahmi, sankhapuspi*
5	41–50	Twaka—skin quality	*Bhringraja, haridra*
6	51–60	Dristi—vision	*Triphala, jyotismati*
7	61–70	Shukra—virility	*Asvagandha, kapikacchu*
8	71–80	Vikrama—physical strength	*Àmalaki, bala*
9	81–90	Buddhi—thinking	*Brahmi, sankhapuspi*
10	91–100	Karmendriya—locomotion	*Bala, sahacara*

During the life span, the body undergoes progressive involution and decay, leading ultimately to senescence and death. Ayurveda describes the process of aging and sequential senile changes in different ways in different contexts. The three *doshas*, namely, *kapha, pitta, and vata*, have been described to dominate specifically during childhood, adulthood, and old age respectively. The *vata dosha*, because of its drying and decaying effect, plays the central role in aging.

Sarangdhara Samhita (SS.6:20) describes a unique scheme of biological aging in a ten-decade frame speculating the specific sequential loss of certain biovalues specific to respective decades of life, opening the possibility of developing specific *rasayanas* to restore the likely biolosses of the particular decade (Table 10.1). If *rasayana* therapy is planned in relation to age, there is a possibility of retarding the aging process. Table 10.1 describes the pattern of age-related biolosses and proposes certain *rasayanas* for the purpose.

10.2.3.2 Tissue- and Organ-Specific *Rasayana*

Rasayana in general is a holistic restorative and rejuvenative modality, but one can visualize some *rasayana* remedies and recipes for specific promotion and protection of certain specific tissues and organs. Such *rasayanas* can be prescribed in need-based manner for promotive or even for curative purposes for organ protection. Some examples are proposed in Table 10.2.

10.2.3.3 Disease-Specific *Rasayana*

Although *rasayana* therapy is primarily a promotive and preventive health care modality, a concept of disease-specific *rasayana* therapy has been projected by Susruta and his commentator Dalhana under the term *naimittika rasayana.* Susruta gives only two examples for *naimittika rasayana*, namely, *silajatu* and *tubaraka rasayana* for *prameha* (diabetes) and *kustha* (leprosy) respectively. However, in the contemporary contexts, one can visualize using a range of other *rasayanas* for different diseases. The *naimittika rasayana* is really not a specific treatment of a disease entity;

Table 10.2 Some tissue- and organ-specific *rasayana* drugs

S. no.	*Rasayana* quality	Purpose	Suggested remedies
1	*Medhya rasayana*	Neuroprotection and cognition	*Brahmi, sankhapuspi*
2	*Hridya rasayana*	Cardioprotection	*Arjuna, puskarmula*
3	*Mutra janana*	Nephroprotection	*Punarnava, guksuru*
4	*Twacya rasayana*	Skin health	*Haridra, somaraji*
5	*Caksusya rasayana*	Eye health	*Triphala, jyotismati*
6	*Kanthya rasayana*	Throat health and speech	*Vaca, yashtimadhu*
7	*Vrishya rasayana*	Virility	*Asvagandha, kapikacchu*
8	*Stanya rasayana*	Promoting lactation	*Shatavari*
9	*Srotoprasadana*	Promoting microcirculation	*Guggulu*
10	*Nasya rasayana*	Helping nose and sinuses	*Katphala, apamarga*

Table 10.3 Some disease-specific *rasayana* drugs

Selected diseases	Suggested *naimittika rasayana*
Diabetes mellitus	*Silajatu, haridra*
Leprosy and dermatoses	*Tubaraka, haridra, somaraji*
Bronchial asthma and allergies	*Haridra, sirisa*
Hypertension and IHD	*Sarpagandha, pushkaramula, arjuna*
Urinary disorders	*Punarnava, gokshura*
Arthritis	*Bhallataka, eranda*
Neurodegenerative diseases	*Brahmi, ashwagandha*
Dementias	*Brahmi, sankhapuspi*
Immunodeficiency	*Àmalaki, guduchi*
Cancers	*Bhallataka, àmalaki, haridra*

rather, it is a *rasayana* for promoting the strength and immunity of a patient to fight with his existing disease in a *rasayana* way. A few *naimittika rasayanas* are suggested in Table 10.3.

10.2.3.4 *Achara* and *Ajasrika Rasayana*

Achara rasayana is a unique concept in Ayurveda which implies that a moral, ethical, and benevolent conduct, namely, truth, nonviolence, personal and public cleanliness, mental and personal hygiene, devotion, compassion, and yogic life bring about rejuvenative state in the mind-body system. A person who adapts such a lifestyle and conduct gains all benefits of *rasayana* therapy without physically consuming any material *rasayana* remedy and *rasayana* recipe. All forms of *sadvritta*, *achara*, and practice of yoga and spirituality produce such a quantum *rasayana* effect in a nonpharmacological way. This can be practiced alone or in a combination with material substance *rasayana* therapy of all range. Similarly, *ajasrika rasayana* refers to daily rejuvenative dietetics with adequate quantity of nourishing *sattvika* elements of diet. *Ajasrika rasayana* is used alone or along with material *rasayana* remedies.

10.2.3.5 *Divya Rasayana*

The Ayurvedic classics as well as the Vedic texts present a unique concept of *divya rasayana* which is claimed to possess divine power to bring about divine transformation in an individual. Caraka, Susruta, and Vagbhatta describe a number of *divya rasayana mahausadhis* with paranormal attributes. They are supposed to grow in *Soumya* Himalayan range and are rarely found. This class of *rasayanas*, which are of plant origin, displays a kind of spiritual pharmacology, and their actions are due to their *divya prabhava*. Caraka Samhita Chikitsa Sthana Chapter 1, Pada-4 (Ayurveda Samutthaniya Rasayana), Susruta Samhita Chikitsa Sthana Chapter 30 (Nivritta Santapiya Rasayana), and Astanga Hridaya Chapter 39 mention a range of *divya ausadhis* such as *brahma*, *subarchala*, *soma*, *padma*, *varahi*, *golomi*, *ajagari*, etc. The identity of these drugs is presently unknown, and this entire context warrants serious research.

10.3 Methods and Effects of *Rasayana* Therapy

Besides *achara* and *ajasrika* components, another important requirement for use of medicinal *rasayana* therapy is *samsodhana or* biopurification of the body through appropriate *panchakarma* procedures. Ayurveda emphasizes that a *rasayana* remedy yields its full effect only when the body has been therapeutically purified by *langhana*, *deepana*, *pacana*, *snehana*, *swedana*, *vamana*, *virecana*, *vasti*, *sirovirecana*, etc. If the *srotamsi*, i.e., microchannels of the body are clean and competent with their physiological integrity at the time of administration of the *rasayana* remedy, it is fully utilized by the system, and its bioavailability is ensured. Hence, *samsodhana karma* should be planned accordingly [15]. The most appropriate choice of age for use of *rasayana* therapy is *purva vaya* or *madhya vaya*, i.e., young or adult age, not the actual old age when irreversible senile changes might have already occurred.

In all procedures of *rasayana* therapy, a physician is expected to take due consideration of many individual and environmental factors while selecting a *rasayana* remedy for a particular patient. Few of the factors to be considered are *prakriti*, *vaya*, *agnibala*, *dhatu* status and *ojabala*, *srotas* status, *agnibala*, *desa satmya*, *ritu satmya*, *vyadhibala*, *manobala*, etc. Persons with different categories and features of the abovementioned factors would need different *rasayanas* in consideration of their biological features to yield best results.

10.3.1 The Rasayana Effect and Rejuvenation

The *rasayana* remedies described in Ayurveda are claimed to possess special nutritional supplement effect. Generally, most of the *rasayanas* are micromolecular

Table 10.4 Antistress activity of some *rasayanas* in terms of Ed 50 in stressed rats

Drugs tested	Swimming performance adrenal wt.	Prevention of ascorbic acid rise	Prevention of adrenal cortisol rise	Prevention of stress ulcers	Antistress zunit/mg/g
Ashwagandha	15.0±1.3	13.0±1.4	14.5±1.5	16.0±1.8	14.9±1.5
Tulasi	13.3±1.2	12.0±1.6	13.0±1.5	13.4±2.0	13.7±1.3
P. ginseng	44.0±3.8	15.0±1.8	24.1±2.1	24.07±2.2	25.2±2.3

Table 10.5 Effect of *ashwagandha* on plasma corticosterone, phagocytic index, and swimming endurance under normal and stress conditions[17]

Observations mean±SE	Control	*Ashwagandha*-treated	Stress (swimming)	Swimming stress+*ashwagandha*
Plasma corticosterone (g/dl)	98.95±0.51	98.95±0.27	107.2±0.38	99.77±0.14 $P<0.05$
Phagocytic index	68.50±0.56	69.60±0.70	78.0±0.58	68.83±1.20 $P<0.05$
Total swim time			5.30±0.24	8.90±0.50 $P<0.05$

Table 10.6 Biological Age Scale (BAS) and Brief Psychiatric Rating Scale (BPRS) scores before and after treatment with *ashwagandha* [21]

Observations	Before treatment	After treatment	*T*	*P*
Total BAS scores	18.77±4.55	14.20±4.37	2.92	<0.01
Total PBRS scores	32.40±5.22	22.93±2.86	6.12	<0.01

nutrients, and they act through nutrition dynamics and not really on pharmacodynamics like other drugs. The *rasayana* drugs are likely to be nutrient tonics, antioxidants, antistress, adaptogen, and immunomodulators. The net effect of all these attributes is the antiaging effect. Certain recent studies on popular *rasayana* remedies like *amalaki*, *ashwagandha*, *guduchi*, *brahmi*, and classical compound *rasayana cyavanaprasa* have shown evidence to suggest their efficacy as antiaging remedies. Tables 10.4, 10.5, and 10.6 are being reproduced here to give a glimpse of such an evidence about the popular *rasayana* drugs, *ashwagandha*, tulasi, and ginseng [2, 16–27].

The above-cited observations indicate that the Indian *rasayana* drug *ashwagandha* has significant antistress effect on notably lower effective dose (Ed^{50}) as compared to popular Chinese herbal tonic *ginseng*. *Ashwagandha* also shows relevant humoral basis for its antistress and anti-inflammatory effect. The clinical trial of *ashwagandha* in elderly volunteers shows significant reduction in the rate of biological aging (BAS) and mental health status as measured by BPRS (Tables 10.4, 10.5, and 10.6). Several clinical and experimental studies have been conducted on the psychopharmacological effects of popular *rasayana* drugs like *ashwagandha*, *brahmi*, *shankhpushpi*, and *mandukaparni*. Kuboyama et al. [23] reported noticeable neuritic regenerative effects of withanolide-A isolated from *rasayana* drug *ashwagandha* in vitro. Chaudhary et al. [20] reported cholinesterase-inhibiting withanolides from *Withania somnifera*. Holcomb et al. [22] reported amyloid-reducing effects in *brahmi* extracts. Earlier, Singh and Dhawan [25], Pathak and Singh [24], and Singh and Singh [26] also reported anxiolytic and memory-enhancing effects in *brahmi*.

Antioxidant role of *rasayana* drugs is one most commonly studied and proposed mechanism behind their action. Over 100 disorders of which most are degenerative and age-related pathogenesis are found to have an association with reactive oxygen species (ROS)–induced oxidative damage to cellular structures. Incidentally, *rasayana* is found to have antagonistic properties against oxidative stressors that eventually lead to the formation of different free radicals. It is noteworthy that this antioxidant effect of commonly used *rasayana* in Ayurveda is found 1,000 times more potent compared to conventional antioxidants like ascorbic acid, α-tocopherol, and probucol [28]. Working through the augmentation of antioxidant enzyme system in body, *rasayana* is found effective even in the oxidative damage caused by radiation [29, 30]. Various herbs have been reviewed for their antioxidant potential in the recent past. Common ones among them are *Acorus calamus*, *Aloe vera*, *Andrographis paniculata*, *Asparagus recemosus*, *Azadirachta indica*, *Bacopa monnieri*, *Desmodium gangeticum*, *Phyllanthus emblica*, *Glycyrrhiza glabra*, *Terminalia chebula*, *Tinospora cordifolia*, and *Withania somnifera* [31]. We are aware that most of these herbs are well known in Ayurveda for their potent *rasayana* actions.

While focusing upon specific mechanisms behind the antiaging properties of *rasayana*, we also need to understand the comprehensive and holistic approach of Ayurveda toward health and disease. While talking of *rasayana*, Ayurveda clearly emphasizes a balanced lifestyle and diet for its potential of ameliorating the aging process—the ultimate *rasayana* effect which is being expected from any specific *rasayana*. Only now, we are aware that even our balanced diet (*satvic* as is specified in Ayurveda) possesses a huge sum of bioactive phytochemicals which are capable of preventing disease and promoting health. Dietary fibers, vitamin E, carotenoids, and phenolic compounds are few such substances which make the natural food a potent health promoter. Out of many proposed mechanisms behind the food-based *rasayana* effects, the most important one is detoxification of chemical toxicants and carcinogens by phytochemicals present in natural food [32].

Besides their tissue-promotive and regenerative effects, *rasayana* is also claimed to possess life span–enhancing potentials as net outcome of its protective and promotive actions. Priyadarshini et al. [33] recently have experimented with *Drosophila melanogaster* by feeding them with a specially prepared *rasayana* diet suitable to insects. An approximate 51–55% increase in life span was observed in the drosophilas that were fed with *rasayana* diet [33].

Detoxifying potentials of *rasayana* drugs are coming in vogue recently. Priyandoko et al. [34], in an experimental study, tried ashwagandha leaf extracts as a detoxifying agent against methoxyacetic acid (MAA),a common industry chemical which is known to cause premature senescence of normal human cells by mechanisms that involve ROS generation and DNA and mitochondrial damage. Withanone, an active component from *Withania*, protects cells from MAA-induced toxicity by suppressing the ROS levels, DNA and mitochondrial damage, and induction of cell defense signaling pathways including Nrf2 and proteasomal degradation. These findings warrant further basic and clinical studies that may promote the use of *rasayana* herbs as health adjuvant in a variety of conditions where the tissue damage has been a matter of concern because of the pollutants, toxins, and industrial waste exposures [34].

10.3.2 Rasayana Therapy in Chronic Disease Management

In view of their nutrition-promoting effect, the *rasayana* remedies have a potential role in the management of all chronic diseases where they act as nutritional support and also help retard tissue damage caused by toxic chemical medications. Some *rasayanas* have been claimed to be chemoprotective as well as radiation-protective agents. Many *rasayanas* are known to be antioxidants.

The possible role of ashwagandha as an adjunct to antitubercular therapy (ATT) is worth mentioning here. Cytokines play an important role in patients with tuberculosis (TB). In one recent study, TB patients were found having an increased level of TNF-α and interferon-γ. After giving an immunomodulator (*Withania somnifera*), a reduction in the levels of TNF-α and interferon-γ was seen. A study indicated that in case of pulmonary-tuberculosis category-1 patients, if *Withania somnifera* is given along with the ATT treatment, it could increase the immunity of the patients [35].

As stated earlier, the term *rasayana* essentially refers to acquisition, movement, or circulation of nutrition and tissue perfusion. Such a phenomenon is considered conducive to the promotion of qualities of *dhatus*, i.e., body cells and tissues. The improved nutritional status and better qualities of *dhatus* lead to a series of secondary attributes of *rasayana* such as longevity, immunity, youthfulness, improved mental and intellectual competence, etc. Considering the Ayurvedic concepts of physiology, it may be presumed that *rasayana* agents promote nutrition through one of the three modes at the level of *rasa*, *agni, and srotas*.

10.3.3 Rasayana in Cancer Management

The author has already suggested in the past that a suitably planned use of *rasayana chikitsa* as an adjunct therapy in cancer management seems to be of fundamental advantage in view of its immunoenhancing and nutrition-promoting potential.

It is known that cancer tissue competes with normal tissue nutrition. Because cancer cells continue to proliferate indefinitely, their number multiplies day by day. So the cancer cells will soon demand essentially all the nutrition available to the body. As a result, the normal tissues gradually suffer nutritive death. Thus, cellular nutrition deficit is always a risk and crisis in cancer patients, and if there is any strategy to sustain this deficit, it will improve the quality of life in these patients. Hence, in view of the known molecular nutrient potential of Ayurvedic *rasayanas*, it is imperative to opt for *rasayana* therapy as an adjunct to the main treatment of cancer. As such, *rasayana* therapy is a positive approach to cancer management as opposed to the negative approach of conventional cytotoxic chemoradiation therapy. Besides their direct nutrient role, all *rasayanas* are classically known to be *ojas* builders and immune enhancers, and hence, *rasayana* therapy would help sustain the patient who is always immunocompromised.

There is a recently growing trend to develop immunotherapy or immune cell therapy in the treatment of cancer as better option than cytotoxic chemotherapy/ radiation therapy. It seems logical to think that Ayurvedic *rasayanas* may be used as a therapeutic tool to amplify the immunity against a particular cancer induced by artificial methods such as active-specific immunotherapy or immune cell therapy in cancer patients.

Thus, *rasayana* therapy seems to have a potential scope of application in management of cancer in the following perspectives: (1) to provide nutritional support to normal cells of a cancer patient to prevent their nutritive death, (2) to provide protection against injurious effect of chemotherapy and radiation therapy, and (3) to amplify the immunity in a patient against cancer, induced by conventional artificial methods such as active-specific immunotherapy or immune cell therapy.

10.3.4 Evidence-Based Rasayana Therapy: Questions To Be Answered

Referring to the rejuvenative effects of *rasayana* therapy, there are certain queries which are required to be taken up on priority. Who are those people from whom a real benefit from *rasayana* therapy is expected? is a crucial question which needs to be resolved before a ground-level application of this hyped therapy can be made. Is it the group suffering from a premature decay of tissue and subsequent loss of function, or is it the group where the loss of function is in connection with their physical age but, because of the importance of those functions, is required to be preserved? *Rasayana* drugs are often referred to have antiaging effects of their own. "*Labhopayo hi shastanam rasadinam Rasayanam*," however, intends to look for the optimization of ways and means which are supportive for the qualitative improvement of the tissue. A qualitative improvement here essentially refers to the functional and constitutional specification of tissue compensated as per the age. A qualitatively improved tissue, besides its optimal functioning, is also supposed to defy the premature aging consequent to its impaired quality. Therefore, antiaging seems to be a secondary function of the *rasayana*, subsequent to qualitative upgradation and stabilization of cells as being its primary function. Sharangdhara's saying of "*Rasayanam cha tajgheyayam yajjaravyadhi vinashanam*" interestingly looks more apt for its depiction of *rasayana* usage in *jaravyadhi* (early aging) besides its use in *jara* (aging) and *vyadhi* (disease) distinctly [36].

It is for this conviction that *rasayana* drugs are said to produce their beneficial effect more promptly in conditions where a suboptimal quality of tissue is leading to its premature aging and suboptimal functioning. In healthy people where the tissue aging is in connotation to the physical age, *rasayana* can offer only a little to help besides further reducing the rate of aging in reference to various degenerative processes. This is an important point to be considered as unless we make it clear as to who are the people benefiting maximally from *rasayana*, we may not be able to make proper use of it.

10.4 Conclusions

The context of *rasayana* therapy and its *ajasrika*, *achara*, and *divya ausadhi* components are largely unexplored parts of ancient wisdom. However, the prevalent *rasayana* procedures and recipes are of great current value in promotive, preventive, and therapeutic aspects of geriatric health care. There is a great need to acquaint the professionals as well as the public about the use of *rasayana* remedies and recipes besides the *prorasayana* dietetic and lifestyle regimen described in Ayurvedic texts. There is also a need to undertake appropriate research strategies in the field for developing an evidence base for the efficacy of *rasayana* remedies and evidence-based Ayurvedic geriatrics and its mainstreaming [37]. It would be seen that few studies conducted on scientific lines in recent times reveal varying degree of immune-enhancing, adaptogenic, antistress, neuroprotective, and memory-enhancing effects besides possibilities of antiaging impact.

References

1. Caraka (700 BC) Caraka Samhita. Sharma PV (ed) Cikitsa Sthana, Chapter I, Pada 1–4. Choukhamba Orientalia, Varanasi
2. Sarangadhara (1300 AD) Sarangadhara Samhita Khand II, Chapter 6, vs. 20. Choukhmbha Prakasana, Varanasi
3. Susruta Samhita, Singhal GD & Associates (eds) Cikitsa Sthana, Chapters 27–30. Choukhamba Surbharati, Varanasi/New Delhi
4. Udupa KN, Singh RH (1974) Science and philosophy of Indian medicine. Sri Baidyanath Ayurveda Bhawan, Nagpur
5. Vagbhatt (300 AD) Astanga Hridaya Uttara Tantra, Chapter 39 on Rasayana. Choukhamba Prakasan, Varanasi
6. Vagbhatta (300 AD) Astanga Sangraha Uttara Tantra, Rasayana Chapter. Choukhamba Publications, Varanasi
7. Singh RH (2005) Advances in Ayurvedic medicine, vol 1–5. Chaukhamba Vishwabharati, Varanasi
8. Singh RH (2005) Kayachikitsa, vol. I, Chap. 13 on Rasayana. Choukhambha Surbharati, Varanasi
9. Singh RH (2005) Swasthavrtta Vigyana, Chaps. 3, 4, 7, 22–23. Choukhamba Surbharati, Varanasi
10. Singh RH (2009) Mind-body-spirit integrative medicine. Choukhamba Surbharati, Varanasi
11. Singh RH and Associates (2008) Advances in Ayurvedic Medicine, vol 1–5. Choukhamba Vishwabharati, Varanasi
12. Singh RH, Narsimhamurthy K, Singh G (2008) Neuronutrient impact of Ayurvedic rasayana therapy in brain aging. Biogerontology 9:369–374

13. Singh RH (2010) Rasayana therapy and rejuvenation. In: Singh RH (ed) Manual of geriatric health care through Ayurveda. Department of AYUSH, Govt. of India, New Delhi
14. Strength of Ayurveda in geriatric health care. Key Note Lecture by Singh RH, Launching National Campaign on Geriatric Health Care, Department of AYUSH, Ministry of Health, Government of India, 2008
15. Singh RH (2005) Pancakarma therapy. Choukhambha Sanskrit Series, Varanasi
16. Agrawal SC, Singh RH (1998) Effect of Medhya Rasayana drug, Mandukaparni (*Centella asiatica*) on cognitive functions and social adaptability in mental retardation. J Res Ayur Siddha 18:97–107
17. Archana R, Namasiwayam A (1999) Antistress effect of Withania somnifera. J Ethnopharmacol 64:91–93
18. Bhattacharya SK et al (1997) Anxiolytic activity of Glyco-withanolides from Withania somnifera (Ashwagandha). J Exp Biol 35:236
19. Caraka (700 BC) Caraka Samhita. In: Sharma PV (ed) Cikitsa Sthana, Chap. I, Pada 1–4. Pub Choukhamba Orientalia, Varanasi
20. Choudhary MI et al (2004) Cholinesterase inhibiting Withanolides from Withania somnifera. Chem Pharm Bull (Tokyo) 52:1358–1361
21. Dwivedi KK, Singh RH (1997) A study on geriatric patients and response of Ashwagandha as anti-aging agent. Ph.D. Thesis, Kayachikitsa, Banaras Hindu University
22. Holcomb L et al (2006) Bacopa monnieri extract reduces Amyloid levels in PSAPP mice. J Alzheimers Dis 9:251
23. Kuboyama T et al (2005) Neuritic regeneration and synaptic reconstruction induced by Withanolide-A. Br J Pharmacol 144:961–971
24. Pathak SR, Singh RH (1986) Study on influence of some plant products on brain function. Ph.D. Thesis (Ayu-Zoology), Banaras Hindu University, Varanasi, India
25. Singh HK, Dhawan BN (1997) Neuropsychopharmacological studies on Brahmi. Indian J Pharmacol 29:5359–5365
26. Singh L, Singh RH (1978) Study on psychotropic effect of Brahmi (Bacopa monnieri). M.D. Ay. Thesis, Banaras Hindu University, Varanasi, India
27. Singh N (1987) Study of Antistress effect of plant drugs. Ann Acad Ind Med 1(1):1–15
28. Sharma HM, Hanna AN, Kauffman EM, Newman HAI (1992) Inhibition of human low density lipoprotein oxidation in vitro by maharshi Ayurveda herbal mixtures. Pharmacol Biochem Behav 43:1175–1182
29. Rekha PS, Kuttan G, Kuttan R (2001) Effect of brahma Rasayana on antioxidant system after radiation. Indian J Exp Biol 39:1173–1175
30. Puri HS (2003) Rasayana—Ayurvedic herbs for longevity and rejuvenation. Taylor and Francis, London
31. Govindarajan R, Vijayakumar M, Pushpagandan P (2005) Antioxidant approach to disease management and the role of Rasayana herbs of Ayurveda. J Ethnopharmacol 99:165–178
32. Narasingarao B (2003) Bioactive phytochemicals in Indian foods and their potential in health promotion and disease prevention. Asia Pac J Clin Nutr 12:9–22
33. Priyadarshini S, Ashadevi JS, Nagarjun V, Prasanna KS (2010) Increase in *Drosophila melanogaster* longevity due to *rasayana* diet: Preliminary results. J Ayur Integr Med 1:114–119
34. Priyandoko D, Ishii T, Kaul SC, Wadhwa R (2011) Ashwagandha leaf derived Withanone protects normal human cells against the toxicity of methoxyacetic acid, a major industrial metabolite. PLoS One 6:e19552. doi:10.1371/journal.pone.0019552
35. Prasad R (2011) Evaluation of immunomodulation by Withania Somnifera used as an adjunct DOTS-RNTCP to chemotherapy for increased effectiveness in pulmonary-tuberculosis patients. Available at http://www.cstup.gov.in/pdfs/MedicalSc.pdf. Accessed on 15 May 2011
36. Rastogi S (2010) Building bridges between Ayurveda and modern science. Int J Ayur Res 1:41–46
37. Balasubramani SP, Venkatasubramanian P, Kukkupuni SK, Patwardhan B (2011) Plant-based Rasayana drugs from Ayurveda. Chin J Integr Med 17:88–94, Epub 9 Mar 2011

Chapter 11
Translational Effectiveness in Ayurvedic Medicine: Implications for Oral Biology and Medicine

Manisha Harish Ramchandani, Mahsa Dousti, Andre Barkhordarian, and Francesco Chiappelli

11.1 Introduction: Oral Health—The Absence of Disease in the Oral Cavity

The World Health Organization (WHO) defends that health is a state of complete physical, mental, and social well-being, not merely the absence of disease or infirmity. From that viewpoint, the clinician works toward assisting the patients regain a state characterized by freedom from disease and of overall well-being of the mind and of the body.

In the Western health care tradition, two fundamental epochs can be roughly traced, which are fundamentally different in philosophical viewpoints and practical implications [1]. At the root of the Western health care tradition, we find the Egyptian, Greek, and Roman cultures, which all emphasized an intimate intertwining between the mind and the body. Alterations in psychocognitive and emotional well-being were believed to have grave consequences on physiological health; alternatively, alterations in physiological balance were recognized to be associated with profound mental ill-health.

These interrelationships are clear and evident in the writings of Aristotle and many of his followers in the Western tradition for centuries. It is not until the seventeenth and the eighteenth centuries, leading to the philosophical writings of Kant and his followers in the modern era, that the view of health and disease, physiology and anatomy, both in the normal health state and in the pathological state, began to be disarticulated, fragmented, and—some would argue—disjointed.

Whereas in the older and traditional models of universities, medicine was taught as a unified concept, now schools of medicine were emerging, endowed with specific faculties of psychiatry, physiology, anatomy, and the like. As our views of

M.H. Ramchandani (✉) • M. Dousti • A. Barkhordarian • F. Chiappelli
Division of Oral Biology and Medicine, UCLA School of Dentistry, Los Angeles, CA, USA
e-mail: rmanisha@ucla.edu; mahsa.dousti@yahoo.com; andreucsb@hotmail.com; fchiappelli@dentistry.ucla.edu

S. Rastogi (ed.), *Evidence-Based Practice in Complementary and Alternative Medicine*, DOI 10.1007/978-3-642-24565-7_11, © Springer-Verlag Berlin Heidelberg 2012

health and disease became more oriented toward understanding the fundamental elemental principles of the scientific mechanisms that underlie health and disease in the West, our perspectives became more reductionistic. That emphasis consequentially engendered a dissociative process between the mind and the body, and no longer was the patient seen as a whole organism, but more often than not, mental diseases were treated separately from endocrine diseases, and from bone diseases, and so forth. Systemic disease, that is, diseased state—essentially—from the neck down, were considered separately from diseased state of the head and neck region, and even within that region, neurologists and psychiatrists typically addressed pathologies within the caudal or cranial aspect of the head and neck, and dentists and specialists in oral medicine concentrated in stomatopathology, that is, oral diseases [2, 3].

The "non-Western" medical dogmas, which in the West is referred to as "complementary and alternative medicine (CAM)"—meaning to say, complementary or alternative to the modern Western medical approach—actually consists of several and distinct traditions, of which Ayurvedic medicine and traditional Chinese medicine are prime examples [1].

Integrative medicine is the combination of the practices and methods of complementary and alternative medicine with conventional Western medicine. Important health benefits and cost savings can be realized throughout the health care system by balancing fundamental integrative strategies, as determined by the needs of the patient, such as integrating lifestyle changes (e.g., mindful stress reduction), integrating East–West interventions (e.g., use of traditional Chinese herbal medicine), and integrating preventive programs that promote wellness (e.g., Qigong).

It is fair to say that all of the "non-Western" viewpoints on health and disease share a commonality, which makes them actually more affine to the first epoch of Western medicine, as briefly outlined above, than its developments in the last two centuries. That commonality, very briefly sketched out, could be summed up as the conceptualization of health as the absence of disease in the patient as a complete psychobiological entity that interacts with its social and physical environment, and that view is akin to the WHO perspective noted above.

In Ayurvedic medicine, as in all other "non-Western" traditions of health care, the patient is not treated for a specific organ disease per se (e.g., "oral" disease), as much as the treatment is designed to heal the patient as a whole: in that medical tradition, it is understood that the manifestation of disease in the oral cavity, for instance, is reflective of a diseased state pervasive to the entire organism, systemically. "Non-Western" health care approaches in general, and Ayurvedic medicine in particular, cannot and does not separate the oral cavity from the rest of the patient and cannot and does not separate the manifestation of loss of balance and health—that is, disease—in the oral cavity from loss of a state of health in the patient as a total person.

The remainder of this chapter continues and expands the concepts introduced in our previous chapter (cf., Chap. 1) and subsequent chapters in this book, and examines these similarities and these distinctions in further details. It then seeks to reconcile pioneering work currently done in Western health care that seeks to emphasize translational effectiveness through research synthesis of the best available evidence, with the fundamental tenets of Ayurvedic medicine, specifically with respect to disease manifestations that primarily erupt in the oral cavity.

11.2 Oral Diseases Across Medical Traditions

11.2.1 Western Oral Medicine: Early Views

In today's parlance, a disease is an abnormal condition that affect the body of an organism and that is construed as a medical condition associated with specific symptoms and signs. Specifically with respect to oral diseases, the anatomical region of interest pertains to the oral cavity, the pharynx, and the larynx. Modern Western medicine attributes diseases to external factors, such as infectious agents, or to internal dysfunctions, including autoimmune diseases. As of late, in the Western view of health care, four main types of diseases can be conceptualized:

- A *pathogenic* disease is caused by a pathogen of some sort
- A *deficiency* disease results from the lack of some essential mineral or nutrient
- A *hereditary* (or genetic) disease
- A *physiological dysfunction* disease

A disease is often associated to collateral conditions, including pain, discomfort, lethargy, mental exhaustion, and psychoemotional difficulties. Similarly, the state of disease often affects people not only physically but also emotionally; contracting and living with many diseases can alter one's perspective on life, personality, and psychoemotional well-being. These interrelationships were well recognized in antiquity and are today in CAM, generally speaking, and in Ayurvedic medicine, in particular.

Ancient documents recognize Hesy-Ra, perhaps the first official physician-dentist thusly recognized in Western history, to have lived during the Third Dynasty of Egypt, under the pharaoh Djoser (cca. 2650 BC). Henceforth, Egyptian medicine incorporated to a large extent supernatural beliefs and credence by the patients and the caregivers, with practical and pragmatic knowledge of anatomy, public health, and clinical diagnostics. The concept and practice of diagnostics was actually developed and elevated to an art form by the Babylonians, such that only well-formed and skilled physicians could engage in this process. This specialty reached its apex during the reign of the king Adad-apla-iddina (1069–1046 BC), with the writing of the *Diagnostic Handbook* by the physician-dentist Esagil-kin-apli in the city Borsippa on the east bank of the Euphrates, in today's Iraq (cf., Chap. 5).

For Esagil-kin-apli and his followers, as for Hesy-Ra and his followers, the recognition of the causes for the loss of health—the concept of "health" being conceived by both doctrines as a state of balance, akin to the concept of homeostasis introduced by the French physiologist Claude Bernard (1813–1878)—must rest on a careful examination of the patient and of the socioenvironmental forces that impinge upon the patient's living conditions, as well as the use of empiricism (that is to say, the *best available evidence* from prior similar occurrences; cf., Chap. 1), logic, and rationality.

About the same time frame (cca. 700 BC), Ancient Greece witnessed the ascend of medicine as well in its first recorded medical school in Knidos, one of the principal metropolis of Caria, southwest of Anatolia, and one of the Greek Dorian Hexapolis. Alcmaeon formulated there the principles of ancient Greek medical intervention based on restoring the balance of humors (Earth—cold, Water—wet, Air—hot, and Fire—dry) within the body. The traditions of medicine in the ancient territories of Armenia and of ancient Greece were henceforth intertwined. Whence, Hippocrates of Kos (460–370 BC) developed his important and influential theory that the body contains within itself the power to rebalance the four humors and the ability to heal itself (*physis*) through rest and cleanliness. Aristotle (384–322 BC) added ether as the fifth essence since fire, earth, air, and water are earthly and thus viewed as corruptible. Aristotle reasoned that since no changes can be perceived in the heavens, therefore, stars must consist of a different, unchangeable, heavenly substance—ether.

The Aristotelian tradition was brought forward by Galen (129–199 AD), whose theories dominated and influenced Western medical science for nearly two millennia, excluding the contributions by Avicenna (980–1037), who was considered the Prince of Physicians in ancient Persia for his introduction of the conceptualization and of many of the protocols that we still used today in clinical trials, in evidence-based medicine, and in the experimental use and testing of drugs. Avicenna laid the foundations for practical and precise experimentation through what is recognized today as the scientific process of discovering and proving the effectiveness of medical treatments ([4]; cf. Chap. 5).

Indeed, Galen's views were not challenged before the great Muslim scientist Ibn al-Nafis (1213–1288), but these criticisms were largely ignored by the European medical elite (e.g., the School of Salerno) for centuries, due to the Crusades and the war of the Catholic Kings against the Moors. Western science had to wait past the Swiss scientist Paracelsus (1493–1541), whose hermetical views held, in brief, that sickness and health in the body rely on the harmony of man (microcosm) and nature (macrocosm). While Paracelsus is considered by many as one of the premier "fathers" of Western medicine, his views supported that because everything in the universe is interrelated, beneficial medical substances are to be found in herbs, minerals, and various alchemical combinations thereof that will benefit in preventing disease and in regaining health. We are part of, Paracelsus argued, the universe, one coherent organism that permeates with one uniting life-giving spirit, and our health derives from and depends upon our interrelationship with its entirety. Within the span of a hundred years, however, Western thought underwent a remarkable transformation with Andreas Vesalius' (1514–1564) *De humani corporis fabrica* (1543), William Harvey's (1578–1657) *De motu cordis* (1628), and Antonie Philips van Leeuwenhoek's (1632–1723) discoveries, and many other luminaries of science.

Meanwhile, the medicinal herbs of the Armenian highland were especially well known and cited by Xenophanes, Tacitus, Galen, Ibn Sina, al-Biruni, and others.

In fact, traditional texts indicate that medicinal plants of Armenia were cultivated in special gardens founded as early as King Vagharshak (cca. 220–150 BC) and at least until the Anatolian king of mixed Greek and Roman heritage, Artaxias III (i.e., Artashes, 18–35 AD) (first century AD), such as in particular the white bryony (*Bryonia alba*), a perennial vine of the cucumber family with characteristically stellate pale-white flowers and berries that induce vomiting, and the black cumin (*Nigella sativa*). The traditional Armenian medical paradigm was described by Eznik (a.k.a. Yeznik), the fifth century Christian writer and historian from Koghb in Northern Armenia, who ascended to become Bishop of Bagrevand and took part in the Synod in the ancient Armenian city of Artashat where the political and religious leaders of Christian Armenia gathered to discuss the threats of the Persian invasion in 449 BC. Eznik depicts a medical model that, as that of the Greek and the Romans described above, was grounded on the ancient theory of the four elements (earth, water, air, fire) and their corresponding four humors (blood, phlegm, yellow, and black bile).

It is clear that these three great cultures of antiquity—Armenia, Greece, and Persia—not only shared geographical proximity, but cultural foundations as well. Their history is intertwined not only in the wars and alliances they forged, but in the profound advances in scientific method and knowledge they proffered.

Within 100 years of Eznik's erudite contributions, however, the Armenian philosopher Davit Anhaght elegantly discussed questions that he attributed specifically to anatomy, biology, pharmacology, pathology, and medical ethics. And by the end of the first millennium, the scholar Hovhannes Sarkavag (1045–1129) vigorously lectured in favor of a separation of science and medicine from religion, and for the necessity for the experimental study of nature, and a systematic process of gathering and analyzing evidence. In that sense, Sarkavag's Armenian school of the biomedical sciences clearly anticipated the developments of scientific thought to occur in the West in the Renaissance and beyond. It is also remarkable, in light of our current understanding of developmental neurology and of biological psychiatry, to note that this scholar also demonstrated the value of learning and teaching that is obtained in an environment created and sustained by the teacher to stress and emphasize not fear and anxiety but care and concern toward the learner.

11.2.2 Western Oral Medicine from 1728 Onward

The Western medicine progressive compartmentalization of systems and organs led to the separation of oral diseases from the larger systemic pathology. As we discussed elsewhere [5, 6], the inception of dentistry and dental treatment modalities can be traced to the French anatomist, medical doctor, and dentist Pierre Fauchard (1678–1761), and his treatise entitled *Le Chirurgien Dentiste* (The Surgeon Dentist, 1728). This work was the first ever compendium of basic oral anatomy and function, oral pathology signs and symptoms, operative methods for removing decay and tooth restoration, periodontal disease, and manifestations associated with pyorrhea, orthodontics, as well as prosthodontic techniques including replacement of missing teeth and tooth transplantation. It signaled the inception of oral biology and medicine as we recognize today in the West and was soon followed in the USA by Harris' work entitled *The Dental Art, a Practical Treatise on Dental Surgery* (1839).

It is notable that Fauchard was among the first to reject the theory that worms cause tooth decay. Rather, he observed that sugar, which was arriving from the New World as a first rate commodity, was detrimental to the teeth structure and the surrounding gingiva. By the turn of the twentieth century, Miller, following on Pacini's groundbreaking work in microscopic anatomy and Koch's discoveries in bacteriology, reported the observations that bacteria inhabited the oral cavity and that they were responsible for the production of acids capable of substantive damage of tooth structures when in the presence of fermentable carbohydrates—what biochemists were by now describing as the glycolytic process by which glucose, fructose, and most commonly sucrose are metabolized into acids, such as lactic acid. These developments in Western scientific thinking established a fundamental change in our conception of the etiology of dental caries shifted from the diet to a "chemoparasitic" model, which was soon confirmed by the studies on plaque and tartar by Black and Williams. By 1921, clinical experimentation by Major Rodriguez Vargas, of Army Dental Corps, established and demonstrated that dental caries was actually a bacterial disease of the oral cavity [6].

In terms of models of treatment interventions for oral diseases, three time periods can describe this process of evolution in the West:

- Initially, and following Fauchard's conceptualization, dental care was envisioned as a form of manipulations aimed at countering the ills consequential to poor oral health and little or no oral hygiene. Stemming from a "drill and fix" reparative mode, the primary goal of dental care was to repair damaged or decayed dental structures or, when all else failed, to perform extractions—often by today's standards, wanton extractions—some would call it a "drill, fix, or *amputate*" model [6].
- Research in physiology and medicine in the late nineteenth century, particularly with Paul Ehrlich's concept of the "magic bullet"—recognized today as antibodies—which earned him the Nobel Prize in medicine and physiology in 1908, the conceptualization of health and disease was fundamentally changed in the West. The "trend" of research permeated health care in general and the dental field in particular. Understanding and describing the fundamental mechanisms of tooth decay, caries, and other oral disease became the object of pursuit and the core of treatment interventions. Research yielded successful observations with respect to certain modes of cure or prevention—case in point, the protective nature of sealants, of water fluoridation, and of simple behaviors and habits of oral hygiene. A second great period of Western care for oral diseases had emerged, which came to be known as the "*prevention*" model [6].
- Based on the insights of Archibald Cochrane, MD in the early 1970s, the field of evidence-based medicine emerged. Within a few decades, the realization that treatment interventions for oral diseases ought to be based on the best available

evidence had been disseminated, and the American Dental Association formally defined evidence-based dentistry (1999) and launched the present-day "*translational effectiveness*" model of dental care [6–8].

It is important to note that from the translational effectiveness viewpoint mandates a systematic perusal of the entire body of available research reports (i.e., the bibliome) on the treatment of a given oral pathology in order to yield a consensus of the best available evidence principally with respect to effectiveness. The model calls for the efficacious translation of these effectiveness findings in specific clinical settings to ensure not only maximizing benefits, while minimizing risks and costs, but also adherence to the patient's clinical case and history, value system and preferences, and overall health literacy ([6–9]; cf., Chap. 1).

11.2.3 Oral Diseases Manifest Systemic Diseases: The Ayurvedic Tradition

As noted in greater details throughout the noteworthy chapters of this book, Ayurveda, believed to be a comprehensive, traditional system of holistic medicine originated from the Vedic civilization of India about 5,000 years ago, is universally accepted as the oldest form of health care on earth. It is often referred to as the *mother of all healing*.

Ayurveda is a Sanskrit term made up of the words *ayu* and *veda*. *Ayu* means life and *veda* means knowledge or science. The term "Ayurveda" thus means "the knowledge of life" or "the science of life" [10]. Ayurveda lays a foundation within a trend of deeply relaxing wellness therapies. The fundamental philosophy of this tradition can be traced to two original schools also about the 1st millennium BC:

- The *Charaka*, initiated by the "father of Indian medicine," Charaka, defended that *ayu* comprises the mind, body, senses, and the soul and, therefore, that health and disease are not predetermined, and life may be prolonged by human effort and attention to lifestyle. In this view, it is more important to prevent the occurrence of disease than to seek a cure (cf., the ancient Ayurvedic treatise Charaka Samhita).
- The *Sushruta*, led by surgeon and physician Sushruta himself along the banks of the Ganges in northern India and based on the Sushruta Samhita, a descriptive text of over 300 surgical procedures,120 surgical instruments, and demonstration and classification for human surgery.

Together, the *Charaka* and the *Sushruta* signify the basis, foundations, and traditions for ensuring the wisdom (*veda*) or longevity (*ayu*). In fact, from these emerged over the centuries the eight primary domains of Ayurvedic medicine:

- *kāyācikitsā*—internal medicine
- *śalyacikitsā*—surgery and anatomy

- *śālākyacikitsā*—medicine specifically for eye, ear, nose, and throat diseases
- *kaumārabhṛtya*—pediatrics
- *bhūtavidyā*—spirit medicine
- *agada tantra*—toxicology
- *rasāyana*—rejuvenation and antiaging
- *vājīkaraṇa*—aphrodisiacs

The Ayurvedic tradition conceives oral diseases, specifically, as diseases of the organisms that happen to manifest in the oral cavity. In Ayurveda, dental health (*danta swasthya* in Sanskrit) is held to be very individualistic, varying with each person's constitution (prakriti) and climatic changes resulting from solar, lunar, and planetary influences (i.e., *kala-parinama*) [10].

Following the fundamental philosophy of Ayurvedic medicine, treatment intervention in general, and modes of treatment specifically directed to oral diseases, must be grounded on the balance of the three elemental humors (*doṣas*, i.e., doshas), which, by their own nature, can and do deteriorate easily. The relative proportion and combination of these humors in any one patient at any given time determines the likelihood, the site, and the severity of disease. That is to say, Ayurveda is a common sense science with a profound knowledge of all the systems and functions of the body; hence, it is important to understand that any imbalance in the doshas is what really triggers the disease process including oral diseases.

To eliminate disease is to reestablish the appropriate balance among these forces, and that is achieved through a systematic process of *Panchakarma* (five detoxification processes). These elemental energies are:

- *Vāta*: air, space—"wind" (i.e., nervous system equivalent)
- *Pitta*: fire, water—"bile" (i.e., venous system equivalent)
- *Kapha*: water, earth—"phlegm" (i.e., arterial system equivalent)

The objective of curative treatment in Ayurveda is to restore the balance of the doshas (i.e., *dhatusamya*), but in malignant tumors, all three systems get out of control (i.e., *tridoshas*) and lose mutual coordination that causes tissue damage, resulting in critical condition. Tridoshas cause excessive metabolic crisis resulting in proliferation [11, 12]. Dhatusamya is essentially obtained by:

- Strengthening the weakened doshas
- Decreasing the increased doshas
- Maintaining the normal levels of doshas [11]

Treatment through Panchakarma is used for deep detoxification. However, Ayurveda encourages the prevention of imbalance and restoration of balance through the management of the doshas with a natural, down-to-earth Ayurvedic regime that includes proper diet and lifestyle, Ayurvedic herbs and herbal preparation, daily healthy routines, yoga, and meditation practices suited to your unique, individual constitution, as well as Ayurvedic therapies for relaxation and rejuvenation. These are the tools to optimal health and long life with Ayurveda [10, 13].

Specifically directed to enhance and maintain oral health and prevent or treat oral diseases, Ayurvedic doctors recommend using warming, astringent, connective-tissue-healing herbs. These herbs can be used as a rinse or applied as packs (a pinch of powder wetted to a mush with a liquid such as water or vitamin E and tucked next to the teeth). Rinses are made by preparing an herb as tea, or by simply stirring herb powder into water, and by holding the rinse in the mouth for a few seconds or up to several minutes before rinsing [10, 13].

For example, Amla (i.e., *Phyllanthus emblica*, *Emblica officinalis*), an herb that works well as a mouth rinse, or 1–2 g per day can be taken orally in capsules for long-term benefit to the teeth and gingiva. Amla supports the healing and development of connective tissue when taken internally and that always benefits the gingiva. Western experimental science has established that Amla extracts induce programmed cell death in vitro (i.e., apoptosis) and modify gene expression in the bone-resorbing cell population known as the osteoclasts, thus preventing or slowing the progression of rheumatoid arthritis and osteoporosis [14].

Moreover, the Ayurvedic text Charaka Samhita refers to the protocol Kavala (i.e., Gandusha: medicinal gargles that can be oleaginous—*snehi*, soothing—*prasadi*, purifying—*shodhi*, or healing—*ropana* in nature and purpose) that involves swishing oil in the mouth for oral and systemic health benefits and that is claimed to cure about 30 systemic diseases ranging from headache, migraine to diabetes and asthma. In the context of oral diseases, this mode of intervention is reputed to prevent decay, oral malodor, bleeding gums, dryness of throat, and cracked lips and for strengthening teeth, gums, and the jaw [10].

11.3 The Purpose and the Process of Evidence-Based Research

Translational effectiveness refers to the translation of the best available evidence gathered in systematic reviews in specific clinical settings [6–9]. These stringent research synthesis protocols [15, 16] proffer recommendations about clinical practice guideline revisions, decisions about standard of care and health information technology policy, new research and funding directions, and to fully empower patients by ensuring patient empowerment and participation through increased health literacy (cf., Chap. 1).

Optimal efficiency and reliability of this process depends critically on the quality of the systematic reviews by means of adherence to fundamental standards of research excellence and the regular update of the consensus of the highest quality evidence. This is the concerted purpose of the work that will enrich an evidence-based conceptualization of Ayurvedic medicine.

The standard protocol of systematic reviews is based largely on the recommendations of the Center for Reviews and Dissemination (crd.york.ac.uk/CMS2Web, cf., 26), the evidence-based dentistry study group (ebd-pbrn.org), the international forum on evidence-based dentistry and comparative effectiveness research (ifebdcer.org), the Agency for Health Care Research and Quality (AHRQ) (ahrq.gov), and similar entities and can be outlined as the following steps [7, 8, 15, 16].

1. The PICO question generally arises from the patient-clinician encounter, and emerges as the patient's characteristics (P), and the possible interventions (I) to be considered and compared (C) are noted in the pursuit of a given clinical outcome (O). The PICO question also generates the keywords necessary to enable an in-depth perusal of the entire body of available evidence [7, 8].
2. The entire bibliome of peer-reviewed literature and gray literature that is available needs to be accessed through multiple electronic databases and by hand in the library stacks, as necessary. The pertinence of the identified bibliome to the PICO question is ensured by the stringency of the inclusion and exclusion criteria [7, 8]. To minimize publication bias, literature must be collected in all languages. Translators and readers in foreign languages must be recruited, trained, and standardized as needed.
3. The resulting literature is analyzed for the level of the evidence and the quality of the evidence reported in each study by means of well-established and standardized checklists (e.g., CONSORT, PRISMA, SORT, STREGA, STROBE), as well as validated instruments to quantify the measurable outcome of evidence quality (i.e., R-Wong and Jadad for primary research, R-AMSTAR for existing systematic reviews) and strength of clinical relevance (i.e., Ex-GRADE) [7–9, 15–18]. The STRICTA instrument was recently developed for the specific purpose of performing evidence-based research of acupuncture [19, 20]. Concerted effort has also been deployed to establish protocols and tools for the pursuit of the best available evidence in Ayurvedic medicine [21–23]. The construct and content validity of these instruments are established based on standard criteria of research methodology, design and statistical analysis, and interrater reliability, and Cohen's κ coefficient agreement reliability must be clearly defined in a manner similar to that we have employed for the validation of the R-AMSTAR [24], which is commonly utilized in clinically relevant complex systematic reviews [25, 26].
4. The data thusly generated are typically summarized and abstracted in appropriate evidence tables and systematically analyzed for the level and quality of the evidence outcomes by means of acceptable sampling statistical analysis ([7, 24]; cf. Chap. 1). Overarching statistical significance among nonheterogeneous outcomes (as determined by the Cochran Q and I^2 statistical test) are tested by fixed, or when appropriate, random effects model meta-analysis [7, 24], using the Cochrane-RevMan or any equivalent appropriate software. L'Abbé, funnel, and forest plots serve to illustrate data patterns. The level of significance is usually set at $\alpha = 0.5\%$, although the variability inherent to complementary and alternative medicine protocols in general and Ayurvedic medicine in particular may dictate a higher level of significance (e.g., 10%). Bonferroni correction is used as needed to control for increased risk of type I error upon multiple comparisons [7, 15, 26, 27].

5. Decision-making of the best available evidence can be both qualitative and quantitative [6–9, 28–30]. Qualitatively, the clinical relevance of the resulting consensus of the best available diagnostic or prognostic evidence is discussed in the framework of the Logic Model and is described along (a) patient-centered criteria of satisfaction and quality of life, (b) practitioner satisfaction of clinical efficacy, (c) patient and clinician satisfaction about cost-effectiveness and risk-benefit ratio effectiveness, and (d) public health values and concerns, such as translation of the findings and the data into the specific clinical setting presently attending to the patient (i.e., translational effectiveness). Quantitatively, the outcomes of the research synthesis process can be utilized in a probabilistic mode of clinical decision-making that is directed to computing the probabilities of cost and risk, compared to benefits in a utilitarian model of decision-making (cf., Markovian tree). Consensus of the best available evidence will be analyzed in light of limitations of each independent systematic review and of threats to internal and external validity of the research synthesis protocol itself (cf., Chap. 1).
6. Based on PRISMA, AMSTAR, R-AMSTAR, and Ex-GRADE criteria (cf., Chap. 1) and the acceptable sampling analysis protocol, metrics are generated that are quantitative in format (rather than being single-word statements such as "good," "limited") and are grounded on statistical percentile (e.g., medians, interquartile intervals) and confidence intervals. The conclusions produced by the graded and ranked systematic reviews are thus be better used as communication materials for helping researchers and research-funding agencies to identify important gaps in our knowledge and for informing the actions of public health officials and other decision-makers [8, 9, 24, 30].
7. For the purpose of dissemination of knowledge, critical summaries (i.e., "evidence reviews") of each generated systematic review are developed in a user-friendly format for the researcher, the clinician, the policymaker, and as much as the patients themselves. These summaries serve as the foundation for recommendations about each intervention reviewed to ensure that practice, policy, research, and funding decisions can be informed by the highest quality evidence. These summaries also become key instruments to empower the patients by raising health literacy [7–9]. Current work in our research group (cf., EBD-PBRN.org) aims at standardizing and validating the quality and value added of evidence reviews recommendations.

11.4 Conclusion: Translational Effectiveness in the Ayurvedic Paradigm

Gargantuan steps have been taken as of late in the process of incorporating the research synthesis protocol for obtaining the best available evidence of efficacy and effectiveness for Ayurvedic medicine interventions and in the generation of systematic reviews in this domain [21–23, 31, 32]. Nevertheless, the complexity of the field of the Ayurvedic perspective on health care, which is presented in this book, and was briefly outlined in the above section, renders the process of research synthesis toward the best available evidence particularly arduous—and that, particularly if one seeks to focus on disease manifestations specific to one or another organ, such as the oral cavity—simply because the fundamental principles of Ayurvedic medicine defends the intimate intertwining among all organs. The Ayurvedic principles defend that a specific anatomic region (e.g., the oral cavity) cannot and must not be considered in and of itself, and precluding its appartenance and interdependence with all other anatomic sites, organs, and physiologic processes.

Certainly, there are certain pathophysiological manifestations of the organism's increasing and overall loss of inner strength (i.e., energy, weakness: *agni*), which is represented as a loss in digestive capacity (i.e., decreased ability to eliminate toxic substances and influences: *mandagni*), that result in increased levels of unwanted "unripe" byproducts of such impaired processing (*ama*), that in turn unleash a response by the organism toward these toxic materials (*amavastha*). A Western view of this process may be akin to an immune or an autoimmune response raised against *amavastha* [11, 33, 34].

Immune activation results in the production of proinflammatory cytokines, which act on the hypothalamus to induce lethargy, nausea, and other alterations in behavior [2, 3, 5]. Similarly, the Ayurvedic principles teach us that the *amavastha* response increasingly leads to increasing impermeability and sluggishness of the srotas (i.e., *srotas*, internal bodily channels [31] that act as conduits for nutrients crucial to physical functioning throughout the human body—not dissimilar to the concepts of meridians in traditional Chinese medicine), resulting in stagnation or accumulation of the humors (i.e., *sanchaya* of *doshas*) and consequently a state of psychophysiological imbalance and morbidity, which can become so acute as to lead to mortality [11, 33, 34].

The following generalization follows, which could be pertinent to most conditions, which, in Western medicine, might be considered "oral pathologies": that is to say, that many, if not most pathologies viewed through the prism of Ayurvedic medicine commence as a state of weakness of *agni* (*mandagni*) that obturates *srotas*, and leads to *doshas* stagnation. Consequently, Ayurvedic intervention is designed to detoxify the *srotas* network (i.e., *samshodhana*) to allow free flow of *doshas* and to strengthen *agni*. *Panchakarma*, as noted above, is the classic example of a set of five therapeutic procedures described for *samshodhana* systemically, as well as specifically for oral diseases [11, 33, 34].

Ayurvedic principles recommend two types of *samshodhana*:

- External purification through diverse means (e.g., oleation, fomentation, massage) to soften and mobilize impurities (i.e., *malas*) and direct them through gross excretory channels (i.e., *kosthas*)
- Internal purification, the principal and most effective Ayurvedic intervention

An excellent brief compendium of Ayurvedic treatment modalities of diseases specific to the teeth, the tongue, the palate, and other structures in the oral cavity is to be found in [11, 35]. For example, in the case of the pathology of the soft mucosa, which in the West is termed oral lichen planus, an Ayurvedic intervention would prescribe the following:

- Oil gargle with either of *Jatyadi taila* (i.e., an herbal oil preparation from jasmine), or *Irimedadi taila* (a mixture of extracts from acacia and 19 other herbs, designed for oral ulcers, bleeding gums, halitosis)
- Possibly, a *Panchakarma* protocol (aimed at pacifying the aggravated *doshas* [the three bodily humors that make up one's constitution according to Ayurveda: wind, *vata*; bile, *pitta*; and phlegm, *kapha*, as noted above] by using appropriate diet, natural herbs and minerals, and at eliminating the increased *doshas* from the body) with virechana (i.e., administration of purgative substances for cleansing—therapeutic purgation)
- *Rasayana* herbs (i.e., tissue rejuvenating, reinvigorating herbs), such as *Tinospora cordifolia* (common name: Guduchi; a "hepatoprotectant" and immunomodulatory herb)

Moreover, from an Ayurvedic perspective, dental problems are linked to poor bone nourishment and related poor diet, with particular reference to taking excess refined foods which remove minerals from the body while passing through the digestive process. For those wishing to strengthen teeth, white sugar and white flour must be removed from the diet as well as any other processed, denatured, and refined foods. Nature gives us wholesome, nutritive foods, and our modern processing methods remove all the nutrition which has its price. There are various formulas in Ayurveda for strengthening bones and subsequently teeth such as coral and pearl powders. *Ayushakti* have a special formula called *Keshiya* and another called *Praval Moti* for this purpose alone which we found in clinical observation to be very effective. If bones are not being adequately nourished, there is often a deeper imbalance in the body which could be addressed by *Panchakarma*, which aims to restore the digestive fire to its full and optimal power so that what is eaten can be transformed into tissues correctly and completely.

What is clear is that the nature of the Ayurvedic process is grounded largely on philosophical principles of physiological models that are untestable by established Western criteria of the scientific method. That is to say, observations, deductions, diagnosis, decision-making for clinical intervention, and ultimately assessment and evaluation of clinical outcome efficacy and effectiveness are relatively more qualitative than in the Western health care paradigm. Therefore, as we push forward toward an evidence-based conceptualization of the Ayurvedic paradigm of health care, and reminiscent of the stringent adherence of evidence-based process upon the scientific method in research synthesis, certain caveats are noteworthy, which bring us beyond the excellent, albeit preliminary attempt to evaluate the best available evidence for translational effectiveness of Ayurvedic interventions [21, 32]:

- Firstly, it is important to recall the fundamental philosophical tenets of the great Ayurvedic school of thought. In brief, Ayurveda describes five ways to acquire knowledge and create an evidence base. Together, they reflect the epistemology of Ayurveda and its robust approach to ensure evidence-based rigor.

  - *Apta* refers to the unbiased and intuitive acquisition of knowledge from the masters.
  - *Pratyaksha* pertains to observational data acquired through the senses or their extensions in the form of actual experimentation.
  - *Anumana* is evidence derived from logical analysis leading to a deduction.
  - *Upamana* concerns the evidence generated by analogy (or similar association between variables).
  - *Yukti* pertains to facts ascertained from a planned intervention to test an idea or evaluate an observation.
- In the performance of systematic reviews of Ayurvedic medicine, considering the complexity of the field, it will be critical to ascertain a comprehensive search of the pertinent bibliome, because, as in other complex domains of health care where systematic reviews are particularly difficult to bring forth, adequate search is key to ensuring high quality of the resultant review. In order to circumvent difficulties such as the fact that much of the clinical observations and even the clinical research is never published or is published in journals that are not indexed on the main databases, it is critical to enhance standard web searches through multiple search engines with hand searches, personal communications, as well as searches beyond medical or dental sources and databases. Specifically, and because much of the pursuit of the best available evidence is directed to improving evidence-based modes of interventions particularly in terms of cost-effectiveness and benefit-effectiveness, it is important to supplement traditional biomedical search modalities, such as the Cumulative Index to Nursing and Allied Health Literature (CINAHL), Evidence-Based Medicine Reviews, EMBASE, International Pharmaceutical Abstracts, and MEDLINE, with business and economics databases, including ABI/Inform, the economics database EconLit, the general database Web of Science, ProQuest Digital Dissertations and Theses (PQDT) database, and the Public Affairs Information Service databases (PAIS International and PAIS Archive) [36, 37].
- In Ayurvedic medicine, as in other areas of health care where the process of retrieval of information and data from the obtained bibliome may be relatively elusive compared to other more scientifically driven areas of clinical medicine, due to the interdisciplinary nature of the field and the lack of a significant body of evaluative literature, certain challenges of methodology arise in relevant literature retrieval for systematic reviews in the pursuit of effectiveness of strategies, which must be carefully addressed and considered [38].
- In most cases, level and quality of evidence assessments and analysis will be limited, and perhaps even data will not be sufficient for stringent meta-analysis. These limitations ought not hinder the pursuit of evidence-based Ayurvedic medicine, since newer models of evaluation of the best available evidence now exists (e.g., thematic analysis) that pertain to synthesizing diverse and perhaps less quantitative and more qualitative evidence. In that view, a conceptual understanding of the causal pathways that influence health is sought, based on the rationale that causal pathways for health and disease spread wider than uniquely

individual determinants of health outcomes, and that they broaden up to population determinants and patterns of health. That is to say, causal pathways of health and disease viewed through the Ayurvedic paradigm embrace a range of phenomena at a variety of different analytic levels including economic, social, political, physical, and biological factors, along four primary theological (i.e., causal) dimensions: population, environment, organization, and society. It is the interaction among these forces within the individual human experience of the patient that determines a state of health or disease [39]. This view is akin to the model of inner world/outer world person-environment fit, which we presented elsewhere in the context of mind-body interactions in general and oral biology and medicine in particular [3, 5, 40].

- The question then becomes not so much whether or not systematic reviews in Ayurvedic medicine will utilize, derive, and depend more from qualitative assessment of the evidence—because clearly they will—but how best is the qualitative evaluation of the best available evidence to be obtained. Novel methodological approaches have been crafted and validated in response to the growing recognition of the need for qualitative modes of research synthesis to facilitate effective and appropriate evidence-based health care. These techniques involve computer-based (e.g., QSR's NVivo software for qualitative data analysis, EPPI-Reviewer) thematic, rather qualitative synthesis and analysis, and consist of three levels: (a) "line-by-line" coding of the text, (b) development of "descriptive/conceptual themes," and (c) generation of "analytical/interpretative themes." Thematic analysis yields meta-synthesis inferences toward a qualitative "theory-driven" conceptualization of the best available evidence [41–43].

References

1. Chiappelli F, Prolo P, Cajulis OS (2005) Evidence-based research in complementary and alternative medicine I: history. Evid Based Complement Alternat Med 2:453–458, PMCID: PMC1297495
2. Chiappelli F (1986) Mental health and physical health: two sides of the same coin. Psyche 5:4
3. Chiappelli F, Abanomy A, Hodgson D, Mazey KA, Messadi DV, Mito RS, Nishimura I, Spigleman I et al (2001) Clinical, experimental and translational psychoneuroimmunology research models in oral biology and medicine. In: Ader R (ed) Psychoneuroimmunology, IIIth edn. Academic, New York, pp 645–670. Chap. 64
4. Huff TE (2003) The rise of early modern science: Islam, China, and the West. Cambridge University Press, Cambridge, p 128 ff
5. Chiappelli F, Prolo P, Cajulis E, Harper S, Sunga E, Concepcion E (2004) Consciousness, emotional self-regulation, and the psychosomatic network: relevance to oral biology and medicine. In: Beauregard M (ed) Consciousness, emotional self-regulation and the brain. Advances in consciousness research. John Benjamins Publishing Company, Netherlands, pp 253–274. Chap. 9
6. Chiappelli F, Cajulis OS, Oluwadara O, Ramchandani MH (2009) Evidence-based based decision making—implications for dental care. In: Taggart JC (ed) Dental care: diagnostic, preventive, and restorative services. NovaScience Publisher, Inc, New York, pp 117–146. Chap. 5
7. Chiappelli F (2008) The science of research synthesis: a manual of evidence-based research for the health sciences—implications and applications in dentistry. NovaScience Publisher, New York

8. Ajaj RA, Barkhordarian A, Phi L, Giroux A, Chiappelli F (2011) Evidence-based dentistry: the next frontier in translational and trans-national dental practice. Dent Hypotheses 2:55–62
9. Chiappelli F (2011) From translational research to translational effectiveness: the "patient-centered dental home" model. Dent Hypotheses 2:105–112
10. Singh A, Purohit B (2011) Tooth brushing, oil pulling and tissue regeneration: a review of holistic approaches to oral health. J Ayurveda Integr Med 2:64–68
11. Amruthesh S (2007) Dentistry and Ayurveda–III (basics-ama, immunity, ojas, rasas, etiopathogenesis and prevention). Indian J Dent Res 18:112–119. PMID: 17687173
12. Jain R, Kosta S, Tiwari A (2010) Ayurveda and cancer. Pharmacognosy Res 2:393–394
13. Patwardhan B (2010) Ayurveda, evidence-base and scientific rigor. J Ayurveda Integr Med 1: 169–170
14. Penolazzi L, Lampronti I, Borgatti M, Khan MT, Zennaro M, Piva R, Gambari R (2008) Induction of apoptosis of human primary osteoclasts treated with extracts from the medicinal plant *Emblica officinalis*. BMC Complement Altern Med 8:59
15. Littell JH, Corcoran J, Pillai V (2008) Systematic reviews and meta-analysis. Oxford University Press, New York
16. Whitlock EP, Lopez SA, Chang S, Helfand M, Eder M, Floyd N (2009) Identifying, selecting, and refining topics. In: Methods guide for comparative effectiveness reviews. Agency for Healthcare Research and Quality, Rockville
17. Little J, Higgins JP, Ioannidis JP, Moher D, Gagnon F, von Elm E, Khoury MJ, Cohen B, Davey-Smith G, Grimshaw J, Scheet P, Gwinn M, Williamson RE, Zou GY, Hutchings K, Johnson CY, Tait V, Wiens M, Golding J, van Duijn C, McLaughlin J, Paterson A, Wells G, Fortier I, Freedman M, Zecevic M, King R, Infante-Rivard C, Stewart A, Birkett N (2009) STrengthening the REporting of Genetic Association studies (STREGA): an extension of the STROBE Statement. Ann Intern Med 150:206–215
18. Thelle DS (2009) STROBE and STREGA: instruments for improving transparency and quality of reporting scientific results. Eur J Epidemiol 24:7–8
19. MacPherson H, White A, Cummings M, Jobst KA, Rose K, Niemtzow RC, STRICTA Group (2002) Standards for reporting interventions in controlled trials of acupuncture: the STRICTA recommendations. J Altern Complement Med 8:85–89
20. MacPherson H, Altman DG, Hammerschlag R, Li Y, Wu T, White A, Moher D, STRICTA Revision Group (2010) Revised STandards for Reporting Interventions in Clinical Trials of Acupuncture (STRICTA): extending the CONSORT statement. Acupunct Med 28:83–93
21. Narahari SR, Ryan TJ, Aggithaya MG, Bose KS, Prasanna KS (2008) Evidence-based approaches for the Ayurvedic traditional herbal formulations: toward an Ayurvedic CONSORT model. J Altern Complement Med 14:769–776
22. Rastogi S, Chiappelli F (2010) Bringing evidence basis to decision making in Complementary and Alternative Medicine (CAM): Prakriti (Constitution) Analysis in Ayurveda. In: Chiappelli F, Brant XMC, Oluwadara OO, Neagos N, Ramchandani MH (eds) Understanding evidence-based practice: toward optimizing clinical outcomes. Springer, Heidelberg. Chap. 7
23. Mathur A, Shanker V (2010) Standards of reporting Ayurvedic clinical trials—is there a need? J Ayurveda Integr Med 1:52–55
24. Kung J, Chiappelli F, Cajulis OS, Avezova R, Kossan G, Chew L, Maida CA (2010) From systematic reviews to clinical recommendations for evidence-based health care: validation of Revised Assessment of Multiple Systematic Reviews (R-AMSTAR) for Grading of Clinical Relevance. Open Dent J 4:84–91
25. Chiappelli F, Ramchandani MH, Phi L, Brant XMC (2011) Clinically relevant complex systematic reviews in endodontics: relevance to comparative effectiveness research and evidence-based clinical decision-making. In: Chiappelli F, Brant X, Cajulis C (eds) Comparative effectiveness and efficacy research and analysis for practice (CEERAP): applications for treatment options in health care. Springer, Heidelberg. Chap. 3. (In Press)
26. Center for Reviews and Dissemination (2009) Systematic reviews: CRD's guidance for undertaking reviews in health care. York University, York, www.york.ac.uk/inst/crd/index.htm

27. Bartolucci AA, Hillegas WB (2010) Overview, strengths, and limitations of systematic reviews and meta-analyses. In: Chiappelli F, Brant XMC, Oluwadara OO, Neagos N, Ramchandani MH (eds) Understanding evidence-based practice: toward optimizing clinical Outcomes. Springer, Heidelberg. Chap. 2
28. Chiappelli F, Danaei S (2011) Evidence-based standard of care: applications for Comparative Effectiveness and Efficacy Research and Analysis for Practice (CEERAP) in developing patient-centered optimal treatment interventions in health care for the next decade. In: Chiappelli F, Brant X, Cajulis C (eds) Comparative Effectiveness and Efficacy Research and Analysis for Practice (CEERAP): applications for treatment options in health care. Springer, Heidelberg. Chap. 12. (In Press)
29. Chiappelli F, Cajulis OS (2009) The logic model in evidence-based clinical decision-making in dental practice. J Evid Based Dent Pract 9:206–210
30. Chiappelli F, Cajulis O, Newman M (2009) Comparative effectiveness research in evidence-based dental practice. J Evid Based Dent Pract 9:57–58
31. Singh BB, Khorsan R, Vinjamury SP, Der-Martirosian C, Kizhakkeveettil A, Anderson TM (2007) Herbal treatments of asthma: a systematic review—more research for effectiveness of Ayurvedic herbal. J Asthma 44:685–698
32. Narahari SR, Aggithaya MG, Suraj KR (2010) A protocol for systematic reviews of Ayurveda treatments. Int J Ayurveda Res 1:254–267
33. Amrutesh S (2003) Dentistry and Ayurveda—1. Indian J Dent Res 14:1–5
34. Amruthesh S (2003) Dentistry and Ayurveda—II. Basic principles. Indian J Dent Res 14:132–140
35. Amruthesh S (2008) Dentistry and Ayurveda—IV: classification and management of common oral diseases. Indian J Dent Res 19:52–61
36. Blackhall K, Ker K (2008) Searching for studies for inclusion in Cochrane Systematic Reviews on injury prevention. Inj Prev 14:137–138
37. Greyson DL (2010) Non-biomedical sources for systematic reviews of pharmaceutical policy. J Med Libr Assoc 98:85–87
38. Beahler CC, Sundheim JJ, Trapp NI (2000) Information retrieval in systematic reviews: challenges in the public health arena. Am J Prev Med 18S:6–10
39. Baxter S, Killoran A, Kelly MP, Goyder E (2010) Synthesizing diverse evidence: the use of primary qualitative data analysis methods and logic models in public health reviews. Public Health 124:99–106, Epub 18 Feb 2010
40. Chiappelli F, Manfrini E, Edgerton M, Rosenblum M, Kristine D, Cajulis KD, Prolo P (2006) Clinical evidence and evidence-based dental treatment of special populations: patients with Alzheimer's disease. Calif Den Assoc J 34:439–447
41. Thomas J, Harden A (2008) Methods for the thematic synthesis of qualitative research in systematic reviews. BMC Med Res Methodol 8:45
42. Dixon-Woods M, Agarwal S, Jones D, Young B, Sutton A (2005) Synthesizing qualitative and quantitative evidence: a review of possible methods. J Health Serv Res Policy 10:45–53
43. Chalmers I, Hedges LV, Cooper H (2002) A brief history of research synthesis. Eval Health Prof 25:12–37

Part IV
Toward Future Perspectives of Evidence-Based Ayurveda

Chapter 12
Safety Aspects of Ayurvedic Drugs

K.K. Pant, C.K. Katiyar, and Arun Gupta

12.1 Introduction

Ayurveda, the science of life, prevention, and longevity, is the oldest and most holistic or comprehensive Indian medical system. This is based upon its own centuries old strong basic principles and philosophy coupled with prolonged documented observations and rich traditional wisdom. Ayurvedic products form only one component to fulfill the desire of achieving long and healthy life. As per Ayurvedic concepts, every material on earth is made up of five basic elements, which are *prithvi* (earth), *jal* (water), *tej* (fire), *vayu* (air), and *aakash* (space). This is true for both plants as well as human beings, thus providing interface between them.

ASU (Ayurvedic, Siddha, and Unani) drugs include herbals, minerals, and metals, intended for internal (except injectables) or external use for or in the diagnosis, treatment, mitigation, or prevention of disease or disorder in human beings or animals, the ingredients of which are described in the authoritative books of Ayurveda as specified in the first Schedule of Drugs and Cosmetics Act 1940 [1].

Though the safety evaluation of modern (allopathic) medicines was being done for a long time, no such procedure existed to evaluate the Ayurvedic medicines. It was usually the view that these medicines have no or minimal adverse effects. However, in the year 1993, the *World Health Organization* (*WHO*) stated that "inappropriate use of traditional medicines or practices can have negative or dangerous effects" and that "further research is needed to ascertain the efficacy and safety" of several of the practices and medicinal plants used by traditional medicine systems [2].

K.K. Pant (✉)
Department of Pharmacology, C.S.M. Medical University, Lucknow, UP, India
e-mail: pant.kamalesh@gmail.com

C.K. Katiyar • A. Gupta
Dabur R&D Centre, Dabur India Limited, Sahibabad, UP, India
e-mail: chandra.katiyar@dabur.com; arun.gupta@dabur.com

S. Rastogi (ed.), *Evidence-Based Practice in Complementary and Alternative Medicine*,
DOI 10.1007/978-3-642-24565-7_12, © Springer-Verlag Berlin Heidelberg 2012

In the present scenario, safety of a medicine has gained utmost importance due to growing global interest, competition, and scientific discovery along with changing regulatory requirements. In USA, Europe, and also in India, many new regulatory notifications have come in recent years, which itself is a regulatory challenge in the field of herbals.

Ayurvedic medicines contain ingredients of plants, minerals, metals, or animal origin. There may be potential risk of toxicity due to contamination or improper manufacturing processes, etc. Saper et al. (2004) questioned the safety of Ayurvedic medicines contaminated with heavy metals [3]. Subsequently, in 2005, *Health Canada* and *UK* banned few Indian Ayurvedic medicines consequent to which the Government of India made testing of heavy metals mandatory for exported Ayurvedic products. These were the triggers which actually led to the setting of heavy metal limits for herbals by Government of India. Herbal materials can be crude herbs or herbal extracts like aqueous extracts, hydroalcoholic extracts, etc. As per a recent notification by Government of India (*GSR 663 (E) August 2010*), other solvent extracts have also been permitted with the condition of safety studies [4].

Evaluation of safety of Ayurvedic medicines is a complicated task. The first question is what to evaluate: the crude formulation or its individual ingredients? While many protagonists of modern medicine are of the view that individual ingredients must be evaluated for safety, followers of Ayurvedic system may argue that separation of ingredients may destroy the basic character of these medicines. We may actually evolve a middle path to avoid any such confrontation—let the multi-ingredient finished product be evaluated first for safety of the Ayurvedic medicines and if found safe, be put to clinical use. The individual ingredients can be studied later in case adverse drug reactions are reported.

Modern medicines may contain potentially harmful chemicals, due to which, a number of safety procedures have been adopted for their evaluation. Phase I of the clinical studies evaluates the intended drug for its safety only. Only after a chemical substance is found safe for clinical use, further studies can be conducted for its clinical applications.

With the Ayurvedic system of medicine, as with all other forms of traditional medicines, no such check point(s) has been suggested till date. This does not imply that Ayurvedic system is not aware of the adverse drug reactions (ADR) associated with these medicines. The pharmacovigilance system for Ayurvedic products has been put in place with functioning ADR monitoring headquarters at Jamnagar (Gujarat) and others at all tertiary Ayurvedic hospitals. However, currently, the process of an ADR data bank of Ayurvedic drug is very much in the offing and is expected to be completed within a few years.

As a result of WHO promotion of traditional medicine, countries have been seeking the assistance of WHO in identifying safe and effective herbal medicines for use in national health-care systems. In 1991, the Director-General of WHO, in a report to the 44th World Health Assembly, emphasized the great importance of medicinal plants to the health of individuals and communities [5]. Earlier, in 1978, the 31st World Health Assembly (WHA) had adopted a resolution (WHA31.33) that called up on the Director-General to compile and periodically update a therapeutic classification of medicinal plants, related to the therapeutic classification of all drugs [6]. Subsequently, resolution of WHA40.33, adopted in 1987, urged member states to ensure quality control of drugs derived from traditional plant remedies by using modern techniques and applying suitable standards and good manufacturing practices [7]. Resolution WHA42.43 of 1989 urged member states to introduce measures for the regulation and control of medicinal plant products and for the establishment and maintenance of suitable standards [8]. Moreover, the International Conference on Primary Health Care, held in Alma-Ata, USSR, in 1978, recommended, inter alia, the accommodation of proven traditional remedies in national drug policies and regulatory measures [9].

WHO (1993) has published guidelines in order to define basic criteria for evaluating the safety and efficacy of herbal medicines aimed at assisting national regulatory authorities, scientific organizations, and manufacturers in this particular area. Originally, WHO guidelines for GCP have been adapted from ICH guidelines. These guidelines specify the requirements for clinical trial protocol and protocol amendment(s), background information about the name and description of the investigational product(s), trial objectives and purpose and trial design selection and withdrawal of subjects, treatment of subjects; assessment of efficacy and safety, statistics, direct access to source data/documents, quality control and quality assurance, description of ethical considerations relating to the trial, data handling and record keeping, financing and insurance if not addressed in a separate agreement, publication policy if not addressed in a separate agreement, pharmaceutical assessment of preparations, and stability and safety aspects [2].

12.2 Department of AYUSH (Ayurveda, Yoga, Unani, Siddha, and Homeopathy), India

Government of India formed department of AYUSH under Ministry of Health and Family Welfare to coordinate its various facets like education, research, and health care through Indian Systems of Medicine, Ayurveda, Homeopathy, Naturopathy, Siddha, and Yoga. This department funds several extramural projects besides having a research council called Central Council for Research in Ayurveda sciences, dedicated to research in Ayurveda, through its several labs. In order to lay down standards on medicinal plants, Department of AYUSH has prepared 540 monographs on individual medicinal plant parts and 152 Ayurvedic formulation monographs, through Ayurvedic Pharmacopoeia Committee [10, 11].

Ayurvedic medicines are regulated by Drugs and Cosmetics Act of India. This Act has recognized the use of toxic substances in Ayurvedic medicines and has given a separate Schedule E (1) for listing of such substances. These toxic substances need to undergo a detoxification process referred to as "*Shodhana Samskara*" in the Ayurvedic textbooks before they can be used as an ingredient in an Ayurvedic formulation. All the Ayurvedic formulations containing such substances need to carry a warning on their labels "to be taken under medical supervision only."

The following preclinical safety evaluation requirements for Ayurveda, Siddha, and Unani drugs and other traditional medicine have been prescribed through the Gazette of India [4].

Safety data required for various ASU products categories in India are summarized below:

1. *Patent or propriety drugs*
   ASU drugs with any of the ingredients of Schedule E (1) (list of poisonous substances under the Ayurvedic (including Siddha) and Unani Systems of Medicine) of Drugs and Cosmetics Act, 1940 with existing indication
2. *ASU drugs for Balya and Poshak*
   If any of the ingredients specified in the Schedule E (1) of Drugs and Cosmetics Act, 1940
3. *ASU drugs for Saundarya Prasadak*
   If any of the ingredients specified in the Schedule E (1) of Drugs and Cosmetics Act, 1940
4. *Medicines based on extracts of medicinal plants* (*dry or wet*)

Hydroalcohol extract for new indications and extracts other than aqueous/hydroalcoholic

For herbal Ayurvedic preparations, only subchronic studies are required except herbal extracts other than aqueous and hydroalcoholic where acute, chronic, mutagenicity, and teratogenicity toxicity studies should be done.

12.3 Evidence of Safety of Ayurvedic Products

Since Ayurvedic product development was based upon wide-ranging experiments and experiences, need to validate the safety of these products was never felt. However, in the current times, quality of drugs has been affected due to several factors such as problem of adulteration, contamination, short cuts being followed instead of following the recommended methods of producing Ayurvedic products by few individuals, and poor implementation of regulatory controls. These factors have led to the need for evidence of safety of Ayurvedic products.

12.3.1 Traditional Use

Ayurvedic medicines have been traditionally used for thousands of years in India. In 1998 as per statistics of Government of India, there were 609,400 physicians of Indian Systems of Medicines and Homeopathy in India, out of which, more than half belonged to the Ayurveda stream [12].

About 80% of the population in India depends on traditional medicine, out of which, almost 70–75% depends on Ayurvedic medicines in one form or the other.

That means if approx. 250,000 Ayurvedic physicians see on an average ten patients per day, it converts to 2.5 million patients per day. Almost equal numbers of people do not go to physician and use these medicines on their own, which means that almost 5 million people use Ayurvedic medicines on daily basis in India in some form or the other. It also includes home Ayurvedic remedies, though.

It is worthwhile to mention that though the Fourth Estate enjoys full freedom in India, even then media reported incidents of side effects related to Ayurvedic medicines are almost nil. This is an important evidence of safety of Ayurvedic medicine going by their traditional usage pattern.

12.3.2 Method of Preparation

The herbomineral products are processed in a way that eliminates the toxic properties of the metals. Most of the minerals/metals are used only after they are converted into *bhasma* by Marana. Prior to Marana, the minerals/metals are thoroughly purified by classical process called Shodhana. By Shodhana processes, minerals/metals lose the physical impurities present in them and become available in pure form for further processing. Apart from getting purified, they are certain modifications done in the properties of these minerals/metals. Specific types of processes with specific materials are advocated in classical texts for each mineral/metal [13].

12.3.3 Adverse Drug Reaction Monitoring

There was no formal system of ADR monitoring of Ayurvedic medicines in India previously. However, recently, Government of India started pharmacovigilance program for ASU drugs. It is yet to see what data are being collected through this formal system of adverse drug reaction monitoring, basis which it will be possible to comment authentically about the safety of Ayurvedic medicines in India. Moreover, India has a free press and very active print and electronic media. So far, cases of adverse drug reaction of Ayurvedic medicine have not been reported.

12.3.4 Toxicity Studies

Manufacturing of Ayurvedic medicine is controlled by Drugs and Cosmetics Act of India. However, there are certain conditions, which a manufacturer has to meet before being granted a manufacturing permission. Toxicity studies and clinical trials are not mandatory for grant of such licenses.

The major issue with the Ayurvedic/herbal medicines is that there is very less scientific data available on their safety. However, it is also a fact that it is difficult to evaluate polyherbal medicines using the conventional array of toxicological methods since these materials consist of hundreds of active ingredients. There are several publications, which state the potential toxicity of the phytomedicines. Contamination of these products by pesticides, herbicides, naturally occurring toxins, microbes, or adulteration by means of synthetic substitutes is a cause for concern. Toxicity manifestations include hepatotoxicity (most prominent—mild elevations of liver enzymes to fulminant liver failure), nephrotoxicity, and neurotoxicity, hematological, mutagenic, and cardiovascular toxicities. Hence, there is a need for a fundamentally different approach for toxicological studies that need to be adopted for Ayurvedic and herbal products. In light of the above stated facts, an integrated approach for safety assessment focused on the hazard identification is imperative. The type, nature, and extent of effects obtained during toxicity studies can help in adequately classifying herbal medicines as nontoxic, moderately toxic, or severely toxic on selected biological systems [14].

It is essential that the literature sources should be reviewed for the toxicities of the herbal products in prior human experiences or existing animal data. The need for additional preclinical studies prior to clinical trials depends on the following considerations:

- Similarities between the new and old preparations, in terms of product characteristics, and usages in clinical settings
- Scale and exposure (dosage/duration) of the proposed new clinical studies
- Frequency and severity of any known toxicity

Thus, in general, requirements for preclinical studies may range from none for early phase, small, studies using the same preparations that have been used extensively and without known safety problems, to a complete set of conventional toxicology studies for relatively new products in large phase III trials. For many herbal products, certain preclinical studies may be necessary but can be conducted concurrently with the proposed clinical trials.

Following preclinical toxicity studies used for conventional medicines may be adopted to suit the needs of traditional medicine on case-to-case basis.

12.3.4.1 Acute Toxicity [15]

Table 12.1 OECD Test Guideline 425 [15]

Species	Rats (female nonpregnant) for oral and inhalation tests
Age	Young adults
Number of animals	5 rats for each sex per dose level
Dosage	3 dose levels recommended; exposures are single doses or fractionated doses up to 24 h for oral and 4-h exposure for inhalation studies
Observation period	≤14 days

12.3.4.2 Subacute Toxicity [16]

Table 12.2 OECD Test Guideline 412 [16]

Species	Rats for oral/diet/drinking water tests
Age	Young adults
Number of animals	5 rats per dose level
Dosage	3 dose levels recommended; exposures are single doses or fractionated
Observation period	14–28 days

12.3.4.3 Subchronic Toxicity [17]

Table 12.3 OECD Test Guideline 413 [17]

Species	Rodents (usually rats) preferred for oral and inhalation studies; rabbits for dermal studies; nonrodents (usually dogs) recommended as a second species for oral tests
Age	Young adults
Number of animals	10 of each sex for rodents, 4 of each sex for nonrodents per dose level
Dosage	3 dose levels plus a control group; includes a toxic dose level plus NOAEL (no observed adverse effect level); exposures are 90 days
Observation period	30–90 days

12.3.4.4 Chronic Toxicity [18]

Table 12.4 OECD Test Guideline 452 [18]

Species	2 species recommended: rodent and nonrodent (rat and dog)
Age	Young adults
Number of animals	20 of each sex for rodents, 4 of each sex for nonrodents per dose level
Dosage	Three dose levels recommended; includes a toxic dose level and NOAEL; exposures generally for 12 months
Observation period	12–24 months

12.3.4.5 Carcinogenicity [19]

Table 12.5 OECD Test Guideline 451 [19]

Species	Testing in two rodent species, the rat and mouse preferred due to relatively short life spans
Age	Young adults
Number of animals	Each dose group and concurrent control group should therefore contain at least 50 animals of each sex
Dosage	Three dose levels recommended; highest should produce minimal toxicity and NOAEL; exposure periods are at least 18 months for mice and 24 months for rats
Observation period	18–24 months for mice and 24–30 months for rats

12.3.4.6 Developmental and Reproductive Toxicity [20, 21]

Table 12.6 OECD Test Guideline 415 and 416 [20, 21]

Species	Rat, dog is recommended
Age	Young adults
Number of animals	20 pregnant females of each sex per dose level
Dosage	Three dose levels recommended; highest dose should produce toxicity but not mortality in parents; lowest dose should not produce toxicity and NOAEL
Observation period	28 days depending on the animal species

12.4 Heavy Metals in Ayurvedic Products

Heavy metals are commonly defined as those having a specific density of more than 5 g/cm. The main threats to human health from heavy metals are associated with exposure to lead, cadmium, mercury, and arsenic. Although adverse health effects of heavy metals have been known for a long time, exposure to heavy metals continues and is even increasing in some areas [22].

Herbs-based Ayurvedic products were the only therapeutic options available to Ayurvedic physicians up to 1000 AD. The dose of such herbal products was very high, the efficacy was low, shelf life was low, and availability of the materials throughout the year was also a problem. These factors were responsible to look for the need of those products, which can be used in low dose, should be quick acting, and for which round the year availability could be ensured. This was the genesis for use of metallic products (*Rasaushadhi*) in Ayurveda.

It is generally believed that herbal and natural products are safer than the synthetic or modern medicines, but some Ayurvedic products may contain heavy metals as essential ingredients. The ever increasing popularity of Ayurvedic medicine has led to concerns relating to its safety, quality, and effectiveness especially for *bhasmas* as these are usually made of metals like mercury (Hg), copper (Cu), iron (Fe), tin (Sn), zinc (Zn), gold (Au), silver (Ag), and arsenic (As). Cadmium (Cd) and nickel (Ni) are not used as starting material, but may come as contaminant.

All these preparations are not recommended for all the patients. The indications, dose, to whom to give and to whom not to give, what should be the vehicle, what are the diseases, where they are not recommended, etc., are major factors always considered by the physician before they recommend these Ayurvedic metallic products to the patients.

Heavy metal limits for true herbal products as followed in some countries have been enumerated in Table 12.7.

The Ayurvedic Pharmacopoeia of India has specified the following permissible limits of heavy metals in Ayurvedic products [10] (Table 12.8).

Most of Rasaushadhis, by design of preparations, form a ligand of organic/inorganic substances; and free metal is converted into organic/inorganic compound. The current method of analysis of heavy metals by atomic absorption spectroscopy involves heating the test substance around up to 700°C to convert the compound into free metal before testing. However, the art of converting toxic metal into nontoxic metal-based Ayurvedic formulation gets lost in the current methods of heavy metal analysis. Therefore, there is a need to develop nondestructive analytic method for testing of such products before branding them toxic merely because of presence of metals. Alternatively, let the finished product be subjected to toxicity studies, and if then it is found to be nontoxic, it should be accepted for clinical use. The toxicity study results of few of Ayurvedic Rasaushadhi products of Dabur India Limited are given in Table 12.9.

Ayurvedic formulations do contain toxic substances, metals etc., which, if not used following Ayurvedic principles, may show symptoms of toxicity. Järup (2003) has elaborated hazards of heavy metals [22]. Some of them are given in Table 12.10.

12.5 Factors Responsible for Side Effects of Ayurvedic Medicines

The following factors are responsible for toxicity of Ayurvedic medicines:

- Known side effects
- Medication errors

Table 12.7 Heavy metal limits in few countries [23]

		Arsenic (As)	Lead (Pb)	Cadmium (Cd)	Chromium (Cr)	Mercury (Hg)	Copper (Cu)	Total toxic metals as lead
For herbal medicines								
Canada	Raw medicinal plant materials	5 ppm	10 ppm	0.3 ppm	2 ppm	0.2 ppm		
	Finished herbal products	0.01 mg/day	0.02 mg/day	0.006 mg/day	0.02 mg/day	0.02 mg/day		
China	Medicinal plant materials	2 ppm	10 ppm	1 ppm		0.5 ppm	20 ppm	
Malaysia	Finished herbal products	5 mg/kg	10 mg/kg			0.5 mg/kg		
Republic of Korea	Medicinal plant materials							30 ppm
Singapore	Finished herbal products	5 ppm	20 ppm			0.5 ppm	150 ppm	
Thailand	Medicinal plant material, finished herbal products	4 ppm	10 ppm	0.3 ppm				
WHO recommendations			10 mg/kg	0.3 mg/kg				
For other herbal products								
National Sanitation Foundation draft proposal (raw dietary supplement)		5 ppm	10 ppm	0.3 ppm	2 ppm			
National Sanitation Foundation draft proposal (finished dietary supplement)		0.01 mg/day	0.02 mg/day	0.006 mg/day	0.02 mg/day	0.02 mg/day		

Table 12.8 Heavy metal limits in Ayurvedic products [10]

Heavy metal	Permissible limits in Ayurvedic product
Arsenic	3 ppm
Lead	10 ppm
Cadmium	0.3 ppm
Mercury	1 ppm

Table 12.9 Summary of toxicity studies conducted by Dabur on Ayurvedic Rasaushadhis [24]

Product name	Type of study	Species/dose	Observation
Vasant Kusumakar Rasa	Acute oral Undue toxicity	Albino mice/oral (2.5, 5, 7.5 g/kg bw); (500 mg/kg IP)	No sign of toxicity or mortality
Laxmi Vilas Ras	Subchronic (90 days) oral Dose-range-finding study (14 days repeated feeding)	Male and female rats/500 mg/kg bw/day; 31.2, 62.5, 125, 250, 500 mg/kg bw	No significant changes
Vasanta Kusumakar Ras	Chronic (180 days) oral	Male and female Sprague Dawley rats/0, 20, 100, 300 mg/kg/day	NOEL 20 mg/kg bw; no significant changes/findings. Incidental findings and not treatment related were liver round cell infiltration, acute lung inflammation, acute kidney inflammation and abscess
Vasant Malati Ras	Acute oral	Male and female Sprague Dawley rats	LD50>2,000 mg/kg body wt in rats and mice
	Repeated dose oral (90 days)		NOEL at 80 mg/kg body wt
Swarna Bhasma	Acute oral	Male and female Sprague Dawley rats	LD50>2,000 mg/kg body wt in rats and mice
	Repeated dose oral (90 days)		NOEL at 10 mg/kg body wt
Siddha Makardhawaj	Acute oral	Male and female Sprague Dawley rats	LD50>2,000 mg/kg body wt in rats and mice
	Repeated dose oral (90 days)		NOEL at 80 mg/kg body wt
Ras Raj Ras	Acute oral	Male and female Sprague Dawley rats	LD50>2,000 mg/kg body wt in rats and mice
	Repeated dose oral (90 days)		NOEL at 160 mg/kg body wt
Chandraprabha Vati	Acute oral	Male and female Sprague Dawley rats	LD50>2,000 mg/kg body wt in rats and mice
	Repeated dose oral (90 days)		NOEL at 1,000 mg/kg body wt

(continued)

Table 12.9 (continued)

Product name	Type of study	Species/dose	Observation
Medohar Vidangadi Lauh	Acute oral	Male and female Sprague Dawley rats	LD50 > 2,000 mg/kg body wt in rats and mice
	Repeated dose oral (90 days)		NOEL at 1,000 mg/kg body wt
Mahayograj Guggulu	Acute oral	Male and female rats	LD50 b/w 300 and 2,000 mg/kg body wt in rats and mice
	Repeated dose oral (30 days)		Tolerance of 10 times of therapeutic dose (875 mg/kg/day)
Mahalakshmivilas Ras	Acute oral	Female Wistar rats and female Swiss mice	LD50 b/w 300–2,000 mg/kg body wt in rats and mice
	Repeated dose oral (30 days)	Female Wistar rats	Tolerance of 10 times of therapeutic dose (175 mg/kg/day)

Table 12.10 Toxicity of heavy metals [22]

Heavy metal	Toxicity signs and symptoms
Cadmium	Inhalation of cadmium fumes or particles can be life threatening, and although acute pulmonary effects and deaths are uncommon, sporadic cases still occur. Cadmium exposure may cause kidney damage. The initial tubular damage may progress to more severe kidney damage. Animal experiments have suggested that cadmium may be a risk factor for cardiovascular disease, but studies of humans have not been able to confirm this
Mercury	Acute mercury exposure may give rise to lung damage. Chronic poisoning is characterized by neurological and psychological symptoms, such as tremor, changes in personality, restlessness, anxiety, sleep disturbance, and depression. The symptoms are reversible after cessation of exposure. Metallic mercury may cause kidney damage. Metallic mercury is also an allergen, which may cause contact eczema. Methyl mercury poisoning has latency of 1 month or longer after acute exposure, and the main symptoms relate to nervous system damage. High doses may lead to death, usually 2–4 weeks after onset of symptoms. However, the general population does not face significant health risks from methyl mercury exposure with the exception of certain groups with high fish consumption
Lead	The symptoms of acute lead poisoning are headache, irritability, abdominal pain, and various symptoms related to the nervous system. Lead encephalopathy is characterized by sleeplessness and restlessness. Children may be affected by behavioral disturbances and learning and concentration difficulties. In severe cases of lead encephalopathy, the affected person may suffer from acute psychosis, confusion, and reduced consciousness. People who have been exposed to lead for a long time may suffer from memory deterioration, prolonged reaction time, and reduced ability to understand. Recent research has shown that long-term low-level lead exposure in children may also lead to diminished intellectual capacity. Acute exposure to lead is known to cause proximal renal tubular damage

Table 12.10 (continued)

Heavy metal	Toxicity signs and symptoms
Arsenic	Inorganic arsenic is acutely toxic, and intake of large quantities leads to gastrointestinal symptoms, severe disturbances of the cardiovascular and central nervous systems, and eventually death. In survivors, bone marrow depression, hemolysis, hepatomegaly, melanosis, polyneuropathy, and encephalopathy may be observed. Ingestion of inorganic arsenic may induce peripheral vascular disease, which in its extreme form leads to gangrenous changes. Populations exposed to arsenic via drinking water show excess risk of mortality from lung, bladder, and kidney cancer, the risk increasing with increasing exposure. There is also an increased risk of skin cancer and other skin lesions, such as hyperkeratosis and pigmentation changes

- Improper manufacturing process
- Contaminants
- Irrational use of Ayurvedic medicine
- Quality of Ayurvedic medicine
- Abuse/adulteration

12.5.1 Known Side Effects

Almost every drug is known to have side effects. An ideal drug should be free from side effects and should not give rise to any other disease. It is hard to achieve targets; however, we should make efforts to keep the undesirable effects as minimum as possible. *Kashyapa* described the minimum side effects of the drugs as *Alpadosa*, *Mandaglaapana*, and *Naatiglapanam* [25].

12.5.2 Improper Manufacturing Process

Certain products contain metallic ingredients which have to be prepared strictly as per the classical Ayurvedic textbooks which include methods to render them nontoxic. Sometimes unscrupulous manufactures may use short cuts, and safety problems may arise. However, if Ayurvedic drugs are prepared properly, this problem does not arise.

To give an example, one of most commonly used Ayurvedic product is *Swarna Vasant Malti*, which contains gold, besides mercury, sulfur, etc. Sharma et al. (2001) published the results of studies with this formulation in 20 volunteers. Blood chemistry profile of these volunteers before and after 3 months of therapy with this drug has shown no statistically significant changes in blood urea, creatinine, bilirubin, SGOT, SGPT, CPK, LDH, and hemoglobin [26].

Government of India has issued guidelines on Good Manufacturing Practices for Ayurvedic medicines, which are already in vogue. This regulatory measure is generally quite effective to tackle with the problem related to improper procedure of manufacturing.

12.5.3 Contaminants

Saper et al. (2008) have reported that 14 out of 70 Ayurvedic products tested were containing heavy metals [3]. Though in some of the medicines mentioned in this chapter had heavy metals present as contaminants, in certain other cases, they are Rasaushadhis prepared as per the Ayurvedic textbooks. The following points need intense scientific debate on this issue:

(a) Various methods used to test heavy metals involve process of digestion, which converts bound metal into free metals, which are then tested using various techniques. Do these products undergo the same process inside the human body and actually release metals from bound to free form?
(b) Does mere presence of heavy metals in plant make it toxic or the presence of heavy metals in plants may be contributing to therapeutic activity as well?
(c) There is a need to conduct a comparative study of a plant material containing heavy metals from the soil vs. the plant material which does not contain heavy metals from the soil, but the similar quantity of heavy metals is added from outside. Both these samples should be subjected to compare their toxicity to answer the above two questions.
(d) In India, we do not have any systematic study basis which the limit of heavy metals can be decided. It is recommended therefore to first screen the plant materials available in India for heavy metal presence from various geographical locations and then decide the limits.

It is also possible that sometimes these heavy metals may come as contaminant during processing in improper vessels or from the water used. These are probable sources of contamination and the Good Manufacturing Practices should be able to take care of it.

12.5.4 Irrational Use of Ayurvedic Medicines

The following factors are very important with respect to rational consumption of Ayurvedic medicines:

(i) **The vehicle**, e.g., honey, water, etc.
(ii) **Relationship with food**

There are ten different timing of taking the medicine as per Ayurveda which are given below:

1. *Abhukta* (early morning empty stomach)
2. *Pragbhukta* (immediately before food)
3. *Adhobhukta* (immediately after food)
4. *Madhyabhukta* (mid way in the meal)
5. *Antarabhukta* (between morning meal and evening meal)
6. *Sabhukta* (with food or mixed in food)

7. *Samudagbhukta* (before and after intake of light meal)
8. *Muhur-muhur* (with food or without food, infrequent intervals)
9. *Sagras* (with every bite or with some of the bites)
10. *Grasantar* (between subsequent bites)

(iii) **Improper dose**

(iv) **Incompatible formulations**

Though Ayurvedic physicians always take care for any incompatible formulations, however, this possibility cannot be overruled in over-the-counter products.

(v) **Individualized medicines**

As per Ayurvedic concepts, one medicine is not suitable for all. To give an example, three patients of common cold will be prescribed different medicines by same physician depending upon their psychosomatic constitution (*prakriti*). The application of this principle of individualized medicines by the trained Ayurvedic physicians is extremely important factor and helps to take care of safety-related aspect of the products as well. With this approach, the patient receives only those products, which are suitable to him.

12.5.5 Quality of Ayurvedic Medicine

Maintaining quality of Ayurvedic medicine is of paramount importance. After almost 30 years of effort, Government of India has developed Ayurvedic Pharmacopoeia of India giving the quality standards of certain raw materials. Since Ayurvedic medicines cover a large number of ingredients and formulations, generation of quality specifications of all the ingredients and formulations is an uphill task and will take its own time. In the meantime, most of the Indian Ayurvedic industries use their own in-house standards to maintain the quality. However, presence of unscrupulous manufacturers cannot be ruled out. GMP guidelines for Ayurvedic medicines in India have recommended implementation of quality control measures as well.

12.5.6 Abuse/Adulteration

The Charaka Samhita has classified physicians into three categories: genuine physician, feigned physician, and pseudo physician. Due to socioeconomic reasons, quackery in the name of indigenous system practitioners is also one important factor in certain parts of India.

Gupta et al. (2000) reported the presence of corticosteroids in some of the Ayurvedic preparations prescribed by the so-called traditional medicine physicians in India. In this study, almost 42% Ayurvedic medicine samples were found to be adulterated with corticosteroids [27].

In another study, Gogtay et al. (2002) reported the presence of phenytoin and phenobarbital in the Ayurvedic tablets given to the patients of epilepsy. This is to be noted that these kinds of malpractices usually happen at the end of the physician rather than at the end of manufacturer [28].

Ayurvedic products sometimes are adulterated with similar-looking cheaper alternatives also. This practice, though not common, can easily be controlled by strict GMP norms implementation.

As mentioned earlier, Ayurveda uses holistic approach of treatment where food, medicine, and nontherapeutic measures like exercise and behavior go together. The use of medicines since thousands of years, without noticeable side effects, should become a criteria for classifying Ayurvedic medicines as generally recognized as safe. The data presented above also suggest that whenever properly processed and manufactured Rasaushadhis were subjected to safety studies, these medicines came out to be safe.

12.6 Issues in Safety Evaluation of Ayurvedic Drugs

In the last 3,000 years, many things have changed, but the basic rules of safety were embedded in the formulae itself as per the classical Ayurvedic texts on herbals, and we are following the same even today. But today, can we say that because of traditional use and because of the formulation being mentioned in the classical texts, toxicity study should not be done? We need to understand that the plants used centuries ago on which the data are available in classical texts might not be the same today because of changes in geographical and climatic conditions; even the inherent genetic makeup of the plants might have changed.

How are modern drugs evaluated for their safety? Can the same parameters be applied to Ayurvedic drugs also or they need a separate form of safety evaluation? These questions need to be answered for developing a safety evaluation procedure for these drugs.

Modern medicines are evaluated for their safety by doing animal studies first. The lethal dose that kills 50% of the animals (usually mice) is called LD_{50}. From this, the effective dose can be calculated using a hit-and-trial method. Toxicity studies are carried out in animals using short and medium tenures (long-term treatment is not recommended in small animals). If the drug is found to be useful, it is then evaluated clinically using human volunteers—normal healthy subjects first and then patients. The drug then enters the market for clinical use, but for the next 5 years, yearly safety evaluation called phase IV or postmarketing evaluation is mandatory. This is done to eliminate any risk that arises after long-term therapy and could not be evaluated at the time of clinical studies.

Can the same parameters be applied to Ayurvedic medicines also? The question is gradually gaining ground, and more and more Ayurvedic physicians are now of the view that they should be applied. The main reason for this is the scientific credibility that it will provide to the Ayurvedic system of medicine as safe and effective drugs. Moreover, today the patient consciousness and legal issues involved make it safe for the practicing physician also to be sure that the medicine he/she is prescribing is a scientifically proven safe medicine.

Herbs are different from chemicals. Single plant has more than one active component or alkaloid or chemicals, which might have different biological activities when used separately. Different compounds have different actions. These chemicals may have synergistic actions. The individual chemicals may counteract the adverse drug reactions of each other. They may have effects on the bioavailability and help in absorption of the other active ingredients of the formulation. So even taking a single plant would mean taking number of chemical constituents, and hence, it becomes a challenge to identify them.

Ayurvedic products differ in their consistency too, e.g., the bulk density, specific gravity, physical form, etc., having direct impact on dose. The dose of Ayurvedic formulations also depends on the fact whether crude herb or herbal extract is used in the formulation. Like the pure chemicals may have a dose range from mcg to mg, the plant as a whole may have a dose range from mg to gm, and the large dose of herbals itself poses logistic challenges for conducting toxicity/safety studies.

Different parts of a single plant might have different actions and might have different toxicity profiles too. The uniformity of the samples used in the formulation is required for standardization of the final formulation. Hence, the selection of the parts of plants itself is a challenge for the safety of the formulation.

Secondary metabolite plays a major role in determining the action of the product. Berberine, an antimicrobial product, has poor absorption when given alone, while extract of Berberis aristata having berberine as major constituent resolves this issue, and bioavailability of berberine gets enhanced. Each extract might have different metabolites, and the absorption of the extract will also depend on it.

The absorption, distribution, metabolism, and excretion of herbs are not fully known. Hence, it remains a mystery how these herbs are acting inside the body. This lack of facts regarding pharmacokinetics itself poses a challenge to determine the safety of the formulation.

As per Schedule Y of Drugs and Cosmetics Act, if a product is used up to 2 weeks, a toxicity study of 4 weeks is required. So, the duration of toxicity studies is linked with durations of its use. According to the OECD guidelines, the NOAEL limitations are 2,000 mg per kg. Moreover, these guidelines are applicable for allopathic medicines. Therefore, these guidelines if used as such for herbal medicines might not actually be giving the validated safety outcomes.

Ayurvedic treatment follows few strict principles and ideologies, which cannot be extrapolated by modern method of toxicity study. Ayurvedic treatment regime typically includes diet, drug, vehicle, and behavioral modalities, but a part of treatment cannot be evaluated by any kind of toxicity. In Ayurveda, not all medicines are prescribed to be taken with water; some are prescribed with honey, and some are given with other vehicles like juices, etc. The herbal practitioner follows the ethics by giving the treatment as described and taught. So, while conducting the toxicity studies, should the medicine samples be given with honey or water, etc.? Therefore, in this complex scenario in herbals, it is advisable, if possible, that one sample should be given with standard vehicle and another sample without standard vehicle, and only then some conclusion about the safety of regime can be drawn. But the concept cannot be established by current methods of toxicity studies. More importantly, Ayurvedic physicians are having their own unique way to prescribe the medicines. One may prescribe different products concomitantly along with some other things like aahar, vihar, and anupana to different patients with same disease depending upon their psychosomatic constituents. Modern toxicity methods would not be able to capture this variable.

Along with the oral preparation, topical formulations are also being described in Ayurveda. There are appropriate methods available to find out the rate of absorption, the depth of absorption, and methods to study whether the topical formulations go and accumulate somewhere inside the skin or do they accumulate in some other organs of the body. By and large, only few toxicity studies such as dermal irritation test and mucosal irritation test are conducted on these products. Therefore, there is a need for some elaborate discussions on the desirability of toxicity and safety studies on topical herbal products.

Allopathic medicines may have a short onset of action, while the onset of action of herbs is not definitely known, and it actually might be much longer say in days or weeks. Therefore, herbal formulation that does not produce effect within a short time, it may not actually produce any toxicity too in a model that has been chosen basis the concept of toxicity studies on Allopathic formulations. Therefore, there is a need to look at a different paradigm, and the guidelines for the toxicity studies in herbals need to be changed accordingly.

To cite the example of lead, if it takes 6 months to produce the clinical symptoms, and while conducting toxicity study on Ayurvedic formulations having lead as an ingredient, it may not actually show any toxicity if the studies are conducted just for 1 month or 3 months. So the question arises then how are we conducting the toxic study with it? Therefore, there is a need to have total new modern protocol for that, but this needs a lot of discussions, because other considerations will be required.

12.7 Way Forward for Safety Evaluation of Ayurvedic Drugs

According to the Drugs and Cosmetics Act and Rules of India, the clinical trials were not mandatory keeping in view the traditional use and the reference of Ayurvedic textbooks. In Ayurvedic literature, a list of toxic substances has been mentioned, which should be used only after detoxification processing. Therefore, the law has been amended in India recently, which says that if the formulations are known to have any of these herbs, which are known to be toxic, the toxicity studies need to be conducted.

Another guideline, which is yet to be published, mentions that a 28-day toxicity study needs to be conducted, and if the product is to be given for a longer period, a 90-day toxicity study is required. And also, if any of the products contains these listed toxic ingredients, then it needs to be mentioned on the label itself as "To be taken under medical supervision only."

According to ICMR (Indian Council of Medical Research) guidelines, every product needs to undergo toxicity study if the product is reported to contain Schedule E (1) drugs, or it is to be given for more than 3 months [14]. The available guidelines for toxicity studies are WHO guidelines, ICH guidelines, OECD guidelines, Schedule Y guidelines, etc. The basic methodologies in almost all these guidelines are more or less same, which revolve around the principles of safety of allopathic medicines.

Nowadays, C. elegans model is also used as a tool of predictive toxicity. This may be useful for herbal drugs as well. Therefore, instead of doing the studies in rat, mice, followed by monkey, which is usually done for unknown medicines, these in vitro models may give fast and expedited results at least from safety screening purpose, and then the herb which is passing in the screen can be subjected to animal models to evaluate its safety. Ayurvedic medicines are not unknown substances, as these have been used since hundreds of years. So, if we still have to conduct toxicity studies in rat, mice, and monkey, probably, we need to find a way and need to debate and discuss on this issue.

As per the recent amendment notification by Government of India dated August 10, 2010 for the manufacturing license requirement, the special class of products, e.g., herbal extracts other than aqueous extracts, need to undergo toxicity studies, or a total safety profile needs to be established [5].

So there is a need to find out alternative means, alternative methods of toxicity safety evaluations other than documented use of traditional practice. One can also use pharmacovigilance as a tool of clinical safety basis documentation of actual clinical practice.

Ayurvedic formulations contain food ingredients, as well as therapeutic food ingredients. Therefore, it is presumed that all other ingredients except published in Schedule E (1) do fall under the list of GRAS, i.e., generally recognized as safe though it has not been notified separately.

A quick review of approx. 100 classical Ayurvedic products reveals that there are several ingredients which are common in more than ten formulations. Such ingredients can also be declared as generally recognized as safe (GRAS). The representative list of few such ingredients is given below. Thorough review of formulations mentioned in the Ayurvedic textbooks shall lead to more than 250 such ingredients (Table 12.11).

Therefore, there is a need to arrive at a criterion to declare a list of generally recognized as safe (GRAS) ingredients as well as products.

Sanjeev Sarmukaddam et al. (2010) proposed "equivalent trials" using modern medicine benchmark as a comparator and a "safety/tolerability index" on this perspective. They proposed that the trials on Ayurvedic medicines can be designed with the hypothesis that Ayurveda interventions are equivalent to conventional medicine for efficacy and superior in terms of safety. The safety index proposed by Sanjeev Sarmukaddam et al. was in light of the hypothesis that equivalence generally pertains to efficacy, but it would be desirable to match the safety and tolerability of the

Table 12.11 Frequency of occurrence of few medicinal plants in classical Ayurvedic medicines

Name of the plant	No. of products
Zingiber officinale	65
Tinospora cordifolia	59
Hedychium spicatum	50
Adhatoda zeylanica	39
Commiphora wightii	32
Mesua ferrea	31
Solanum xanthocarpum	27
Curcuma longa	25
Withania somnifera	25
Nardostachys jatamansi	23
Picrorhiza kurroa	20
Nymphaea stellata	19
Solanum indicum	17
Oroxylum indicum	17
Stereospermum suaveolens	14
Gymnema sylvestre	12
Premna integrifolia	11
Vitex negundo	10

investigational drug with that of comparator. They proposed safety index was to capture the burden of adverse events at any point in a trial subject. This type of safety index will allow making comparison between two arms for adverse events more methodological and robust. It might be difficult to establish the validity criteria for such an index as there are no gold standards to compare with, but it is not impossible. As safety is of paramount importance and an inherent strength of Ayurveda, such an index may be explored in real-life drug evaluation system [29].

12.8 Conclusions

The interest of consumers has been increasing in Ayurvedic/herbal products over the decades. One of the reasons is increasing awareness of the consumers about the side effects of the traditional medicines and chemical ingredients. Consumers perceive Ayurvedic/herbal options safer, though may not be validated scientifically due to their traditional use among the large masses, especially in traditional-medicine-rich countries like India and China. However, this increasing interest of consumers has also invited scientific scrutiny of these products, not so much for efficacy but certainly for safety. Probably, this was the reason that Saper et al. (2004, 2008) tested some of the Ayurvedic products available in US market for the presence of heavy metals and published in the *Journal of American Medical Sciences* [3, 30]. Being negative, these articles were picked up by the media with a view to shatter the miss of safety around these products. One of the points, however, missed by the authors of these articles was the Ayurvedic process of detoxification of some of the poisonous substances including heavy metals used in Ayurvedic medicines. The biggest drawback of this negative publicity was the reaction of the Western Government in banning the use of some Ayurvedic products. However, it needs to be addressed that "does mere presence of certain heavy metals in these products which are consumed at very very low dose makes them toxic" Some of the Indian companies have conducted toxicity studies of herbometallic products following OECD guidelines, and their data are contrary to the views put forward by Saper et al. to scrutinizing the safety of these products. The issue of safety of traditional medicines be it Ayurvedic, herbal, or traditional Chinese medicine products needs to be viewed with caution, and centuries of their safe use cannot be discarded. As far as certain reports of toxicity of lead due to Ayurvedic medicines are concerned, it appears that out of millions of consumers, only one to two such cases have been reported. Therefore, unless blood levels of controlled population are compared with the blood levels of patients consuming these products, reaching any conclusion shall be premature and should not be supported by the scientists.

One area of concern of proving safety of Ayurvedic drugs by traditional use is lack of system of pharmacovigilance. Government of India has initiated an action in this regard in 2009 by documenting the actual use of Ayurvedic medicines. The data have yet to come, and whenever they come, they will provide the directions of the level of safety of such products. Till that time, there is a need of developing optimum scientifically validated methods of safety evaluation of such products being used in the holistic manner as they were in actual clinical practices along with their do's and don'ts.

References

1. Malik V (2010) Drugs & Cosmetics Act, 1940 and Rules 1945. In: Law relating to Drugs & Cosmetics. Eastern Book Company, Lucknow
2. WHO Research guidelines for evaluating the safety and efficacy of herbal medicines (1993) World Health Organization, Geneva
3. Saper RB, Kales SN, Paquin J, Burns MJ, Eisenberg DM, Davis RB, Phillips RS (2004) Heavy metal content of Ayurvedic herbal medicine products. JAMA 292:2868–2873
4. GSR 663(E) (2010) Gazette notification of Government of India
5. WHO report of the 44th World Health Assembly (1991) World Health Organization, Geneva
6. WHO report of 31st World Health Assembly (1978) World Health Organization, Geneva
7. WHO report of the 40th World Health Assembly (1987) World Health Organization, Geneva
8. WHO report of the 42nd World Health Assembly (1989) World Health Organization, Geneva
9. The International Conference on Primary Health Care (1978) Alma-Ata, USSR
10. The Ayurvedic Pharmacopoeia of India. Part I; Volumes I–VII. Government of India, Ministry of Health and Family Welfare, Department of Ayurveda Yoga & Naturopathy Unani Sidha and Homeopathy (AYUSH), New Delhi
11. The Ayurvedic Pharmacopoeia of India (formulations). Part-II; Volumes I–III. Government of India, Ministry of Health and Family Welfare, Department of Ayurveda Yoga & Naturopathy Unani Sidha and Homeopathy (AYUSH), New Delhi
12. Indian Systems of Medicine and Homeopathy in India (1999) Planning and evaluation cell, Department of ISM & H, Ministry of Health & Family Welfare, Government of India, New Delhi
13. Bhaishajaya Ratnavali (1961) Ed. Rajeshwar Dutt Shastri. Chowkhamba Sanskrit Sansthan, Varanasi

14. Ethical Guidelines for Biomedical Research on Human Subjects (2006) Indian Council of Medical Research, New Delhi
15. OECD (2001) Guidelines for testing of chemicals: Test No. 425. Acute oral toxicity
16. OECD (2009) Guidelines for the testing of chemicals, section 4: health effects, Test No. 412: Subacute inhalation toxicity: 28-day study
17. OECD (2009) Guidelines for the testing of chemicals, section 4: health effects, Test No. 413: Subchronic inhalation toxicity: 90-day study
18. OECD (2008) OECD guideline for the testing of chemicals test guideline 452: Chronic toxicity studies
19. OECD (2008) OECD guideline for the testing of chemicals test guideline 451: Carcinogenicity studies
20. OECD (1983) Test guideline 415. One-generation reproduction toxicity study. In: OECD guidelines for the testing of chemicals. Organisation for Economic Cooperation and Development, Paris
21. OECD (2001) Test guideline 416. Two-generation reproduction toxicity study. In: OECD guidelines for the testing of chemicals. Organisation for Economic Cooperation and Development, Paris
22. Järup L (2003) Hazards of heavy metal contamination. Br Med Bull 68:167–182
23. WHO Guidelines for assessing quality of herbal medicines with reference to contaminants and residues (2007) World Health Organization, Geneva
24. Data on Dabur R&D Files, Dabur India limited, Sahibabad, Ghaziabad, India
25. Savarikar SS, Safety of Ayurvedic Drugs (2011) Ayurvedic perspective in relation to current drug safety design. International conference on recent advances in safety and efficacy of Ayurvedic formulation: 33–44
26. Sharma DC, Jha J, Sharma P (2001) Evaluation of safety and efficacy of a gold containing Ayurvedic drug. Indian J Exp Biol 39:892–896
27. Gupta SK, Kaleekal T, Joshi S (2000) Misuse of corticosteroids in some of the drugs dispenses as preparations from alternative systems of medicine in India. Pharmacoepidemiol Drug Saf 9(7):599–602
28. Gogtay NJ, Bhatt HA, Dalvi SS, Kshirsagar NA (2002) The use and safety of non-allopathic Indian medicines. Drug Saf 25(14):1005–1019
29. Sarmukaddam S, Chopra A, Tillu G (2010) Efficacy and safety of Ayurvedic medicines: recommending equivalence trial design and proposing safety index. Int J Ayurveda Res 1(3):175–180
30. Saper RB, Phillips RS, Sehgal A, Khouri N, Davis RB, Paquin J, Thuppil V, Kales SN (2008) Lead, Mercury, and Arsenic in US- and Indian-Manufactured Ayurvedic medicines sold via the internet. JAMA 300(8):915–923

Chapter 13
Toward Evidence-Based Practice of Ayurveda: Extrapolating the Challenges in the Current Decade

Sanjeev Rastogi

13.1 Contemporary Ayurveda: Causes of Concern

In one of its recent series titled as *India: Towards Universal Health Coverage,* Lancet tried to focus upon health-care fallacies, needs, and plans relevant to contemporary India. The series presented evidences to show a high burden of infectious diseases [1], reproductive and child health problems, nutritional deficits [2], chronic diseases, and injuries [3] upon existing health-care delivery system practiced in India. This series further identified issues like equity in health care [4], human resource management [5], and health-care financing [6] as area of concern to optimize Indian health-care delivery. As an outcome, this series proposed a comprehensive "Integrated National Health System" plan to care for existing deficits in Indian health care essentially through effective utilization and mobilization of available resources operating under a continuously upgrading and accountable model. A focus on primary health care with better community participation to ensure a health equity remained the core position in this plan proposition.

At the outset, the series remained successful in identifying the gaps between need and reality in contemporary Indian health care and also in successful drafting of an action plan to cut into the ice. Nevertheless, despite its comprehensiveness, unfortunately, the elaborate "Integrated National Health System" plan for some reasons failed to identify the possible role of complementary stakeholders of Indian health care on an equity basis. It advocated for strengthening of diversity in health-care delivery by allowing integration between existing medical and non-medical health providers on a regulatory basis but at the same time limited this integration to public–private sector and allopathic system of medicine only [7].

S. Rastogi
PG Department of Kaya Chikitsa, State Ayurvedic College, Lucknow University, Lucknow, Uttar Pradesh, India
e-mail: rastogisanjeev@rediffmail.com

S. Rastogi (ed.), *Evidence-Based Practice in Complementary and Alternative Medicine*,
DOI 10.1007/978-3-642-24565-7_13, © Springer-Verlag Berlin Heidelberg 2012

Traditional Indian health care including Ayurveda could not seemingly find a place to this integration plan aiming ambitiously toward radical corrections into Indian health-care scenario. Though, at some places of the series, physicians trained in Ayurveda, Yoga, and naturopathy were considered as important resource to universal health care in India [5], this recognition was rather more in reference to the existing deficits in the human resource pertaining to health care in rural India and not in true spirit of recognizing these sciences as a potential mean of health-care provision.

There are two learnings which can be had from this Lancet series. First, Ayurveda, including other traditional health-care practices prevalent in India, is still out of focus as a dependable stakeholder to health care, and thereby, it does not earn a sizable concern among policy makers who are busy designing the health-care models suiting to the contemporary needs of India. The eventual result is the exclusion of these systems from any possible integration plan to improve existing health-care delivery in India. Second and even more important learning is the observation about failure of Ayurvedic fraternity (including its policy makers) in recognizing the issues of concurrent national and global interest and in finding their prospective roles to the corresponding national health care.

Ayurveda, for most recent years of its practice, is passing continuously through a bewildering phase. In lack of effective training, research, and unmonitored accountability, Ayurvedic clinical practice largely suffers with subjective interpretations eventually limiting its becoming into a dependable stakeholder to health care. There are soaring deficits on account of Ayurveda planning and policy making. In want of effective and goal-oriented directives suiting to the contemporary needs, Ayurveda is succumbing to its own fallacies in the form of its under-, ineffective and improper utilization. Situation of contemporary Ayurveda in India is expressed pathetically by David Eisenberg who headed a US delegation (2010) to India aiming at exploration of the possibilities of introducing Ayurveda into western biomedical curriculum. Eisenberg expressed his discontent by observing paucity of evidence-based approach in Ayurveda and a lack of formal interaction between allopathic and Ayurvedic medicine. David Eisenberg, who also had served as adviser to NIH with regard to CAM expresses,

> "I was struck by the observation that formal interaction between allopathic and Ayurvedic clinical researchers, basic scientists, and their respective institutions is limited in India at this point of time",
> "Learned of no prospective research documenting the inter-rater reliability of Ayurvedic diagnostic procedures nor did we learn of any ongoing studies to test the sensitivity of specificity of Ayurvedic diagnostic categories",
> "With few exceptions, there was little evidence of authoritative, multidisciplinary research involving Ayurvedic medicinal plants, their safety, reproducibility, quality assurance, mechanism of action, efficacy or cost effectiveness in the treatment of common medical conditions",
> "There was also little evidence of strategic partnering involving Ayurvedic medical experts, Ayurvedic pharmacy experts, botanical authorities across India, agricultural and environmental experts, drug discovery experts, medicinal chemists, clinical trial experts, large pharmaceutical companies, major universities as well as relevant governmental agencies and ministries". [8]

Echoing to the global viewpoint about contemporary Ayurveda in India, these expressions may serve as an eye opener although there are meager evidences that the gaps and limitation of contemporary Ayurvedic practices are being cared by means of finding the effective ways for its improvement. Recognizing and reacting to the global calls of bringing evidence base to Ayurveda pertaining to its effectiveness and safety, some novel initiatives are taken by the Government of India. Setting up of an independent department of Ayush to steer the traditional health-care planning and execution was one such mega initiative. Since its inception, Ayush, through many of its collaborative mechanisms and with involvement of many apex biomedical research organizations in India, laundered substantial budget to bring out the scientific and evidence base to Ayurveda. "Golden Triangle Project," "Millennium Project," "Human Genome Project," and "Science in Ayurveda" are few ambitious projects who tried to add substantially to the scientific understanding of Ayurveda. Launch of national campaigns to promote Ayurvedic therapies of *panch-karma* and *kshar-sutra* is of the efforts taken to make Ayurveda accessible and available at primary health-care level. Launch of National Pharmacovigilance movement pertaining to Ayurveda, Siddha, and Unani drugs in 2008 is an initiative taken to establish the safety of drugs belonging to these systems. National Rural Health Mission (NRHM), a most comprehensive health mission launched in India since independence, in principle, also recognizes mainstreaming of Ayurveda as one of its objective. Ayurveda practitioners are also proposed to be made available at every secondary and tertiary care center to make these therapies available to everyone. Various new centers pertaining to Ayurveda education and practice are proposed and are being executed. An overview of these initiatives gives us a feeling of solace for acting substantially toward the ultimate objective of exploring Ayurveda in scientific vigor.

At this point of time, we may think that we did substantially to bring Ayurveda and contemporary science together to synthesize an integrated approach of health care where modern technology meets traditional wisdom without compromising the values inherent to them [9]. It is however important to identify if this interfacing is equity and respect based or if it is favoring one at the cost of the other. Unfortunately, observations to various ongoing ambitious and cost-intensive projects commissioned to trace a scientific basis to Ayurveda find the later to be true. At many places, the interface is like meeting of a rich prince and an ordinary citizen where the prince, by virtue of his position, is allowed to choose the bargains. In our case, it is easy to speculate who bargains better [10].

At the same time, it is also important to see what has made the ordinary citizen so docile that it is not able to argue even for its genuine requirements. Public sector Ayurvedic hospitals in many states of India are facing a crisis of inpatients to the extent that any need of inpatient facility in Ayurvedic hospitals has been brought under interrogation. Ayurvedic hospitals in Uttar Pradesh (one of the most populous state in India),who have a capacity of 10,288 beds, are reported to have a bed occupancy which is less than 1% [11]. Although certain surveys show a compatible outpatient increase at Ayurvedic hospitals at the same time and argue it to be a reflection of changing pattern in medical care seeking behavior (MCSB) of patients, the claims are simply refuted if the data are adjusted to the population increase in corresponding years [12]. Undoubtedly, the consumer base and corresponding support system to Ayurveda in India shrunk considerably over the period of time. The reasons partly are the advent of more reasonable, quicker, and attractive packages of relief offered through modern medicine but at the same time also the failure of Ayurvedic fraternity to change as per need in presumption that the last word in their medicine has already been said [13].

For many past decades of its growth, Ayurvedic fraternity by and large failed to perceive the contemporary needs and consequently failed to react proactively. In lack of well-defined goals and effective planning to commission them, Ayurveda as a system remained destined to a mere survival marked with a severely compromised growth. In lack of an effective support system, works done by individual institutions or people, despite their importance in terms of relevance and timeliness, could not gather a wave of change in Ayurveda [14].

Presence of Ayurveda in global academic publishing is equally gloomy. Reflecting the poor strategic positioning and work culture of Ayurveda in India, Ayurveda articles, comparing to other CAM modalities, are poorly visible at important indexing databases including PubMed [15]. A quantitative and qualitative deficit concerning the Ayurvedic manuscript preparation is among important limiting factors, affecting their ultimate visibility. Ayurvedic scholars are poorly acquainted with research methods suiting to their needs and also have poor access to knowledge of converting a research into publication. There also been a poor motivation among Ayurvedic scholars toward documentation. A documentation is neither practiced in clinic nor is visible at research. The results are huge anecdotal claims about Ayurvedic interventions, albeit unverifiable in most instances. In absence of rigorous research, an anecdotal claim can never turn into a dependable observation having an external validity.

Training and education programs of Ayurveda are equally inefficient. There had been a huge debate on the structure and composition of syllabus to Ayurveda undergraduates and postgraduates, but it was rarely thought how this utopist training would practically be imparted [16].

13.2 Evidence-Based Ayurveda: Constraints and Corresponding Remedies

EBM is based upon the fundamental principle of utilizing evidences generated through practice and research as a dependable tool to help in a decision making referring to a clinical condition. It is evident here that in contemporary sense, an evidence has to come primarily through observations furthered through research. It is therefore easy to infer that, for evidence-based Ayurveda, Ayurvedic clinics are to be focused initially for their observations and are to be substantiated further through research in order to verify the observations coming through practice.

Evidence-based practice is the final outcome of a systematic approach that brings out the best among the available information to make clinical decisions

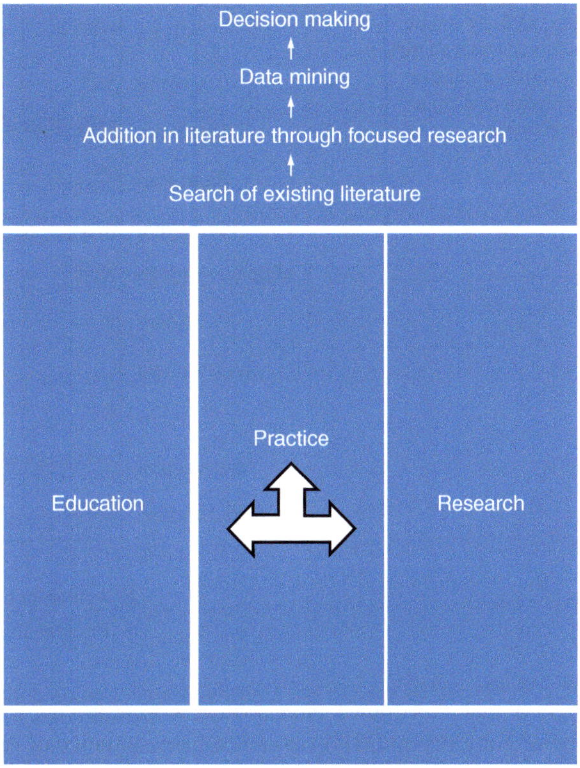

Fig. 13.1 Constructing the model of evidence-based practice in Ayurveda

more transparent and outcomes more predictable. It is evident that to reach at this outcome, we need to have strong foundation of researches oriented pragmatically toward real-life situations. In conditions where research models are not adequately addressing to the clinical needs, they are needed to be substantiated with new research models to fill the gaps. Further to this, we need to find tools for an effective data mining through which the clinical quarries may be addressed quickly, adequately, and efficiently. We need to understand clearly here that EBM and EBA are essentially the outcome of many well-defined steps constituting a process operating at multiple levels defining the comprehensive medical practice. Unless these steps and eventually the ultimate process are admired and adopted carefully, we cannot think of an evidence-based medicine.

13.2.1 Building Up the Foundation of EBA

The construct of EBA is essentially founded upon three pillars, namely, education, practice, and research in Ayurveda (Fig. 13.1). More strong these pillars are built, more smooth would be the erection of EBA. For their fundamental importance and also for their obvious limiting role toward EBA, it is important to consider them in

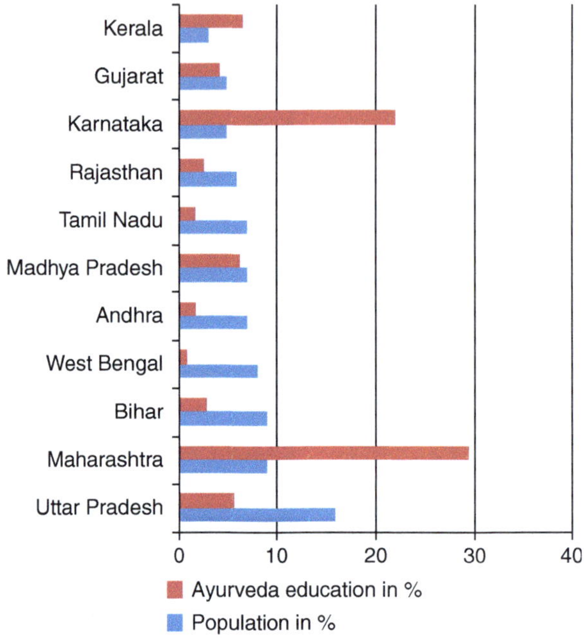

Fig. 13.2 Statewise Ayurveda educational facilities in India in comparison to state population

light of their constraints and also in view of removing them to bring a uniform foundation for a strong EBPA (evidence-based practice of Ayurveda).

13.2.1.1 Ayurvedic Education: Lagging Behind the Global Needs

India has approximately 240 and 62 colleges imparting undergraduate and postgraduate education in Ayurveda [11]. Approximately 11,225 graduates and 991 postgraduates in Ayurveda are produced from these colleges every year. Interestingly, these educational facilities are found grossly disproportionate when compared to the statewise population in India. Uttar Pradesh, one most populous state in India, is ranked fifth in order of providing Ayurveda education, whereas Maharashtra and Karnataka ranked highest in providing Ayurveda education despite that their population is much lesser than Uttar Pradesh (Fig. 13.2) [17].

In lack of clear identification of role of Ayurveda in national health care, a quantitative estimation of its educational as well as treatment facilities has never been speculated. As per 2007 census data, India has 453,661 registered practitioners of Ayurveda. With an estimated population of 1,155,347,700 (2009 World Bank data), one Ayurvedic physician is found to cater the needs of 2,545 people. Comparing to 6.0 allopathic physicians per 10,000 people, Ayurveda has 3.9 physicians for an equal population [18]. It is clear that if Ayurveda is to be brought on equal footing, its education facilities are required to be enhanced quantitatively in geographical areas where it is underrepresented.

Besides quantitative increase, Ayurveda education also needs a major upheaval in terms of its quality. Ayurvedic education, which currently follows the pattern of education primarily developed for conventional medicine lacks severely in terms of producing sufficient textual and practice-based knowledge [16]. In lack of such knowledge, Ayurvedic physicians are often found admixing modern medicines to their prescriptions in order to make it more workable. Despite its huge dependence upon the fundamentals, the fundamentals of Ayurveda are poorly taught and rarely practiced in clinics of Ayurvedic teaching hospitals. *Prakriti, dosha* estimations, examination of a pathogenesis in terms of *dosha*, the primary site of their origin and the secondary site of their presentation, feature in case of a single- or poly-*dosha* pathogenesis, and choosing a drug in terms of its specific effects upon presumptive pathogenesis are the questions that, despite their innate importance to the practice of Ayurvedic medicine, rarely get answered in formal Ayurvedic education.

Admixture of components of conventional basic and clinical medicine into Ayurvedic curricula as an attempt to update Ayurvedic graduates into contemporary medical science presumably did more harm than good to the mental makeup of Ayurveda students. By intruding into two polar streams of medicines simultaneously, in the absence of any knowledge of making the advantage of this admixture, Ayurveda graduates usually land up to a split and disarrayed mind affecting eventually the quality of Ayurvedic practice.

Despite its beautiful textual elaboration, a logical didactic approach of reaching at a diagnosis and then to the treatment is not adequately taught in Ayurvedic institutions. This results in empirical treatment approaches in most cases where *dosha–dushya* didaction does not find a place of concern in prescription writing.

In the absence of appropriate teaching and its practice, Ayurvedic graduates are not adequately trained in evidence-based, logical, and accountable approaches of practicing medicine. The results are poor, unaccountable, and nondependable forms of practices marked in concurrent Ayurveda.

It is observed that the poor status of education in Ayurveda may largely be attributed to inadequate training of its mentors into the methods of teaching, practice, and research [19]. Ayurvedic teaching faculties are found grossly in updated toward recent researches, treatment protocols, and research methodologies. There are insufficient mechanisms operating to translate researches into practice and their addition into academic curricula.

In the current scenario of Ayurvedic education, looking at evidence-based Ayurveda is impossible unless the points raised are adequately taken care of.

13.2.1.2 Ayurvedic Clinical Practice: A Resistant Intervention Model

Resistant intervention model (RIM) tries to explain the rigid and nonflexible model of traditional Ayurvedic practice which offers little room for improvements based upon contemporary experiences and experiments. Despite the goodness of the traditional protocols, RIM adopts them as a ritual without allowing for an open-ended discussion aiming at further improvements to whatever is already known.

Till recently, Ayurvedic practice used to follow a rigid resistant intervention model which is now gradually becoming more flexible and is ready to adopt contemporary ideas.

As per 2007 data given by Dept. of Ayush, India has 2,402 Ayurvedic hospitals and 13,913 dispensaries with a cumulative bed capacity of 43,751. Comparing the bed capacity with Indian population, we find that one bed in an Ayurvedic hospital is available to 26,407 people. This makes it a soaring low 0.4 bed per 10,000 people ratio against 9 beds per 10,000 people in modern medicine [18]. Unfortunately, despite this low bed ratio of Ayurveda, Ayurvedic hospitals are often found to have a poor bed occupancy ratio which again reflects even poorer utilization of meager infrastructural facilities available. Undoubtedly, clinical practice in Ayurveda by and large is a reflection of its education system as we discussed in Sect. 13.2.1.1.

In India, we can trace two distinct schools of Ayurveda practice. Based upon thoughts of practicing Ayurveda within classical or integrated purview contextual with current medical knowledge and tools, these schools are seen continuously claiming their superiority over the other. Unfortunately, when it comes to evidence-based practice models, neither survives to the minimum requirements essential to make a medical intervention reproducible, dependable, and accountable. Classical Ayurvedic practice is often mystified by many subjective approaches like pulse diagnosis, disguised formulations, self-dispensation and no documentations, and prescription writings. Despite their possible importance in producing therapeutic responses in a given condition, these methods are having no role in EBA where a decision is transparent as it is typically drawn through the available evidences helping in reaching toward a clinical judgment.

Ayurvedic physicians are rarely found updated about advances in system of their medicine as they have a poor access or interest to acquire knowledge through medical journals, organizations, or scientific congregations [20].

Ayurvedic clinical practice is also marked by a near-absent documentation in clinic. Prescriptions generated are often found devoid of diagnosis, clinical findings, proper dose schedules, and specified vehicles of drug intake. *Prakriti* and *dosha–dushya* analyses, despite their critical importance to Ayurvedic diagnostics and therapeutics, rarely find a mention in institutionally generated Ayurvedic prescription.

It is clear that in absence of clear and elaborate documentation, we cannot think of building a base on which evidence-based practice can be erected. Quality of drugs and standardization of various treatment protocols and procedures are further issues required to be handled efficiently as a prerequisite to EBA.

13.2.1.3 Ayurvedic Research: Inappropriate Methods and Unfocused Targets

For the large part of late decades in the past century, researches in Ayurveda remained focused upon reverse pharmacology where, on the basis of clues identified in Ayurvedic texts, trials upon Ayurvedic drugs were made upon known clinical conditions. Unfortunately, because of using the research protocols primarily designed to evaluate new chemical entities (NCE) [21], this approach focused on isolated compounds, single herbs, and their combinations in a controlled condition and thereby could not be translated to the practice of Ayurveda where the drugs are used in conjunction with many more pharmacologically active components including the vehicles, food, and spices. A complex matrix of Ayurvedic understanding of a disease and complex real-life interventions suggested render the stereotypical RCT models of research misfit to research needs of Ayurveda. It is argued many times that for Ayurvedic research needs, a whole system research (WSR) model is required to be developed where complete Ayurvedic regimens can be tested for their potential effectiveness on patients. Despite their own complexities of finding a suitable and valid model of research addressing to all the research needs and also addressing to the mystery of Ayurveda, whole system research seems superior in terms of external validity when the same is compared to RCT. Taking the clues from the real-life practice, whole system research identifies the package of individual treatments used together to the patients as per their Ayurvedic diagnosis. A double diagnosis method may be used here to provide a better external validity to the model where a modern diagnosis may follow an Ayurvedic diagnosis [22]. Considering the *dosha–dushya–prakriti* matrix of Ayurvedic diagnostics and therapeutics, we are aware that despite its symptomatic similarity, a same package of treatment may not be applicable to every patient. WSR model may have an advantage of identifying various subgroups of such patients with variables like *dosha* intensity, *dushya* involvement, *prakriti*, and other patient-centered factors affecting the therapeutic response that may be contrasted and compared for treatment responses in similar and variable treatment packages.

While choosing a model in WSR, it is however important to judge its validity on various criteria including representativeness, equipoise and credibility, congruity, and context [23]. Verhoef [22] has proposed various variations to the classical RCT design of clinical research to suit the CAM needs. These variations are *pragmatic trials* allowing the assessment of individualized approach, *factorial designs* comparing single modalities with a group of modalities, and *preference trials* where patient preference may be considered in treatment allocation and outcome is compared with no treatment preferences. *N-of-1 trials* are single-patient trials where the same patient is subjected to various treatment modalities and crossovers over a long period of time. A cumulative data comparing many similar n-of-1 trials may prove useful in terms of its external validity.

In Ayurvedic research, outcome measurement is also a matter of great concern. It is of common observation that usual endpoints and primary and secondary outcome measures as are utilized in conventional medical research do not match to the requirement of Ayurveda. A most feasible outcome measure in Ayurveda research could be the monitoring of changes in objective or subjective features observable or perceivable in research subjects during intervention. A quality of life improvement has been stressed as one important parameter to assess the effectiveness of an intervention [24]. This has a great relevance to Ayurveda as most people who receive Ayurvedic therapy feel better irrespective of their disease status.

Qualitative researches are largely ignored in Ayurveda. For CAM researches, however, a justifiable mixed approach with due combination of quantitative and qualitative researches is most relevant. A patient preference is found to play a crucial role in treatment outcomes and thereby should play an important role in medical decision making [25]. Incidentally, we have observed that the people who visit Ayurvedic hospital for their respective illnesses choose the Ayurvedic therapy as the most preferred one if given an opportunity to choose among various systems of medicine including the conventional one [12, 26]. It is important to validate the Ayurveda researches in context to real-life need with due consideration of sociocultural and economic factors in order to increase their external validity and subsequent applicability in specified populations.

Individualization of therapies, despite its clinical importance, has been considered as one significant hurdle toward evaluating the Ayurvedic therapies in conventional RCT model. Furst et al. [27] recently have shown a way to deal with complexities associated in blinding of Ayurvedic regimens by proposing a multiple-placebo model [27]. Incidentally, the study suggests that individualization can be incorporated in an otherwise standard RCT design and that blinding can be successful if more than one placebo preparation is required. The study might therefore be used as a blueprint for testing the efficacy on interventions that present similar problems [28].

13.2.1.4 Safety Perspectives of Ayurvedic Drugs

An issue which has attained maximum attention in the past few years pertaining to the practice of Ayurveda is no other than its safety perspectives. Ayurvedic drugs are repeatedly challenged for their safety profiles which are largely unproved in a variety of vulnerable population including the elderly, infants, and pregnant and lactating women [29]. Out of the total repertory of Ayurveda, a huge number of herbs are found common to many preparations. Examples are *triphala, trikatu*, and many more. Due to their common usage and unnoticed adversities, these drugs are labeled as generally regarded as safe (GRAS) drugs. The cause of concern in Ayurvedic drugs is more with compounds containing heavy metals [30]. These herbometallic compounds of Ayurveda often deliberately contain metal components with a projection that they possess pharmacological properties rendered to them through Ayurvedic methods of drug preparation. Interestingly, despite a huge global outcry on heavy metal components of Ayurvedic medicines, National Pharmacovigilance Resource Center for Ayurveda, Siddha and Unani drugs (NPRC-ASU), during the past 3 years of its functioning, did not come across a countable number of ADRs where a heavy metal component of Ayurvedic drugs could be incriminated for drug-related adversity [31].

On the contrary, recently, metal-containing Ayurvedic drugs are reported for their corrective effects in conditions of substantial systemic compromise [32]. The "biotransformation" argument of Ayurvedic fraternity, endorsing a therapeutic value to metal components of many Ayurvedic preparations, deserves a merit when we see that conventional know-how which estimates the heavy metals in a preparation is not able to make a qualitative estimation of the incriminated metal. Atomic absorption spectroscopy (AAS), the commonly employed technique of heavy metal estimation in a compound, is found unable to discriminate between various compounds of heavy metal found in an Ayurvedic preparation. Unless a heavy metal in an Ayurvedic drug is identified for its actual compound, and unless these drugs are found to give a corresponding increase of the incriminated metal in plasma of the consuming population, it is unjust to question the safety of Ayurvedic drugs. It is however also important to note at this point that besides heavy metal, there are many other issues which are repeatedly challenging the safety of Ayurvedic drugs. Counterfeit drugs, adulterations, contaminations, poor storage, and indiscriminate usage are few issues which are raised repeatedly against the safety of Ayurvedic drugs and are still waiting for suitable answers [33].

13.3 Conclusions

Ayurveda is witnessing a global resurrection since the past few decades. The issues that seem to be most pertinent to Ayurveda in the current decade are safety, standardization, and efficacy of Ayurvedic medicine as a matter of primary concern to its consumers, practitioners, and policy makers. Besides this, there are also the concerns like evidence base search and practice, research methodology, and improving the quantum of research for a better translation of Ayurvedic theory into practice [34]. Undoubtedly, all these issues are intertwined together to the extent that they cannot be looked in isolation without affecting the impact of others. This looks to be the high time to investigate our limitations and fallacies and also to think pragmatically toward the best utilization of Ayurveda as a dependable and predictable intervention in human health care.

At the time when we point out the limitations in the current practices of Ayurveda, it is also important to notice that Ayurveda is fast gaining trust among its users which is repeatedly reflected in global surveys pertaining to the use of CAM. Ayurveda has become a fast-resurging traditional system of health care which is based on its own unique pro-nature holistic principles and which are deeply pro-science and are getting rapidly autoproved through the newer developments in the field of science of today. There is a fast-accumulating new scientific evidence for its validity in the form of thousands of doctoral theses and lakhs of research papers awaiting a scientific review and critical examination which has not yet happened because the new science base of Ayurveda is not easily accessible to the reviewers because of language barriers and also because of barriers of sectarian publications. It also needs to be kept in mind that Ayurveda is a fully operational traditional system of medicine enjoying a huge infrastructure in India standing almost parallel to conventional medicine serving a big proportion of the population of this most populous country of the world. Unfortunately, the government and the policy makers have not extended adequate support to Ayurveda in India today, resulting into its obvious weaknesses. It is worth mentioning that Ayurveda is provided only about 5% of the total health budget of India for its development and maintenance.

Further, it needs to be emphasized that Ayurveda has rich primary evidence (textual, experience-based, massive acceptability) for its utility which does warrant new supportive evidence on scientific line which is being genuinely attempted now, and a reasonable scientific evidence is gradually accumulating.

A cautious yet pragmatic step would therefore be required to bring the best part of Ayurveda endorsed with scientific evidences but essentially without tempering to the holism and user-friendly, pro-nature approach of it which happen to be the soul of this ancient yet contemporary wisdom in terms of its applicability in the current decade.

References

1. John TJ, Dandona L, Sharma VP, Kakkar M (2011) Continuing challenge of infectious diseases in India. Lancet. doi:10.1016/S0140-6736(10)61265-2
2. Paul VK, Sachdev HS, Mavlanker D et al (2011) Reproductive health and child health and nutrition in India: meeting the challenges. Lancet. doi:10.1016/S0140-6736(10)61492-4
3. Patel V, Chattarjee S, Chrisholm D et al (2011) Chronic diseases and injuries in India. Lancet. doi:10.1016/S0140-6736(10)61188-9
4. Balarajan Y, Selvaraj S, Subramanian SV (2011) Health care and equity in India. Lancet. doi:10.1016/S0140-6736(10)61894-6
5. Rao M, Rao KD, Shiva Kumar AK, Chattarjee M, Sundaraman T (2011) Human resources for health in India. Lancet. doi:10.1016/S0140-6736(10)61188-0
6. Shiva Kumar AK, Chen LC, Chaudhari M et al (2011) Financing health care for all: challenges and opportunities. Lancet. doi:10.1016/S0140-6736(10)61884-3
7. Reddy KS, Patel V, Jha P, Paul VK, Shiva Kumar AK, Dandona L (2011) Towards achievement of universal health care in India by 2020: a call to action. Lancet. doi:10.1016/S0140-6736(10)61960-5
8. Haniffa A (2010) Ayurveda needs more evidence based approach. Downloaded from http://news.rediff.com/special/2010/jun/30/ayurveda-needs-more-evidence-based-approach-says-us-team.htm (Last accessed on 15 December 2010)
9. Rastogi S (2010) Building bridges between Ayurveda and modern science. Int J Ayurveda Res 1:41–46
10. Capsi O, Baranovitch O (2009) When science meets medical tradition: what is needed for a dialogue on integrative medicine? J Altern Complement Med. 15:579–583. doi:10.1089/acm.2008.0503, 15:579–583
11. AYUSH in India 2007, Planning and evaluation cell, Department of Ayurveda, Yoga & Naturopathy, Unani, Siddha and Homeopathy (AYUSH), Ministry of health and Family Welfare, Government of India
12. Rastogi S, Hem C, Rastogi R (2008) Practice of the Ayurvedic system of medicine: a pilot study. New Appr Med Health 15:19–38
13. Das S (2008) Foreword. In: Rastogi S (ed) Principles and practice of Ayurvedic rheumatology. Chaukhambha Sanskrit Pratishthan, Delhi
14. Singh RH (2010) Exploring issues in the development of Ayurvedic research methodology. J Ayurveda Integr Med 1:91–95
15. Preliminary draft of Guidelines for Manuscript Writing in Ayush Research, WHO draft document meeting on 22 Jan 2011, State Ayurvedic College, Lucknow

16. Patwardhan K, Gehlot S, Singh G, Rathore H (2010) Global challenges of graduate level ayurvedic education: a survey. Int J Ayurveda Res 1:49–54
17. Census India, http://censusindia.gov.in/2011-prov-results/data_files/mp/04population.pdf%2050%20No23.4.pdf
18. http://www.who.int/whosis/whostat/EN_WHS2011_Part2.pdf
19. Rastogi S (2010) Global challenges of graduate level Ayurvedic education. Int J Ayurveda Res 1:133
20. Rastogi S (2010) Identifying attitudes about drug safety: a sample survey of Ayurvedic physicians. Int J Risk Safety Med 22:93–101
21. Patwardhan B (2011) Ayurveda GCP guidelines: need for freedom from RCT ascendancy in favor of whole system approach. J Ayurveda Integr Med 2:1–4
22. Verhoef MJ, Lewith G, Ritenbaugh C, Boon H, Fleishman S, Leis A (2005) Complementary and alternative medicine whole systems research: beyond identification of inadequacies of RCT. Compelement Ther Med 13:206–212
23. Lewith G, Walach H, Jonas WB (2002) Balanced research strategies for complementary and alternative medicine. In: Lewith G, Walach H, Jonas WB (eds) Clinical research in complementary therapies: principles, problems and solutions. Churchil Livingstone, Edinburg, pp 1–27
24. Berlim MT, Fleck MPA (2003) Quality of life: a brand new concept for research and practice in psychiatry. Rev Bras Psiquiatr 25:249–252
25. Shannon S, Weil A, Kaplan BJ (2011) Medical decision making in integrative medicine: safety, efficacy and patient preference. Altern Complement Ther 17:84–91
26. Rastogi S (2011) Panchakarma: exploring through evidences. Light Ayurveda J 9:30–36
27. Furst DE, Venkatraman MM, McGann M, Ram Manohar P, Booth-LaForce C, Sarin R, Sekar PG, Raveendran KG, Mahapatra A, Gopinath J, Krishna Kumar PR (2011) Double-blind, randomized, controlled, pilot study comparing classic Ayurvedic medicine, methotrexate, and their combination in rheumatoid arthritis. J Clin Rheumatol 17:185–192
28. Ernst E, Furst DE (2011) A blueprint for placebo-controlled double-blind studies of complex, individualized interventions. Focus Altern Complement Ther 16:49–50
29. Rastogi S (2011) Why and how? Addressing to the two most pertinent questions about pharmacovigilance in Ayurveda. Int J Ayurveda Res 2:47–51
30. Saper RB, Kales SN, Paquin J, Burns MJ, Eisenberg DM, Davis RB et al (2004) Heavy metal contents of Ayurvedic herbal medicine products. JAMA 292:2868–2873
31. Baghel MS (2010) The national pharmacovigilance program for Ayurveda, Siddha and Unani drugs: current status. Int J Ayurveda Res 1:197–198
32. Rastogi S, Srivastav PS (2011) Ayurveda in critical care: illustrating Ayurvedic intervention in a case of hepatic encephalopathy. Ayu 32: (in press)
33. Gogotay NJ, Bhatt HA, Dalvi SS, Kshirsagar NA (2002) The use and safety of non allopathic Indian medicines. Drug Saf 25:1005–1019
34. Patwardhan B (2010) Ayurveda for all: 11 action points for 2011. J Ayurveda Integr Med 1:237–239

Index

A
Abhyanga, 114
Acetyl salicylic acid (ASA), 168
Achara and *Ajasrika Rasayana*, 182
Achillea millefolium, 91
Adana, 56
ADR. *See* Adverse drug reactions (ADR)
Adverse drug reaction monitoring, 215
Adverse drug reactions (ADR), 212
Age-specific *Rasayana*, 180–181
Agni, 53, 144, 179
Agnikarma, 131–132
AGREE. *See* Appraisal of Guidelines and Research and Evaluation, Europe (AGREE)
Agricultural Online Access (AGRICOLA), 21
Alfalfa, 85
Algae, 88
Allied therapies, 113–135
Allium sativum, 87
Aloe (*Aloe vera*), 85–86
Altered state of consciousness (ASC), 130
Alternative medicine, 4
Althadin, 86
Ama, 38, 39, 53, 141–146
Amavata, 141–146, 150
American Dental Association, 197
Amla, 199
AMSTAR. *See* Assessment of multiple systematic reviews instrument (AMSTAR)
Animal studies, 12
Anumana, 204
Anuphatya, 55
Anuvasana, 116
Apathya, 60–61
Appraisal of Guidelines and Research and Evaluation, Europe (AGREE), 19
Apta, 204
Arctium lappa, 86
Aristotelian concept, 3
Aristotle, 3, 194
ASA. *See* Acetyl salicylic acid (ASA)
ASC. *See* Altered state of consciousness (ASC)
Ashtanga Hridaya, 114, 163
Ashwagandha, 186
Assessment of multiple systematic reviews instrument (AMSTAR), 15
Asthapana basti, 116
Asya madhurya, 37
Atharvaveda, 160
Avicenna, 80
A-vyakta, 160
Ayurveda for future, 47
Ayurvedic biology, 47
Ayurvedic diet, 57–59
Ayurvedic pharmaceutics, 39
Ayurvedic research, 240–242
Ayurvedic, Siddha, and Unani (ASU) drugs, 211

B
Basti, 114, 116
Bee pollen, 86
Bernard, C., 193
Best case series, 41
Bhutagni, 144
Bioenergetic medicines, 25
Biomarkers, 37
Biomedicine, 37

S. Rastogi (ed.), *Evidence-Based Practice in Complementary and Alternative Medicine*,
DOI 10.1007/978-3-642-24565-7, © Springer-Verlag Berlin Heidelberg 2012

Biopurification, 168
Biotransformation, 242
Bloodletting, 114
Brihattrayi, 177
Bronchial asthma, 39
Buerger's disease, 128
Burdock, 86

C
CAM. *See* Complementary and alternative medicine (CAM)
The Canon of Medicine, 80–81
Capsella bursa-pastoris, 90
Carbohydrates, 52
Cardiovascular diseases, 159–173
Case series, 41–42
Catnip, 86
CDC. *See* Centers for Disease Control and Prevention (CDC)
C. elegans model, 229
Centers for Disease Control and Prevention (CDC), 52
Chamomile, 86
Chance effect, 71–73
Charaka Samhita, 114
Choleric, 82
Choose My Plate, 54
Classification of *Rasayana*, 180–183
Clinical outcomes, 17
Clinical research, 13
Clinical trials, 12
Cloves, 86
Cochrane, A., 196
Cochrane Centre, 13
Cochrane Collaboration, 22
Cochrane Library, 170
Cochrane reviews, 170
Cohen's kappa coefficient, 106
Comfrey, 86–87
Commiphora guggulu, 170–171
Commiphora myrrha, 89
Commiphora wightii, 170–171
Complementary and alternative medicine (CAM), 8
Consensus inference, 18–20
Consolidated standards of reporting trials (CONSORT), 13
CONSORT. *See* Consolidated standards of reporting trials (CONSORT)
Construct validity, 106
Cumulative Index to Nursing and Allied Health Literature (CINAHL), 204
Cyt P450, 42

D
Dandelion, 87
Das pranaytananani, 163
Department of AYUSH, 213–214
Detoxification, 116
Dhatusamya, 198
Dhatvagni, 144
Dhooma, 116
Dhumapana, 40
Dipana, 156
Disease-specific *Rasayana*, 181–182
Dissociation, 156
Divya Rasayana, 183
Documentation *(apta)*, 36
Dosha, 38
Dosha-dhatu-mala, 113–114
Dosha–dushya, 239
Dosha–dushya–prakriti matrix, 241
Dosha pratyaneek, 171
Dracocephalum kotschyi, 87
Dragonhead, 87
Duchenne's muscular dystrophy, 133

E
Eastern purple coneflower, 87
EBA. *See* Evidence-based Ayurveda (EBA)
EBPA. *See* Evidence-based practice of Ayurveda (EBPA)
Echinacea, 87
Effectiveness, 9
Efficacy, 9
Ehrlich, P., 196
Emblica officinalis, 199
Emesis, 114
Equisetum telmateia, 88
Equivalent trials, 229
Eucalyptus, 88
Evidence-based Ayurveda (EBA), 33, 236–243
Evidence-based decision-making, 100
Evidence-based dentistry, 197
Evidence based panchakarma, 119–133
Evidence-based practice of ayurveda (EBPA), 238
Experimentation *(yukti)*, 36

F
Factorial designs, 241
Fasting, 155
Fats, 52
Fennel, 87
Foeniculum vulgare, 87

Food classification, 52–53
Four *purusharthas*, 99
Frequently recommended foods (FRF), 56
Fume inhalation, 40

G
Garlic, 87
GCP, 213
Generally regarded as safe (GRAS) drugs, 242
Geriatric health care, 179
Global health-care scenario, 68
Glutathione, 42
Glycyrrhiza glabra, 88–89
GMP, 226
Goldenseal, 87
Golden Triangle Project, 235
Grades of Recommendation, Assessment, Development, and Evaluation (GRADE), 19
The grandfather of herbs, 88–89
GRAS drugs. *See* Generally regarded as safe (GRAS), drugs
Guava, 87–88
Gum tree, 88
Guru (complex), 55

H
Healing robot, 130
Heavy metals, 218
Herbal enema, 114
HerbMed, 22
Hippocrates, 6
HLA gene polymorphism, 101
Horsetail plant, 88
Human Genome Project, 235
Hydrastis canadensis, 87

I
ICMR. *See* Indian Council of Medical Research (ICMR)
Ignition, 156
Incompatible diet, 58
Indian Council of Medical Research (ICMR), 37
Indian Council of Medical Research (ICMR) guidelines, 229
Individual body types (*prakriti*), 52
Innate immunity, 56
Integrated National Health System, 233
Integrative medicine, 5, 192
Inter-rater, 15
Intra-rater reliability, 15
Inverted intestine loop model, 42
Invisible, 160
"Iran," 79
Iran's traditional medicine (ITM), 79
Irimedadi taila, 203
ITM. *See* Iran's traditional medicine (ITM)

J
Jadad scale, 15
Jalaukavacharana, 116
Janubasti, 117

K
Kapha, 38
Kashaya vasti, 126
Katibasti, 117, 131–132
Kavala, 199
Kayachikitsa, 177
Kayakalpa, 180
Kelp, 88
Khavaigunya, 53
Krimija hrida roga, 167
Kshar-sutra, 235

L
Labiatae, 89
Laghu, 154
Laghu (simple), 55
Lagvasana, 155
Langhana, 155
Lavandula angustifolia, 88
Lavender, 88
Leech therapy, 127
Lemon balm, 88
Leukoderma, 127
Leukorrhea, 132
Level I, 14
Level II, 14
Level III, 14
Levels of evidence, 13, 14, 75
Licorice root, 88–89
Loka-purusha samya theory, 160

M
Macrocosm, 160–161
Madanaphala, 119
Madhava nidana, 141
"Magic bullet" concept, 196

Mahabhuta, 160
Mahamula, 163
Mahaphala, 163
Mandagni, 149–152, 150, 156–157
Mandagni (hypodigestive state), 144–146
Marigold, 89
Marma, 165
Matra, 54
Matra vasti, 126
Matricaria chamomilla, 86
Medical care seeking behavior (MCSB), 235
Medicago sativa, 85
Melaleuca oil, 90
Melancholic, 82
Melissa officinalis, 88
Mentha piperita, 90
Meta-analyses, 16, 17
Meta-systematic, 21
Methodology, 10
Microcosm (theory of *loka-purusha samya*), 160–161
Millennium Project, 235
Mind–body interaction, 6
Minerals, 52
Miswak, 89
Multiple-placebo model, 242
My Pyramid, 54, 59
Myrrh, 89
Myrtle, 89
Myrtus communis, 89

N
Nanomedicine, 39
Nasya, 114, 116
National Cancer Institute (NCI), 41
National Center for Complementary and Alternative Medicine, 19
National Institute of Health (NIH), 170
National Library of Medicine, 19
National Pharmacovigilance Resource Center for Ayurveda, Siddha and Unani drugs (NPRC-ASU), 242
National Rural Health Mission (NRHM), 235
NCCAM, 21
NCE. *See* New chemical entities (NCE)
NCI. *See* National Cancer Institute (NCI)
Nepeta cataria, 86
New chemical entities (NCE), 241
NIH. *See* National Institute of Health (NIH)
Niruha, 116
Nischalata, 149–152
NLM, 21
N-of-1 trials, 241
Non-Western health care, 192
Not recommended food (NRF), 56
NPRC-ASU. *See* National Pharmacovigilance Resource Center for Ayurveda, Siddha and Unani drugs (NPRC-ASU)
NRF. *See* Not recommended food (NRF)
NRHM. *See* National Rural Health Mission (NRHM)

O
Oaksatmya, 57
Observations *(pratyksha)*, 35
Occasionally recommended food (ORF), 56
OECD guidelines, 231
Optimal medical therapy (OMT), 173
Oral Biology and Medicine, 191–205
Oral Health, 191–193
Oregano, 89
ORF. *See* Occasionally recommended food (ORF)
Origanum vulgare, 89
Otostegia persica, 89

P
Pachana, 156
Padanshik, 57
Panchakarma, 42, 113
  *a*yurvedic detoxification, 113–135
  protocol, 203
Panch-karma, 235
PAQ. *See Prakriti* analysis questionnaire (PAQ)
Paschat karma, 114
Pathogenesis, 171
Pathya, 60–61
Patient, interventions under consideration, outcomes (P.I.C.O.), 9
Patra pinda sweda, 126
PCI. *See* Percutaneous coronary intervention (PCI)
PDCAAS. *See* Protein digestibility corrected amino acid score (PDCAAS)
Pearson's correlation coefficient, 106
Peppermint, 90
Percutaneous coronary intervention (PCI), 173
Pharmacovigilance program, 215
Phlegmatic, 82
Phyllanthus emblica, 199
P.I.C.O. *See* Patient, interventions under consideration, outcomes (P.I.C.O.)

Pinda sweda, 133
Placebo, 34
Plantago, 90
Plantain, 90
Point-of-care, 37
Poorva karma, 114
Prabhava, 171
Pracchana karma, 116
Pradhana karma, 114
Pragmatic trials, 241
Prakriti, 35, 38, 45, 63, 100, 160, 161
  analysis, 99–110
  diagnosis, 106
Prakriti analysis questionnaire (PAQ), 106–107
Prameha, 37
Pratiniyamiki Siddhi, 71
Pratyaksha, 204
Prayoga, 72
Preference trials, 241
Preferred Reporting Items for Systematic Reviews and Meta-analyses (PRISMA), 16
Primary evidence base, 46
"Prince of Physicians," 80
PRISMA. *See* Preferred Reporting Items for Systematic Reviews and Meta-analyses (PRISMA)
Prorasayana, 188
Protein digestibility corrected amino acid score (PDCAAS), 55
Proteins, 52
Psidium guajava, 87–88
PubMed, 21, 69
Purgation, 114, 115
Puta, 39

Q
Qigong, 192
Quality assessment of studies of diagnostic accuracy included in systematic reviews (QUADAS), 15
Quality of reporting of meta-analyses (QUOROM), 16

R
Raktamokshana, 114, 116
Randomized clinical trials, 34
Rapidly digestible starch (RDS), 55
Rasaushadhi, 218
Rasayana
  in cancer management, 186–187
  effect, 183–186
  herbs, 203
  therapy, 177–188
Rauwolfia serpentina, 170
RDS. *See* Rapidly digestible starch (RDS)
Real effect, 71–73
Rejuvenation, 177–188
Relative fasting, 155
Reporting single cases, 41–42
Research designs, 12
Research meta-synthesis, 21
Research methodology, 7
Research question, 9
Research synthesis, 8–20, 11
Resistant intervention model (RIM), 239
Resistant starch (RS), 55
Resources, 11
Retrospective approach, 103
RIM. *See* Resistant intervention model (RIM)
Robotic *shirodhara*, 130
Rosemary, 90
Rosmarinus officinalis, 90
RS. *See* Resistant starch (RS)

S
Safety/tolerability index, 229
Sage, 90
Salivary diagnostics, 37
Salvadora persica, 89
Salvia officinalis, 90
Samprapti, 171
Samsarjana, 61–62
Sanguine, 82
Sarpagandha, 170
Satureja khuzistanica, 90
Science in Ayurveda, 235
SDS. *See* Slowly digestible starch (SDS)
Sensory-specific desire (SSD), 54–55
Sensory specific satiety (SSS), 54
Shamana, 113
Shamana chikitsa, 120
Shepherd's purse, 90
Shirobasti, 117
Shirodhara, 117, 129–131
Shirovasti, 131
Shirovirechana, 116
Shodhana, 113, 116
Shodhana chikitsa, 120
Shodhana Samskara, 213
Siddhabheshaja, 71

Siravyadha, 116
Siwak, 89
Slowly digestible starch (SDS), 55
Snehana, 114–115
Snehapana, 114
Special action, 171
Speculation *(anumana)*, 36
Srotoprasadana effect, 179
Srotus, 45
SSD. *See* Sensory-specific desire (SSD)
SSS. *See* Sensory specific satiety (SSS)
Standards for reporting interventions in clinical trials of acupuncture (STRICTA), 13
Sushruta, 163
Susruta Samhita, 114
Svetapradara, 132
Svritra, 127
Swedana, 114–115
Symphytum officinale, 86–87
Systematic reviews, 14, 23
Systems biology, 5
Syzygium aromaticum, 86

T
Tagetes, 89
Tai Chi, 5
Taraxacum officinale, 87
Tea tree oil, 90
Teleology, 3
Terminalia arjuna, 42, 170
Test–retest reliability, 106
"Therapeutic emesis," 115
Thyme, 91
Thymus vulgaris, 91
Tissue-and organ-specific *Rasayana*, 181
"Torched City," 79
Total quality of life (TQL), 159
Traditional Indian health care, 234
Traditional Persian Herbal Medicine, 84–91
Traditional Persian medicine, 79–94
Translational effectiveness, 191–205, 199
"Translational effectiveness" model, 197
Tridosha, 45, 100, 198
Trikatu, 61
Trip database, 23

U
The United States Department of Agriculture (USDA), 54
Upakarmas, 117
Upamana, 204
USDA. *See* The United States Department of Agriculture (USDA)
Uttara vasti, 132

V
Vaca, 119
Vaitarana vasti, 126
Vamana, 114, 115
Vamana (emesis), 40
Vasantic vamana, 119
Vasti, 114, 116
Vata, 38, 141–146
Vataja hrida roga, 166–167
Vata vikara, 119
Virechana, 114, 115
Viruddha ahara, 58, 148, 149–152, 150, 151
Viruddh-ahara, 142, 146
Visarga, 56
Visible, 160
Vital seat, 165
Vitamins, 52
Vyadhi pratyaneek, 171
Vyakta, 160

W
Water, 52
Western medicine, 4, 5
Western Oral Medicine, 193–195
WHA. *See* World Health Assembly (WHA)
WHO. *See* World Health Organization (WHO)
Whole system research (WSR) model, 241
World Health Assembly (WHA), 212
World Health Organization (WHO), 93, 211
WSR model. *See* Whole system research (WSR) model

X
Xenobiotics, 42

Y
Yadrcchiki Siddhi, 71
Yarrow, 91
Yastimadhu, 119
Yukti, 204

MIX
Papier aus verantwortungsvollen Quellen
Paper from responsible sources
FSC® C105338

If you have any concerns about our products,
you can contact us on
ProductSafety@springernature.com

In case Publisher is established outside the EU,
the EU authorized representative is:
Springer Nature Customer Service Center GmbH
Europaplatz 3, 69115 Heidelberg, Germany

Printed by Libri Plureos GmbH
in Hamburg, Germany